Isokinetics
Muscle Testing, Interpretation and Clinical Applications

Zeevi Dvir PhD LLB

Department of Physical Therapy, Sackler Faculty of Medicine, Tel-Aviv University

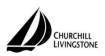

CHURCHILL LIVINGSTONE

EDINBURGH
LONDON
MADRID
MELBOURNE
NEW YORK
AND
TOKYO
1995

CHURCHILL LIVINGSTONE
Medical Division of Pearson Professional Limited

Distributed in the United States of America by Churchill
Livingstone Inc., 650 Avenue of the Americas, New York,
N.Y. 10011, and by associated companies, branches and
representatives throughout the world.

First published 1995
  Reprinted 1996

ISBN 0 443 04794 4

British Library Cataloguing in Publication Data
A catalogue record for this book is available from the British
Library.

Library of Congress Cataloging in Publication Data
Dvir, Zeevi.
    Isokinetics: testing, interpretation, and clinical applications /
Zeevi Dvir.
        p.   cm.
    Includes index.
    ISBN 0-443-04794-4
    1. Isokinetic exercise.   I. Title.
    [DNLM: 1. Isometric Contraction.   2. Physical Therapy--methods.
WE 500 D988i 1994]
RM725.176D85 1994
615.8'24--dc20
DNLM/DLC
for Library of Congress   94–17531
                                                    CIP

The
publisher's
policy is to use
**paper manufactured
from sustainable forests**

Produced by Longman Publishers Singapore Pte Ltd
Printed in Singapore

Isokinetics

To Miki, Dotan, Yuval and Noam with all my love

For Churchill Livingstone

Publisher: Mary Law
Project Editor: Dinah Thom
Copy Editor: Teresa Brady
Indexer: Monica Trigg
Design direction: Judith Wright
Project Manager: Neil Dickson
Sales Promotion Executive: Maria O'Connor

Contents

Preface

It is now slightly over 25 years since isokinetic dynamometry was first introduced into clinical practice and exercise science. Physical therapy, in particular, has benefited significantly from this technology, which rapidly became the tool of choice in hundreds of research papers as well as the cornerstone of quantitative muscle performance assessment in the clinical setting. About a decade ago, the technology behind isokinetic dynamometry made considerable progress when computers were incorporated to control the hardware, that is the integral power sources and the on-line processing of mechanical signals. This enabled users to establish a common basis for carrying out eccentric contractions and to obtain comprehensive information on muscle strength immediately.

My own experience of isokinetic dynamometry did not start when I first switched on the system my department acquired in 1986. For a period of about 2 years from 1980 I approached a number of independent manufacturers of high-tech medical equipment in my country with a proposal for constructing an active dynamometer, based on a design I then had. The result was disappointing, and as a result I abandoned the idea. Thus, although the advent of active dynamometry, at a later date, did not surprise me, the feeling of having missed an exclusive opportunity was very acute.

Hence, when the next opportunity in isokinetics arose years later—to write a book about isokinetic dynamometry—I decided to be more tenacious. The need for such a reference source was very obvious. In spite of the fact that there were thousands of users of isokinetic dynamometers in the US alone, the number of books whose main subject was isokinetics could be counted on the fingers of one hand. Moreover, I felt that there was a conspicuous lack of texts defining the main methodological and procedural problems surrounding this technology. This book does not pretend to cover all the topics that have been examined under isokinetics. Nor is it intended to be a quick and superficial introduction to clinical applications. Rather, it is aimed at those who have at least some experience and are at a stage where they are beginning to ask some very serious questions, and would not necessarily be happy with very simple answers.

In this book I have attempted to draw an unbiased picture of isokinetics. The source material used throughout the book is based exclusively on papers which appeared in peer review journals. Published abstracts are referred to in only a few cases. The first four chapters cover relevant biomechanical and physiological issues, aspects of operation, measurement, validity and reproducibility, and isokinetically-based muscle conditioning methods. The other five chapters describe the use of isokinetics on the major joint systems of the body: the hip, knee, ankle, spine and shoulder. I decided not to deal with the elbow and wrist joints in separate chapters as the database was insufficiently comprehensive.

The section on the medicolegal applications of isokinetics, perhaps the most involved and fascinating aspect of this technology, is not based exclusively on published material. I decided to include this topic, not only because of its increasing importance, but also because it reflects my personal experience with a wide spectrum of legal cases.

Finally, I would like to thank Mr Angus Strover FRCS of the Droitwich Knee Clinic, UK, for his thoughtful reflections on the chapter on the knee, and Mr Asher Pinchasoff from the Sackler Faculty of Medicine, Tel Aviv University, for the photographic work. However, this book is first and foremost a tribute to the exquisite patience, encouragement and love shown and given to me by my beloved ones throughout the long period of writing.

Tel Aviv 1995   Z.D.

Physiological and biomechanical aspects of isokinetics

This book deals with the measurement and conditioning of dynamic muscle performance, primarily in the clinical setting. 'Dynamic' here refers to a specific situation in which a muscle or muscle group contracts against a *controlled accommodating resistance*, which is moving at a *constant angular velocity*. Isokinetic dynamometry is concerned with the provision of this resistance and the measurement of the moment exerted by the muscle against the resistance. In this chapter some independent physiological and biomechanical issues concerning the use of isokinetic systems are discussed.

BASIC PRINCIPLES

LENGTH–TENSION RELATIONSHIP

Voluntary and involuntary muscle performance

Isokinetic dynamometry has been employed almost exclusively for assessing the performance of voluntarily contracting muscles. This means that besides the physiological and mechanical factors, psychological factors are also involved. Indeed, motivation and cooperation are essential components in isokinetic testing. However, it is also possible to use isokinetic dynamometers for measuring muscle performance which may be initiated involuntarily, for instance in patients suffering from spastic paresis following stroke.

The fundamental relationship

The most basic relationship governing muscle performance is perceived as the association between the length of the muscle and the magnitude of the corresponding tension. Our understanding of this relationship is almost exclusively based on animal preparations. In those few instances where human experimentation has been allowed, the findings, in volunteers who underwent cineplastic amputation (Ralston et al 1949), proved to be in close agreement with the principles established from animal experiments.

Principles of isometric contractions

Investigation of isometric contractions is based on an experimental set-up in which the length of the muscle is set by the experimenter 'the independent variable', and the tension under passive pull or electrical stimulation ('the dependent variable') is recorded by a force-measuring device. (Hill 1953).

Starting in a slack position so that the distance between the ends of the muscle is shorter than its total length, the muscle is tetanized using electrical simulation. The tension developed is measured by a load cell connected in series with the muscle. The distance between the ends of the muscle is then increased by small amounts and at a certain point, passive resistance is recorded by the load cell even before stimulation. The process is repeated until no increase in tension is apparent.

The tension recorded by the dynamometer reflects two independent sources (Fig. 1.1):

1 the active tension produced by the contractile elements in the muscle
2. the passive tension produced by the noncontractile elements.

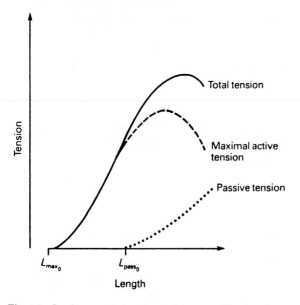

Fig. 1.1 In vitro muscle length–tension curve. The dotted line represents the resistance to stretch contributed by the passive elastic elements of a denervated muscle. The solid line represents the total tension contributed by active and passive elements during stimulation which produces maximal tetanic tension. (From Kandel et al 1991.)

As the two components are physically intertwined it is impossible to simultaneously measure their independent contributions. However the active tension is found by subtracting the value of the passive tension, as recorded before stimulation, from the corresponding value of the total tension. The curve describing the active component then has an almost perfectly symmetrical inverted 'U' shape (Fig. 1.1).

The muscle length corresponding to the maximal active tension is known as the 'resting length' which should not be confused with the length of the muscle at the 'anatomical position'. Furthermore, the strength (see below) developed by the muscle at the resting length is unlikely to be its maximal.

The length–tension relationship of the whole muscle reflects the mechanical behavior of the muscle fiber (Gordon et al 1966). The amount of tension developed is related to the number of cross-bridges between the actin and myosin filaments in the fibers, which in turn is related to their degree of overlap.

STRENGTH IN LIVE SUBJECTS

The maximal moment

The techniques, be they isometric, isokinetic or other, employed to measure muscle 'force' in live subjects, are based on a different method. Instead of force, which is basically a linear entity, the appropriate term is strength. This is defined as *the rotational effect of the force*, generated by a single muscle or a muscle group, about the joint under consideration, and is also called the *maximal moment*. Thus strength introduces the concept of synergy, reference being made, where applicable, to the combined action of a number of muscles rather than of a single muscle (Herzog et al 1991).

Disregarding, for a moment the effect of gravity (see below) strength is measured by recording the force exerted on the sensor of the dynamometer by the body segment distal to the joint, and multiplying the value obtained by the length of the force sensor's lever-arm (Fig. 1.2) to give a moment, M. In other words the mechanical potential of the muscle is only inferred rather than measured

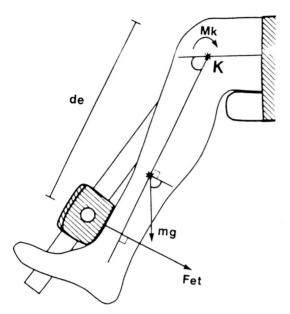

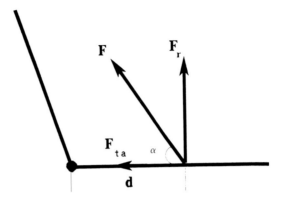

Fig. 1.3 The total muscle force, F, is a vector with two components: F_r, the rotatory component and F_{ta}, the transarticular component. α, angle of application (AOA); d, lever of F_r

Fig. 1.2 In an isometric or isokinetic gravity-free situation the moment M_k, generated by the muscle (the quadriceps femoris in this case) would be equal to the distance between the force resistance pad and the instantaneous center of rotation of the knee, d_e, times the force recorded by the sensor, F_{et}. (Adapted from Nisell et al 1989.)

directly. Moreover, simple mechanical considerations indicate that the amount of force exerted on the force sensor is inversely proportional to the distance between the joint axis and the point of force application. Since the length of body segments is generally small, a deviation of even 1 centimeter from the original placement of the sensor may, upon retesting, introduce errors of approximately 2.5–5% with a corresponding effect on the reproducibility of the test findings.

Total force and measurable force

There is however another fundamental difference between the direct and the usual methods namely that in the latter only a fraction of the total muscle force is measurable. For instance consider Figure 1.3 a schematic, planar view of the elbow joint. The force, F, developed by the brachialis, which here represents the total flexor force, is a vector with two components, the transarticular, F_{ta} and the rotatory, F_r. The transarticular component acts to stabilize

the joint but does not contribute to generating the moment about the elbow. In dynamic situations, this function of flexing or controlling the extension of the forearm is performed by the rotatory component of the brachialis force. The value of the moment, M, is obtained through multiplying the rotational component, F_r (Fig. 1.3) by the length of the lever, d, which is the perpendicular distance from F_r, to the center of rotation (the elbow joint).

$$M = F_r d$$

From trigonometry:

$$F_r = F \sin \alpha$$

where α is the direction in which F is being applied or the 'angle of application' (AOA) (Fig. 1.3). It follows that:

$$M = dF \sin \alpha$$

The moment–angular position curve

Therefore, as well as increasing with the length, d, the muscular moment depends on two factors: the muscle force and the sine of its angle of application ($\sin \alpha$). These variables behave in a somewhat opposite manner. When the muscle is at its most stretched position the AOA is very small and hence the sine of the angle is minimal, tending to reduce the value of M. As the muscle becomes shorter, its tension generating capacity diminishes, i.e. F decreases, but the corresponding AOA, and hence sin α, becomes greater.

Since during the initial sector of the total range of motion (ROM) the rate of increase of sin α is much faster than the corresponding rate of decrease in the muscle force, F, the moment, M, generated by the muscle tends to increase in this sector. This is the reason for the observed rise in muscle strength from the so-called 'outer end' to the 'middle range' position. The opposite may generally prevail in the later sector, from the 'middle range' to 'inner end position', leading to a decrease in the moment, M. The shape of the resulting moment–angular position curve, is illustrated in Figure 1.4 which is based on an isokinetic test of the elbow supinators and pronators.

The gravitational correction

In dynamic contractions, the external moment, namely the moment which has to be overcome by the muscle, is normally generated by three distinct elements:

1. the individual weight of the segment/s distal to the joint
2. the load against which one acts, for instance lifting an object
3. the acceleration components involved in performing the motion.

Since the majority of isokinetic tests consist of angular motions and motion proceeds at a constant angular velocity (at least during the larger sector of the tested range of motion at slow to medium

velocities) the dynamic equations governing isokinetic exertions ignore acceleration components. Therefore in order to determine the net muscle force it is necessary to incorporate the effect of weight. Consider Figure 1.5 which refers to the isometric measurement of the strength of the knee extensors and flexors, in the seated position.

The extensors act in the opposite direction to the weight of the leg and the resistance of the dynamometer. The moment exerted by the extensors, M_e (anticlockwise in Figure 1.5) must be equal to the moment of weight of the leg (shank and foot), M_l plus the moment exerted by the resistance of the dynamometer, M_d, (both clockwise in Figure 1.5). This relationship is given by the equation:

$$M_e = M_d + M_l$$

On the other hand, when the flexors contract isometrically, the moment they generate, M_f, and the moment exerted by the weight of the leg act in the same direction (clockwise, in Figure 1.5), and hence the equation is:

$$M_f + M_l = M_d$$

Or by rearranging:

$$M_f = M_d - M_l$$

Thus, in the 'gravitational position' the strength of the extensors may be underestimated and that of the flexors overestimated by an amount equal to the gravitational moment.

In isokinetic testing the above argument is valid for the analogous case of extensor and flexor concentric (see below) contractions, i.e., where the muscle is overcoming the weight of the limb and

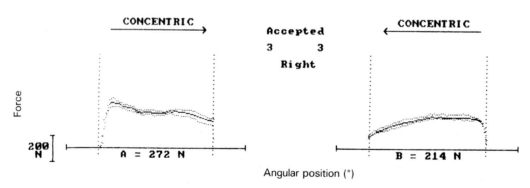

Fig. 1.4 Isokinetic strength curves: left, supinators; right, pronators; multiplication by the lever-arm length results in moment rather than force units. A and B are the average force (in N).

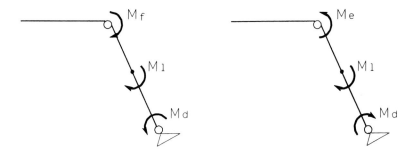

Fig. 1.5 Moment configuration simulated during flexors' (M_f) and extensors' (M_e) isokinetic testing. M_d, moment generated by the dynamometer's lever-arm; M_l, gravitational moment of the leg.

the resistance of the dynamometer. In order to obtain the true value of the muscle strength it is therefore necessary to perform the so-called 'gravity correction' procedure.

The agonist/antagonist strength ratio

Clearly failure to account for gravitation in calculating the net moment developed by tested muscles is particularly conspicuous in terms of agonist/antagonist moment (strength) ratio. This statement is generally valid in the case of those muscles which move the limbs in the frontal and sagittal planes but not in rotations.

Consider for instance the case of the strength ratio between the hip extensors and flexors, *Ext/Flx*, where *Ext* and *Flx* are the respective muscular moments. Let us assume that the weight of the limb exerts, at a certain point in the tested ROM, a moment of 20 N m, and that each muscle exerts a maximal 'uncorrected' moment of 60 N m at this point. (For a detailed discussion of units of measurement see Chapter 2.) Based on these 'uncorrected' values:

$$Ext/Flx = 60/60 = 1.0$$

If however the gravitational moment is added to the extensors and subtracted from the flexors the result is:

$$Ext/Flx = (60 + 20)/(60 - 20) = 2.0$$

This is a very significant difference which may reach much higher values in other instances (Winter et al 1981, see also Chapters 6 and 8 for detailed discussion).

INSTRUMENTED AND MANUAL STRENGTH ASSESSMENTS

A fundamental consideration, intimately related to the issue of gravity correction and surprisingly overlooked by most students of isokinetics, is the correspondence between manual and instrumental strength assessment. The large majority of human movements involve antigravitational exertions where the main challenge to the muscles derives directly from the weight of the limb segments, or the trunk. When the strength of a muscle/muscle group is assessed, the sine qua non for a nonzero measurement is the development of a muscular moment in excess of what is required to balance the gravitational moment.

For instance assume that the maximal moment which can be generated by the hip flexors in the standing position is just sufficient to hold the thigh at an angle of 20° flexion. If a force sensor is placed against the anterior aspect of the thigh at this position, no force will be recorded. On the other hand, if the sensor is sufficiently sensitive, some force will be recorded between the neutral position and the above angle.

The significance of this observation is that if any moment (force) is recorded, the corresponding manual strength rating which is commonly based on a 0–5 scale cannot, by definition, be less than 3. The only way to circumvent this problem, is to test the relevant muscle/s in a nongravitational position. This indeed has been done with respect to both the knee and trunk muscles, employing the side-lying position (Thorstensson & Nilsson 1982, Smidt et al 1983). The advantage of this method is the ability to detect forces that may be much smaller than are demanded in normal activity. However this testing position is nonfunctional and requires special and cumbersome equipment. It should be emphasized that all commercially available systems are based on the assumption that the subject/patient is capable of exceeding the countergravitational moment and thus only two grades, 4 and 5, correspond to the full range of force (moment) that a given muscle may generate.

Consider, for example, the case of knee extensor strength. The average figure in men, tested at a low velocity, is in the neighbourhood of 180 N m (Freedson et al 1993). This means that in a seated test position, a normal subject may generate about 600 N of force (approximately 60 kgf) against a sensor placed immediately above the ankle. This figure serves to define, in terms of manual test, the range 3–5, exposing a severe deficiency in the manual (clinical) strength rating system regarding subjects whose muscular strength is isokinetically measurable in antigravity positions.

This deficiency may work in a number of ways. It may underestimate a true gain in strength or overestimate a stagnant muscle potential. The former scenario is the most common since human sensitivity in assessing force is generally poor. However overestimation also occurs. This does not mean that the examiner judged more sensitively than the instrument but probably erred in assuming the existence of a change. A study by Rabin & Post (1990) compared manual and isokinetic evaluation of shoulder flexor and external rotator strength before and after surgery. With the manual method, strength was judged to have improved significantly, but no such effect was evident using the isokinetic technique.

THE MOMENT–ANGULAR VELOCITY RELATIONSHIP IN DYNAMIC CONTRACTIONS

MUSCLE TENSION AND SPEED OF CONTRACTION

If the relationship between force and length (moment–angular position) is the most basic physiological parameter of skeletal muscle, the other basic parameter is the relationship between the force, or tension, developed by the muscle and its velocity or speed of contraction. Dynamic muscle performance may be measured by:

1. controlling the external load and measuring and/or calculating the resulting velocities and accelerations, or
2. controlling the velocity and measuring the force (moment) output.

The second approach, for which isokinetic dynamometers are particularly suitable, has been adopted for quantifying muscle performance since the late 1960s.

In discussing the tension–velocity of contraction relationship, findings based on isolated muscle preparations and those based on live subject experiments should be distinguished. In the latter instance, the term 'moment–angular velocity relationship' should be used.

Mathematical description

A formula which describes the force–velocity relationship has been proposed by Hill (1953):

$$(T + a)(v + b) = (T_o + a)/b$$

where T is the tension, T_o is the isometric tension, v is the speed of shortening, and a and b are constants, such that $v_{max} = bT_o/a$, where v_{max} is the speed of shortening with no load.

This equation may also be expressed in a normalized form, namely:

$$v' = (1 - T')(1 + T'/k)$$

where $v' = v/v_{max}$, $T' = T/T_0$, and $k = a/T_0 = b/v_{max}$.

Power output

The power output, P, available from the muscle is given by (McMahon 1984):

$$\text{Power} = \text{Tension} \times \text{speed of shortening}$$

or

$$P = Tv$$

Using Hill's formula, this may be expressed as:

$$P = v(bT_o - av)/(v + b)$$

Its maximal value is reached when the speed of shortening is 25–33% of v_{max}.

The above equations are depicted graphically in Fig. 1.6 (McMahon 1984), which is based on $k = 0.25$. It should be noted that the force–velocity equation allows for active lengthening (where 'active' refers to a contractile state). In this case the rise in muscle tension as a function of the imposed active stretching velocity is dramatically steeper than in the corresponding case of shortening.

MUSCLE MOMENT AND ANGULAR VELOCITY

In studies based on live subjects the terms 'force' and 'velocity' are no longer appropriate. The former is replaced by the moment (strength) and angular velocity of the joint replaces the linear velocity of shortening (lengthening) of the muscle. In addition,

Box 1.1   Concentric and eccentric contractions
• Concentric contraction occurs when active muscle undergoes shortening while overcoming external resistance • Eccentric contraction occurs when active muscle undergoes lengthening while being overcome by an external resistance

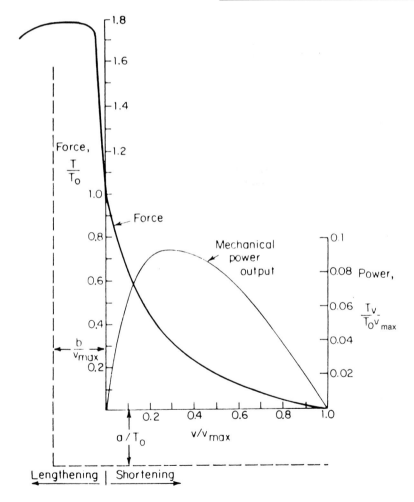

Fig. 1.6 Hill's force–velocity curve. The shortening part of the curve was calculated with $k = 0.25$. The asymptotes for Hill's hyperbola (broken lines) are parallel to the T/T_o and v/v_{max} axes. Near zero shortening velocity, the lengthening part of the curve has a negative slope approximately 6 times steeper than the shortening part. The externally delivered power was calculated from the product of tension and shortening velocity. (From McMahon T A Muscles, reflexes and locomotion. Copyright © 1984 by PUP. Reproduced by permission of Princeton University Press.)

the terms shortening and (active) lengthening are replaced by 'concentric' and 'eccentric contractions'. (see Box 1.1).

Applicability of in vitro muscle behavior

Numerous studies based on isokinetic measurements of various muscle groups, have confirmed that the principles governing in vitro muscle behavior namely the force–velocity relationships are generally also valid for moment–angular velocity relationships. However there are some exceptions mainly with regard to concentric activity at very low velocities (Perrine & Edgerton 1978, Froese & Houston 1985) and in eccentric contractions (see below).

The above-mentioned principles may be summarized as follows. When the imposed test velocity is increased:

1. For concentric contractions, there is a parallel decrease in the maximal moment developed by the muscle/muscle group (Figs 1.7–1.9).
2. For eccentric contractions, the maximal moment may rise initially but at higher velocities it plateaus (Figs. 1.10, 1.11).

Order of strength

Additionally, the principles mentioned above are supplemented by:

1. For the same velocity, the ecccentric strength is greater than the concentric strength.
2. According to the principle proposed by Elftman (1966), the order of strength, dependent on contraction mode, is: eccentric > isometric > concentric.

Range of test velocities

As is evident from Figures 1.7–1.11 which refer to concentric contractions, the range of test velocities can reach 500°/s. The use of such a high velocity may sometimes be only of academic value as not many subjects, particularly those suffering from some movement dysfunction, will be able to generate a sufficient moment to move the distal segment faster than the preset velocity. Neither are such velocities relevant to all joints. A corresponding velocity range for eccentric contractions has never been reported simply because no available isokinetic system can impose velocities of this order of magnitude.

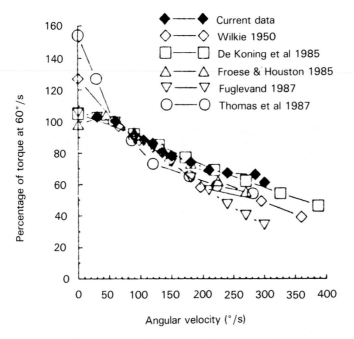

Fig. 1.7 Gravity-corrected, normalized angle-specific moment–velocity relationships for arm flexion, ankle plantar flexion and knee extension. 'Moment' here is referred to as 'torque'. (From Taylor et al 1991 copyright © Springer-Verlag.)

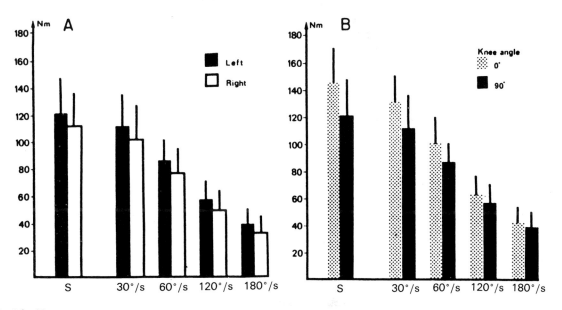

Fig. 1.8 Moment–angular velocity relationship in ankle plantar flexion. **A** Right and left knees flexed at 90°. **B** Knee at either 90° or 0° flexion. (From Fugl-Meyer et al 1979.)

Furthermore, stretching active muscles at very high velocities, poses a serious threat to the integrity of the muscles and hence should not be even tried. Hence Figures 1.10 and 1.11 which depict eccentric moment–angular velocity curves are based on the low–medium spectrum of velocities, i.e., up to 120°/s.

Interestingly, the inverse relationship between the moment and the velocity, characteristic of concentric contractions, is not confined to the case

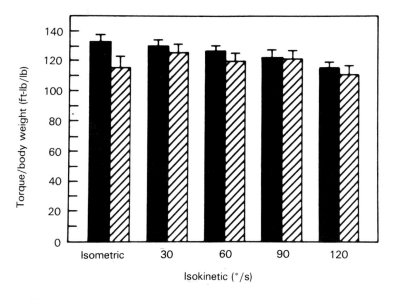

Fig. 1.9 Isometric and multispeed isokinetic extensor moment/bodyweight ratios for 18–29 (solid bars) and 30–44 (hatched bars) year-old male subjects. (From Smith et al 1985.)

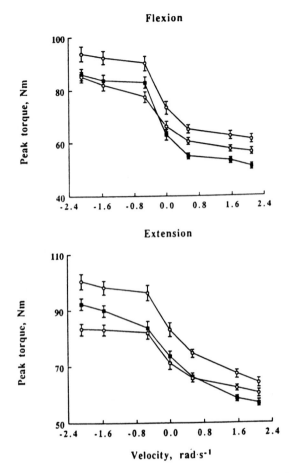

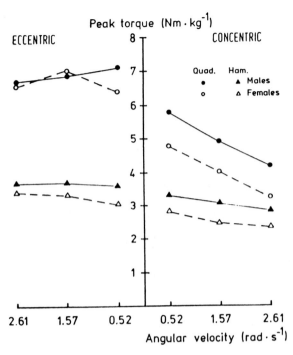

Fig. 1.11 Bodyweight-normalized moment–angular velocity curves for concentric and eccentric contractions of the quadriceps (circles) and hamstring (triangles) in males (solid symbols) and females (open symbols). (From Colliander & Tesch 1989 copyright © Springer-Verlag.)

Fig. 1.10 Moment–angular velocity curves for concentric and eccentric forearm flexion and extension. Solid squares, peak moment; open circles, angle-based moments. Moment is referred to as 'torque' and angular velocity is in radians/second. (From Hortobagyi & Katch 1990 copyright © Springer-Verlag.)

of a single joint. It is valid for two-joint muscles like the hamstring and, in a more global form, to multijoint muscles like the extensors of the trunk (Timm 1988).

Increased moment of eccentric contractions

The increased moment, observed during eccentric contractions, deviates from both the theoretical model and the in vitro findings. It is shown by the levelling off of the moment–angular velocity curve which takes place even at relatively low velocities. This finding has been confirmed in a number of studies of the elbow (Griffin 1987, Hortobagyi & Katch 1990), shoulder (Shklar & Dvir 1994) and,

particularly, the knee (Rizzardo et al 1988, Colliander & Tesch 1989, Ghena et al 1991).

The explanation for this phenomenon which probably has the widest acceptance posits a negative feedback loop which involves peripheral and spinal regulation in order to avoid excessive stresses on the muscle itself (Stauber 1989). According to this explanation the central nervous system monitors total tension over the time concerned (the tension–time integral, or impulse), and limits the eccentric potential of the muscle which could exceed the isometric strength by about 100% (Edman et al 1979). Indeed, when this loop fails to operate properly, as might occur in sudden and vigorous stretching of an active muscle, tear of the musculotendinous unit could result. A typical example is the rupture of the Achilles tendon during an unexpected forward fall.

Though in these instances the eccentric activity of the muscle is interpretable in terms of a defensive action, the end result might be a direct insult to the defender.

THE E/C RATIO

The contraction mode-dependent order of muscle strength mentioned earlier has been confirmed in a number of studies referring to muscles of the elbow (Rodgers & Berger 1974, Griffin 1987), hip (Olson et al 1972) and knee (Smidt 1973). An important result of this principle is expressed in the ratio:

$$\frac{\text{Maximal eccentric moment}}{\text{Maximal concentric moment}}$$

which is also known as the E/C ratio.

Since the magnitude of the moments generated in both contraction modes are velocity-dependent (though less so with respect to the eccentric) this ratio is by definition velocity-dependent. Moreover, in view of the shape of the moment–angular velocity curve, E/C should increase proportionately with the test velocity. Current knowledge regarding the range of this ratio refers mostly to the low–medium sector of the velocity spectrum, since the use of high velocities for the study of eccentric muscle performance is not free of risk, as emphasized before. Table 1.1 shows the consistent findings for the E/C ratio in normal individuals. Some exceptions have been noted, with a general tendency towards higher values, but the upper limit has remained by and large at 2.0.

E/C ratio and isokinetic leg-press

Interestingly, these typical figures of the E/C ratio may not necessarily be confined to single joint instances. Recently, muscle performance in isokinetic leg-press has been studied with a particular focus on the variations of the ratio (Dvir 1994). The leg-press was performed in the supine position with the hip and knee initially at 90° and involved simultaneous concentric extension of the joints through an ROM of about 30°. The return movement consisted of resisted (eccentric) flexion of the knee and hip.

Although these motions called for different muscles to act at possibly different phases, the overall ratios between the forces exerted against the foot attachment were 1.56 and 1.68 for the velocities of 8 and 15°/s respectively. Though these values are exceedingly high for such very low velocities, it should be borne in mind that first, force rather than moment was measured, and second, at this angular sector of knee motion, the passive tension developed in the hamstring during the forced stretching could add considerably to the eccentric moment generated by this muscle. On the other hand, the fact that the higher velocity resulted in a higher E/C ratio is in accord with findings relating to single joint exertions.

Range of the E/C ratio

It is therefore proposed that, with respect to single joint testing, particularly the knee and shoulder, the E/C value derived from low–medium test velocities is very likely to be within the range 0.95–2.05. This conclusion has been debated in probably only one paper. Trudelle-Jackson et al (1989) challenged the lower end of the proposed range, claiming that 35–54% of normal subjects had an E/C of less than 0.85. On the other hand, many other papers have consistently shown the proposition to be valid, sometimes even in the presence of a pathology (Conway et al 1992).

Table 1.1 The range of the maximal eccentric moment/maximal concentric moment (E/C) ratio

Joint	E/C range	Angular velocity range (degrees/sec)	Author(s)
Knee	1.1–1.5	45–180	Kramer & McDermid 1989 (based on data in the text)
	1.3–1.7	60–180	Rizzardo et al 1988
	1.2–1.6	30–150	Colliander & Tesch 1989
Elbow	1.1–1.3	30–120	Griffin 1987
	1.4–1.7	30–120	Horobagyi & Katch 1990
Shoulder (all six common motions tested independently)			Dvir & Shklar 1993
Minimal (internal rotation)	1.1–1.2	60–180	
Maximal (adduction)	1.2–1.7	60–180	

However, deviations from the above range, related to pathological conditions have been reported. A particularly low E/C (less than 0.85), was proposed as a potential source in patellofemoral problems by Bennett & Stauber (1986). This proposition, which was based on 'an error in the neuromotor control' of the quadriceps, is discussed at length in Chapter 6. An alternative explanation proposes a selective inhibition of eccentric performance due to pain. This theory relies on the high stresses produced during eccentric contractions as well as the opposite motion of the patella (see also Chapter 6).

Pathological increases in the E/C ratio

Spastic paresis

A less controversial example of an unusually high E/C ratio, which is also neurophysiologically mediated, is the case of quadriceps performance in patients with spastic paresis (see below). In these patients, eccentric contractions are not supposed to trigger antagonistic spastic responses, since the resulting motion works to relax the antagonists rather than stretch them. Furthermore, there is pro-

bably an increased output from the primary endings of the spindles in the agonist (Knutsson 1987).

Figure 1.12 depicts the concentric and eccentric strength curves of the quadriceps in a patient with spastic paresis. There is a very sharp decrease in the concentric strength (the paresis) to about 10% of normal (for the appropriate gender and age). On the other hand, the eccentric strength is within the normal range. The E/C ratio is therefore strikingly high: between 4 and 5.

Beta-thalassemia major

The phenomenon of a sharp increase in the E/C ratio has also been demonstrated in another clinical group, where there may not be neurological involvement. These are patients suffering from beta-thalassemia major, a severe form of hereditary anemia which leads, among other complications, to scarring and degeneration of muscle tissue.

These patients who have an acute concentric strength deficiency retain an eccentric strength which, although not on a par with the norm, leads to a ratio which is far in excess of the normal (Fig. 13, Dvir & Dagan 1994). The excessive connective tissue component may be the reason for this phenomenon.

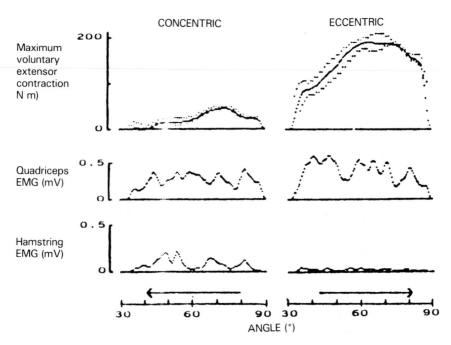

Fig. 1.12 Abnormal eccentric/concentric strength ratio (test velocity, 180°/s) in the knee extensors of a patient with spastic paraparesis. (From Knutsson 1987.)

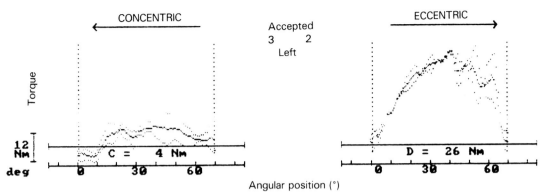

Fig. 1.13 Abnormal eccentric/concentric strength ratio (test velocity, 30°/s) in a patient with beta-thalassemia major. C and D are the avereage moment (in Nm).

THE MOMENT–ANGULAR VELOCITY RELATIONSHIP IN PASSIVE STRETCHING

Passive stretching in healthy individuals

When a limb segment of an healthy individual is moved passively in such a way that a gravitational component acts on the segment, the resisting moment may be attributed to the force of gravity, and also to the viscoelastic characteristics of the muscle and its associated connective tissues. However, since the second element starts to exert an appreciable force only after the resting length has been reached, a position well into the far ROM of the joint, it is unlikely to play a decisive role in mediating the moment.

Another factor is the reflex contraction in some muscles which normally move the segment in the opposite direction ('antagonist activation'). This phenomenon seldom occurs in normal subjects, and then only when passive motion is performed at the highest velocities (Thilmann et al 1991).

Restraint of antagonist activation

Indeed, one characteristic of a well coordinated neuromuscular system is its ability to perform smoothly even in extremely high velocities, by virtue of restraining antagonist activation. For instance in a highly trained baseball pitcher, concentric contraction of the glenohumeral depressors may proceed from late cocking to acceleration (Glousman et al 1988) at maximal force, resulting in arm angular velocities in the order of thousands of degrees per second without provoking appreciable antagonist activity. (*Cocking* means the pull back of the arm before its forceful forward movement, a concept based on the action of the cock of a gun.)

One of the reasons an untrained athlete, with equivalent dynamic performance of the former muscles, may find it difficult to generate the same arm angular velocity, is the reciprocal activation of the latter muscles. This 'deactivation' of antagonists is acquired following intensive specific training.

SPASTICITY AND PARESIS

Antagonist activity

Without elaborating on the complex mechanisms which underlie the phenomenon of spasticity, antagonist muscle performance is clearly impaired in some patients with neurological involvement. It is most conspicuous in those presenting with spastic paresis following a lesion in the central nervous system. Spasticity is described as 'a motor disorder characterized by a velocity-dependent increase in tonic stretch reflexes (muscle tone) with exaggerated tendon jerks, resulting from hyperexcitability of the stretch reflex, as one component of the upper motor neuron syndrome' (Lance 1980).

The component of paresis or weakness is evident in the voluntary, as well as in the automatic or semiautomatic, movements of daily living such as walking (Knutsson 1987). One source for this weakness may be the spastic restraint exerted by the antagonist activity mentioned earlier. In such a case, agonist performance may be intact but the countermoment may result in an overall reduction in strength.

Evaluation using isokinetic dynamometers

The exact evaluation of spasticity and paresis is essential for the determination of the patient's clinical and disability status. Common methods are based on clinical scales (manual), electrophysiological and mechanical instruments (Katz & Rymer 1989). In the latter, the role of isokinetic dynamometers is unique. These instruments are also capable of passively moving a limb segment at a predetermined velocity and consequently enable a systematic measurement of involuntary muscular resistance. Indeed, this was one of the first applications of the KinCom system, which was the prototype of active systems.

Although the velocity dependence of spasticity has been challenged (Katz & Rymer 1989), the ability of these dynamometers to accurately measure the 'spastic resistance' with regard to the angular position in the total available ROM, render them an important tool in this field.

Demonstration of abnormal antagonist activity

Active isokinetic systems have been used in the pioneering studies of Knutsson and his colleagues, at the Karolinska Institute in Sweden, to demonstrate the effect of abnormal antagonist activity (Knutsson & Martenssen 1980, Knutsson 1987). Figure 1.14 depicts the flexor strength curve during a voluntary contraction of the hamstring in a patient with spastic paresis. The sharp decrease in the moment at 120°/s was associated with greatly increased electromyographic activity in the quadriceps. Activity of this magnitude does not occur in normal subjects at such a relatively low velocity. In the opposite motion, the hamstrings are activated both in passive and active extension of the knee (Fig. 1.15).

Variability of spasticity measurement

Though the application of isokinetic dynamometers to measuring spasticity is obvious, studies using them have generally confirmed the agreement that this condition is highly variable among, and often within subjects (Knutsson 1987, Dvir & Panturin 1993). Moreover, though spastic restraint may be clinically felt by the examiner, isokinetic measurements have failed to corroborate this impression in one group of paraplegic patients (Zelig 1992).

Whether this finding reflects a different source of spasticity, i.e. predominantly from a spinal or a higher CNS lesion, or a residual drug effect even after wash-out, or an improper test velocity range, is

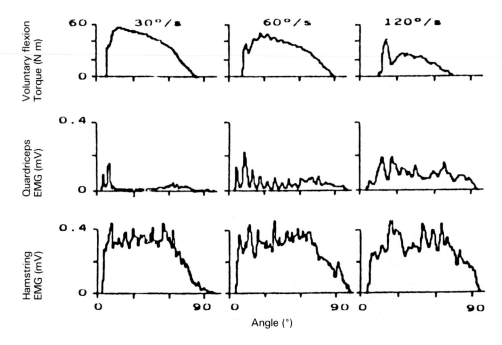

Fig. 1.14 Strength curves and rectified EMG from the quadriceps and the hamstring in a patient with spastic paraparesis at angular velocities of 30, 60 and 120°/s. (From Knutsson 1987.)

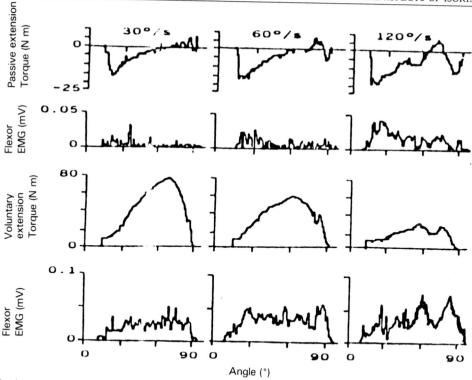

Fig. 1.15 Passive extension and strength curves in isokinetic knee extensions at three different angular velocities. Rectified EMG traces from knee flexors stretched during extensions. (From Knutsson 1987.)

at present difficult to determine. For instance, Thilmann et al (1991) have suggested that in moderately involved patients, the critical velocity required to elicit enhanced stretch reflex was around 100°/s. Nevertheless, in some of our patients, a velocity of even 180°/s was not sufficient to elicit the expected response.

Clearly the use of isokinetic instruments in this field is still at a very early, albeit promising, stage.

CLOSED VERSUS OPEN KINETIC CHAINS
MULTIJOINT MOTION

The design of almost all commercially available isokinetic dynamometers is based on rotational motion of the lever-arm. Since the force sensor is attached (in most systems) to the lever-arm, it means that the measured forces are tangential to the arc of motion. This configuration is particularly suitable for assessing planar, single joint motion or the so-called hinge movements, whose typical example is the knee. It is also the case that the number of muscles involved in executing suchmotion is normally minimal.

However in all other instances, joint motion is multiplanar and, even more importantly, combined harmoniously with other joints. In this case, though the total moment output may be isokinetically measurable, the individual contributions of the muscles/muscle groups responsible for executing the motion may not be directly determined, or at least not in the way possible for planar, single-joint motion.

The analysis and practical use of multijoint motion are of considerable interest in rehabilitation, because of the growing awareness of the need to integrate motions and emphasize the whole rather than the part. Isokinetic dynamometers can play an important role in this respect but the advantages and limitations must be clearly stated. For this purpose it is necessary to define and describe the concepts of closed and open kinetic chains.

OPEN AND CLOSED KINETIC CHAIN (OKC AND CKC)

Open kinetic chain (OKC) This is defined as a sequence of articulated segments: the 'tail' of the

nth segment is connected to the $(n-1)$th and its 'head' is connected to the $(n+1)$th segment. The first segment is commonly regarded as stationary, and is called the 'frame' whereas the end segment is free to move. A classical example for an OKC is the upper limb, where the frame is the ribcage and the distal link is the hand.

Closed kinetic chain (CKC) This is an arrangement of sequentially articulated segments in which the distal segment and the frame are also articulated, thus closing the otherwise open chain.

The motion of the end-segment in an OKC is not constrained whereas in a CKC any segment may be considered 'end' or 'tail'. Thus OKC and CKC are frequently described as distal-end-free or distal-end-fixed respectively. An example of a CKC is the configuration of the whole body in a hand-assisted rise from a seat. As long as the hands grip the forearm rests, the chain consists of the 'articulation' between the floor and the feet, the other body articulations leading to the hands, and back to the floor via the chair.

OKC or CKC?

The human body presents an intricate array of OKCs and CKCs. For instance although bringing the hand to a specific location may be an OKC activity, a function like pinching an object, performed by two fingers, is typically characterized as a CKC activity. The swing phase of gait finds the foot of the swinging leg in an OKC state but once ground contact is established (double support) a CKC is formed. Thus, when the distal segment is constrained to move in a certain fashion (and so are the other segments) the system behaves like a CKC, while when the distal segment is unconstrained the movement is characteristic of OKC.

It is therefore the temporary set-up of the joints/segments rather than their anatomical articulations that decides whether the configuration is OKC or CKC.

Single joint testing

Common isokinetic testing is erroneously understood to be conducted in an OKC mode. Referring for instance to the knee, assuming that the leg and foot are 'free' to move ignores their firm harnessing to the lever-arm, which in turn is part of the dynamometer. Since the thigh is also stabilized, the configuration is a CKC rather than an OKC. A more appropriate term would therefore be 'single-joint-testing' mode. The same applies to isokinetic testing of other major joint systems.

Physiological demands

Single joint testing, however, does not always simulate physiological demands. Consider for instance the dynamics of the lower extremity during stair climbing or descending. During the 'swing' phase which in this case means the process of transferring the lower extremity from one step to the next, the thigh, leg and foot are free to move in space, and therefore motion is taking place in an OKC mode. However, as soon as contact is made with the step, and before the contralateral extremity disengages from the step, i.e. during the weight acceptance phase, motion of all joints becomes interdependent as both feet are 'connected' to the step which constitutes a common segment in this CKC. The same reasoning applies in seat rise, bicycle pedalling, lifting of objects etc.

Therefore, from the functional point of view, conditioning of muscles can significantly benefit from multiple joint, CKC activity. The advantages of CKC conditioning have recently been highlighted in relation to anterior cruciate ligament (ACL) surgery and rehabilitation (Shelbourne & Nitz 1990). The significant advantage of CKC versus OKC activity in ACL reconstruction is that full activation of the quadriceps need not result in considerable tibiofemoral shear forces. Rather, due to coactivation of the hamstring (posterior shear) and larger compressive forces, the strain of the reconstructed ACL is kept at a lower level.

CKC PERFORMANCE AND ISOKINETIC TESTING

Limitations

The measurements of muscle performance in CKC mode using isokinetic dynamometers is not as straightforward as it is in the single-joint-testing mode. This is because the lever-arm turns about a fixed axis whereas CKC motion is simultaneously taking place in a number of joints. Consider the leg-press test, a simple CKC motion involving predominantly the thigh and leg (see Fig. 6.8), which is effected using a conventional isokinetic dynamometer.

In this configuration:

1. Motion of the thigh relative to the frame is radial but not isokinetic.

2. Motion of the leg relative to the frame involves linear as well as radial components but it is not isokinetic.

3. Since the force transducer is sensitive to stresses acting at a right angle to the lever arm, and assuming a fixed neutral ankle joint position, there is only one angular position in the test ROM at which the recorded force reliably represents the combined moments generated by the acting muscles. Therefore, reference to moment values recorded elsewhere in the test ROM is irrelevant. This, incidentally, does not deny acceptable reproducibility for this test (Levine et al 1991).

To solve part of the above difficulty, either a linear isokinetic dynamometer or a biaxial force transducer is required. Neither of these are commercially available, at the time of writing, though specific attachments offered by some manufacturers are intended to provide linear motion. It should also be emphasized that though it is possible, using mathematical modelling, to calculate the forces and moments acting on the knee and hip, the available software does not cater for these mechanical parameters.

Total lower extremity strength

Though isokinetic CKC contractions pose a maximal challenge to combined muscle activity, it is interesting to note that the strength of muscles with respect to the individual joints, namely in OKC mode, may not be closely related to the total (CKC) output.

In a recent study, a group of healthy individuals were tested concentrically and eccentrically, using the leg-press and knee extension tests (Dvir 1994). In order to reliably measure the force exerted against the lever-arm the test ROM was limited to an angular sector of about 30°, arranged symmetrically about the thigh vertical position. Because of

this limited ROM, test angular velocities were set at the very low values of 8 and 15°/s, to allow for proper tension generation. The strength of the quadriceps was measured using the same test conditions in the seated position.

It was discovered that the correlations between the force output in the CKC configuration and that of the quadriceps were low, 0.15–0.44 and not significant. This finding applied to both contraction modes, and for the peak and average moments alike. Consequently, if the concept of total lower extremity strength is perceived as an independent parameter rather than the sum of the strengths of individual muscle groups, the former may not be directly predictable using the latter.

JOINT LOADING DURING DYNAMIC EXERTIONS

It is one of the basic tenets of isokinetics that the muscular force level generated during a maximal contraction isokinetic test performed in an 'OKC' (single-joint-testing) mode is the maximum possible. This, apart from the rate at which the joint moves, is basically what distinguishes isokinetic from the so-called isotonic or isoinertial contractions.

Even in the absence of any external load, i.e., during pure antigravity motions, the force generated by muscle is much larger than the weight (which is also a force) of the relevant segment/s. This situation is due to the conspicuous mechanical disadvantage of muscles which derives from their comparatively very short levers. For example if the weight of the upper limb is 60 N (9.81 N = 1 kgf), the deltoid force needed to maintain the limb in 90° elevation could reasonably exceed 600 N. Ultimately, only a relatively small percentage of the muscle force is used to counteract the external load; the rest is transmitted through the joint articular surfaces or taken up by anatomical structures such as the ligaments and capsule.

Magnitude of forces in isokinetic exercise

Obviously when loads are to be moved, supported or resisted, the muscular forces increase both in proportion to the magnitude of the load and its distance from the instantaneous joint axis. Hence, it is expected that exertions under isokinetic conditions will result in considerable joint forces.

It should be emphasized that these forces are not necessarily the largest that a particular joint may be called to support. These may occur in the course of strong impact loading, due to force absorption in the course of landing, or during simultaneous contraction of antagonistic muscles.

Also if different models are used for prediction of joint forces, significantly different results may be obtained. Nevertheless, those models which have been applied in the case of the knee, give an idea of the magnitude of the relevant forces.

Knee joint forces

Kaufman et al (1991) have used a complex isokinetic set-up in order to study the tibiofemoral and patellofemoral forces that act on the knee during maximal isokinetic exercise.

Their findings indicated that the average tibiofemoral force was four times bodyweight (4 bw), approximately equal to that obtained during walking except that it was reached at a different, and much higher, knee angle. The anterior and posterior shear forces (resisting the anterior and posterior drawer forces respectively) were on average 0.3 and 1.7 bw. The anterior shear force was larger than what would be expected during walking, whereas the posterior shear force was much larger than in walking but on a par with the posterior shear in stair climbing.

Very high patellofemoral forces, reaching 5.1 bw at 60°/s, were calculated as acting during isokinetic exercise. This force should be compared with only 0.5 bw during walking and 3.3 bw in ascending or descending stairs, but 7.6 bw in squat descent (Dahlqvist et al 1987) or 20 bw during jumping (Smith 1975).

Nisell et al (1989, 1992) have used other models in their analysis of the knee joint and have obtained much higher forces: 9 bw and 12 bw in the tibiofemoral and patellofemoral joints respectively.

Implications of high isokinetic forces

Notwithstanding the large differences in the above findings, it is clear that isokinetic exertions may result in considerable knee joint forces. The significance of such high forces hardly needs further elaboration especially where pain, articular surface derangement or recent surgical intervention are involved.

Though analogous forces have not so far been calculated for other joint systems, it would not be unreasonable to assume that equivalent conditions prevail. An indication of this may be found, for example, with the shoulder, where maximal isokinetic exertions are not tolerated in many patients who suffer from some joint dysfunction. Thus although isokinetically-related joint forces may not be comparable to those obtained during specific athletic activities, their magnitude must be allowed for in the planning of testing and muscle conditioning of normal subjects and, especially patients.

ECCENTRIC–CONCENTRIC COUPLING

The phenomenon of concentric contraction potentiation following eccentric contraction ('prestretching') of the same muscle is well established (Cavagna et al 1968, Komi & Bosco 1978, Bosco & Komi 1979, Bosco et al 1987). This phenomenon, which has been termed the 'stretch–shortening cycle' or 'plyometric' contraction, is based primarily on the mechanical behavior of the series elastic element which is found in both the contractile elements and the tendons (Svantesson et al 1991). In eccentric contractions energy is accumulated in the muscle in both mechanical and chemical forms.

Coupling time and extent of stretch

The factors of coupling time (CT) and extent of stretch have been studied with regard to the efficiency of potentiation. (*Coupling time* is the transition period between the eccentric and concentric contractions (Bosco et al 1981). This period is commonly measured in milliseconds.) It has been suggested that the average duration of the cross-bridge, between the actin and myosin, is 15 ms (Stienen et al 1978). Since during active stretch the heads of the myosin filaments are rotated backwards (Huxley & Simmons 1971) it is possible that with a prolonged stretched position, these attachments will detach (Cavagna & Citterior 1974). A short CT is closely related to the extent of stretch of the muscle. A relatively large range of stretch can result in 'slipping' of the sarcomeres (Flitney &

Hirst 1978) and loss of the potentiation effect. Conversely, a limited ROM in the involved joints can contribute to a large eccentric force and, by utilizing the principle of short range stiffness (Rack & Westbury 1974), to a short CT.

Neurological aspects

The neural component in plyometric contraction or stretch reflex potentiation, is modulated via the Ia afferents from the muscle spindle, and possibly assisted by cortical loops (Iles 1977). Reflex potentiation and the increased motorneuron activity to the contracting muscles considerably amplifies the force at the end of the eccentric phase. This leads to an increase in muscle stiffness, which in turn renders the condition favorable to short coupling time.

In controlling the tension level in the muscle, the central nervous system utilizes three mechanisms: it may vary the number of active motor units (Milner-Brown et al 1973a), their rate of firing and level of synchrony (Milner-Brown et al 1973b).The extent to which the neural component influences the end result is not clear but it does not seem to play the primary role.

In vivo studies

Prestretching and vertical jump

In a study by Bosco et al (1981), vertical jump scores were compared in subjects who performed with and without preliminary countermovement (eccentric contraction). With prestretching the force and power were significantly higher, 66 and 81% respectively. The mean CT was 23 ms (SD = 14.7 ms) and the prestretch angular velocity of the knee was 252°/s (SD = 107°/s).

Contraction order

The effect of contraction order on concentric elbow flexor output was studied by Vyse & Kramer (1990). Subjects were tested using two protocols: two cycles of concentric-eccentric contractions, or two cycles of eccentric-concentric contractions. Each protocol was performed at 60 and 150°/s and the criterion parameters consisted of the peak and average moments. It was indicated that although these parameters were about 8% higher in the first protocol

(concentric-eccentric) compared with the second, this enhancement was not significant. On the other hand, the concentric-eccentric protocol resulted in a 10% reduction in the eccentric scores which was attributed to deactivation of the contractile mechanism during the concentric phase and apprehension.

It is however highly significant that the findings failed to reveal a difference, in terms of the performance criteria, between the two test velocities. Therefore the results of this study may be viewed as inconclusive, because the elbow flexors may require higher velocities in order to realize concentric potentiation; the findings of Bosco et al (1981), mentioned earlier, used a much higher angular velocity in knee plyometrics.

Angular velocity and plyometrics

The significance of angular velocity was indicated in a study, which analysed ankle plantarflexor strength during concentric potentiation compared with concentric contraction alone (Svantesson et al 1991). Two test positions, knee at full extension and knee at 90°, and two velocities, 120 and 240°/s were used.

It was shown that the moment generated during a concentric action which was preceeded by an eccentric contraction, was on average 100% larger than that generated during concentric contraction without the preceding stretch. Moreover, the percentage increase in the plyometric (concentric) moment at the higher velocity was larger than in the lower velocity (by a factor of about 3:2 at 90–99° of plantarflexion), and more pronounced at the knee position of full extension. It was also observed that the CT was 30 ms, well within the acceptable range of efficient potentiation.

It should also be noted that, in terms of performance potentiation, the findings of Svantesson et al (1991) correlated with those obtained by Bosco et al (1981), although the mechanical parameters which were used to measure the gain were different.

Simulation of realistic conditions

It is clear that in order to predict effectively the extent of prestretch potentiation, the isokinetic conditions must closely simulate the realistic ones.

This point was made in a study which compared the mechanical output about the ankle joint in isokinetic plantarflexion with that achieved during one-legged vertical jump (Bobbert & Van Ingen Schenau 1991). Isokinetic concentric contractions which were not preceded by eccentric contractions were performed in a velocity range of 30–300°/s. It was indicated that at any given angular velocity of plantarflexion above 60°/s, subjects produced much larger moments during jumping than during maximal effort isokinetic plantarflexion.

Relevance to isokinetics

The issue of plyometric contractions may become relevant in an isokinetic setting where there is continuous activation of a muscle group, using first eccentric and then concentric contractions. As testing protocols develop, the exact method of incorporating eccentric exertions becomes important. Moreover, the possibility of simulating plyo-metric conditions using isokinetic systems is very tempting, especially with regard to the conditioning of athletes, in whom shock absorption through the feet, characteristic of the prestretch phase in the vertical jump event, constitutes a serious risk. The experimental findings on the use of isokinetics in effecting plyometric contractions are somewhat controversial.

On balance, it seems that isokinetic dyna-mometary may be used for simulation of stretch–shortening cycles, although the ideal conditions are still undefined regarding the specific joint, the test (conditioning) position, the mode of operation (OKC or CKC) and the imposed stretch velocities. For instance, since cortical mediation may have an effect on the mechanical output, positioning of the subject should be investigated. Likewise, although the experimental set-up in Svantesson et al (1991) was based on identical eccentric and concentric velocities, this need not necessarily be the case.

REFERENCES

Bennett G, Stauber W T 1986 Evaluation and treatment of anterior knee pain using eccentric exercise. Medicine and Science in Sports and Exercise 18: 526–530.

Bobbert M F, van Ingen Schenau G I 1990 Mechanical output about the ankle joint in isokinetic plantar flexion and jumping. Medicine and Science in Sports and Exercise 22: 600–668

Bosco C, Komi P V 1979 Potentiation of the mechanical behavior of human skeletal muscle through prestretching. Acta Physiologica Scandinavica 106: 467–471

Bosco C, Komi P V, Ito A 1981 Pre-stretch potentiation of human skeletal muscle during ballistic movements. Acta Physiologica Scandinavica 111: 135–140

Bosco C, Tarkka J, Komi P V 1987 Effect of elastic energy and myoelectric potentiation of triceps surae during stretch-shortening cycle exercise. International Journal of Sports Medicine 2: 137–143

Cavagna G A, Citterio G 1974 Effect of stretching on the elastic characteristics and the contractile component of frog striated muscle. Journal of Physiology 239: 1–14

Cavagna G A, Dusman B, Margaria R 1968 Positive work done by a previously stretched muscle. Journal of Applied Physiology 24: 21–30

Colliander E B, Tesch P 1989 Bilateral eccentric and concentric torque of quadriceps and hamstring muscles in females and males. European Journal of Applied Physiology 59: 227–232

Conway A, Malone T R, Conway P 1992 Patellar alignment/tracking: effect on force output and perceived pain. Isokinetics and Exercise Science 2: 9–17

Dahlqvist N J, Mayo P Seedhom B B 1987 Forces during squatting and rising from a deep squat. Engineering in Medicine 11: 69–76

De Koning F L, Blinkhorst R A, Vos J A, van't Hof M A 1985 The force velocity relationship of arm flexion in untrained males and females and arm-trained athletes. European Journal of Applied Physiology 54: 89–94

Dvir Z, Dagan I 1994 Muscle performance in patients with beta-thalassaemia major. Submitted

Dvir Z, Panturin E 1993 Measurement of spasticity and associated reactions in stroke patients before and after physiotherapeutic intervention. Clinical Rehabilitation 7: 15–21

Dvir Z 1994 A preliminary study of isokinetic leg press. Submitted

Edman K A, Elizinga G, Noble M I 1979 The effect of stretch on contracting skeletal muscle fibers. In: Sugi H, Pollack G H (eds) Cross bridge mechanism in muscle contraction. University Park Press, Baltimore, pp 297–309

Elftman H 1966 Biomechanics of muscle. Journal of Bone and Joint Surgery 48A: 363–373

Flitney F W, Hirst D G 1978 Cross-bridge detachment and sarcomere give during stretch of active frog's muscle. Journal of Physiology 276: 449–465

Freedson P S, Gilliam T B, Mahoney T, Maliszewski A F, Kastango K 1993 Industrial torque levels by age group and gender. Isokinetics and Exercise Science 3: 34–42

Froese E A, Houston M E 1985 Torque-velocity characteristics and muscle fiber type in human vastus lateralis. Journal of Applied Physiology 59: 309–314

Fuglevand A J 1987 Resultant muscle torque, angular velocity and joint angle relationships and activation patterns in maximal knee extension. In: Jonsson B (ed) Biomechanics X-A. International series on biomechanics. Human Kinetics, Champaign, Illinois, pp 559–565

Fugl-Meyer A R, Sjostrom M, Wahlby L 1979 Human plantar flexion strength and structure. Acta Physiologica Scandinavia 107: 47–56

Ghena D G, Kurth A L, Thomas M, Mayhew J 1991 Torque characteristics of the quadriceps and hamstring muscles during concentric and eccentric loading. Journal of Orthopaedic and Sports Physical Therapy 14: 149–154

Glousman R E, Jobe F W, Tibone J E, Moynes D, Antonelli D, Perry J 1988 Dynamic electromyographic analysis of the throwing shoulder with glenohumeral instability. Journal of Bone and Joint Surgery 70A: 220–226

Gordon A M, Huxley A F, Julian F T 1966 The variations in isometric tension with sarcomere length in vertebrate muscle fibers. Journal of Physiology 1984: 170–192

Griffin J W 1987 Differences in elbow flexion torque measured concentrically, eccentrically and isometrically. Physical Therapy 67: 1205–1208

Herzog W, Hasler E, Abrahamse S 1991 A comparison of knee extensor strength curves obtained theoretically and experimentally. Medicine and Science in Sports and Exercise 23: 108–114

Hill A V 1953 The mechanics of active muscle. Proceedings of the Royal Society 141B: 104–117

Hortobagyi T, Katch F I 1990 Eccentric and concentric torque-velocity relationships during arm flexion and extension. European Journal of Applied Physiology 60: 395–401

Huxley A F, Simmons R M 1971 Proposed mechanism of force generation in striated muscles. Nature 233: 533–538

Iles J F 1977 Response in human prefibiae muscles to sudden stretch and to nerve stimulation. Experimental Brain Research 30: 451–470

Kandel E R, Schwartz J H, Jessell T M 1991 Principles of neural science, 3rd edn. Elsevier, New York

Katz R T, Rymer Z 1989 Spastic hypertonia: mechanisms and measurement. Archives of Physical Medicine and Rehabilitation 70: 144–155

Kaufman R K R, An K-N, Litchy W J, Morrey B F, Chao E Y 1991 Dynamic joint forces during knee isokinetic exercise. American Journal of Sports Medicine 19: 305–316

Knutsson E 1987 Analysis of spastic paresis. In: International Congress of the World Confederation for Physical Therapy, Sidney

Knutsson E, Martensson A 1980 Dynamic motor capacity in spastic paresis and its relation to prime mover dysfunction, spastic restraint and antagonist coactivation. Scandinavian Journal of Rehabilitation Medicine 12: 93–106

Komi P V, Bosco C 1978 Utilization of stored elastic energy in leg extensor muscles by men and women. Medicine and Science in Sports and Exercise 10: 261–265

Kramer J F, McDermid J 1989 Isokinetic measures during concentric-eccentric cycles of knee extensors. Australian Journal of Physiotherapy 35: 9–14

Lance J W 1980 Symposium synopsis. In: Feldman R G, Young R R, Koella W P (eds) Spasticity: disordered motor control. Year Book Publishers, Chicago, pp 485–494

Levin D, Klein A, Morrissey M 1991 Reliability of isokinetic concentric closed kinematic chain testing of the hip and knee extensors. Isokinetics and Exercise Science 1: 146–152

McMahon T A 1984 Muscles, reflexes and locomotion. Princeton University Press, Princeton, New Jersey

Milner-Brown, Stein R B, Yemm R 1973a The orderly recruitment of human motor units during voluntary isometric contractions. Journal of Physiology 230: 359–370

Milner-Brown, Stein R B, Yemm R 1973b Changes in firing rate of human motor units during linearly changing voluntary contractions. Journal of Physiology 230: 371–390

Nisell R, Ericson M 1992 Patellar forces during isokinetic extension. Clinical Biomechanics 7: 104–108

Nisell R, Ericson M, Nemeth G 1989 Tibiofemoral joint forces during isokinetic knee extension. American Journal of Sports Medicine 17: 49–54

Olson V L, Smidt G L, Johnston R 1972 The maximum torque generated by the concentric, isometric and eccentric contractions of the hip abductor muscles. Physical Therapy 52: 149–155

Perrine J J, Edgerton V R 1978 Muscle force–velocity and power–velocity relationships under isokinetic loading. Medicine and Science in Sports and Exercise 10: 159–166

Rabin S I, Post M 1990 A comparative study of clinical muscle testing and Cybex evaluation after shoulder operations. Clinical Orthopaedics and Related Research 258: 147–156

Rack P M, Westbury D R 1974 The short range stiffness of active mammalian muscle and its effect on mechanical properties. Journal of Physiology (Lond) 240: 331–550

Ralston H J, Pollissar M J, Inman V T, Close J R, Feinstein B 1949 Dynamic features of human isolated voluntary muscle in isometric and free contractions. Journal of Applied Physiology 1: 526–533

Rizzardo M, Bay G, Wessel J 1988 Eccentric and concentric torque and power of the knee extensors in females. Canadian Journal of Sports Science 13: 166–169

Rodgers K C, Berger K A 1974 Motor unit involvement and tension during maximum voluntary concentric, eccentric and isometric contractions of the elbow flexors. Medicine and Science in Sports and Exercise 6: 253–259

Shelbourne K D, Nitz P 1990 Accelerated rehabilitation after anterior cruciate ligament reconstruction. Americal Journal of Sports Medicine 18: 292–299

Shklar A, Dvir Z 1994 Representative values of shoulder muscles performance. Submitted 1994

Smidt G L 1973 Biomechanics of knee flexion and extension. Journal of Biomechanics 6: 79–92

Smidt G L, Hering T, Amundsen L R, Rogers M, Russsel A, Lehmann T 1983 Assessment of abdominal and back extensor function: a quantitative approach and results for chronic low-back patients. Spine 8: 211–219

Smith A J 1975 Estimates of muscle and joint forces at the knee and ankle during jumping activities. Journal of Human Movement Studies 1: 78–86

Smith S, Mayer T G, Gatchel R J, Becker T J 1985 Quantification of lumbar function. Part I: isometric and multispeed isokinetic trunk strength measures in the sagittal and axial planes in normal subjects. Spine 10: 757–764

Stauber W T 1989 Eccentric action of muscles: physiology, injury and adaptation. Exercise and Sports Science Review 19: 157–185

Stienen G J, Blange T, Schnerr M 1978 Tension response of frog sartorius muscle to quick ramp-shaped stimuli and some effects of metabolic inhibition. Pflugers Archives European Journal of Physiology 376: 97–104

Svantesson U, Ernstoff B, Bergh P, Grimby G 1991 Use of a Kin-Com dynamometer to study the stretch-shortening cycle during plantar flexion. European Journal of Applied Physiology 62: 415–419

Taylor N A, Cotter J D, Stanley S N, Marshall R N 1991 Functional torque-velocity and power-velocity characteristics of elite atheletes. European Journal of Applied Physiology 62: 116–121

Thilmann A F, Fellows S J, Garms E 1991 The mechanism of spastic muscle hypertonus: variations in reflex gain over the time course of spasticity. Brain 145: 233–244

Thomas D O, White M J, Sagar G, Davies C T 1987 Electrically evoked isokinetic plantar flexor torque in males. Journal of Applied Physiology 63: 1499–1503

Thorstensson A, Nilsson J 1982 Trunk muscle strength during constant velocity movements. Scandinavian Journal of Rehabilitation Medicine 14: 61–68

Timm K E 1988 Isokinetic lifting simulation: a normativedata study Journal of Orthopaedic and Sports Physical Therapy 9: 155–166

Trudelle-Jackson E, Meske N, Highenboten C, Jackson A 1989 Eccentric/concentric torque deficits in the quadriceps muscle. Journal of Orthopaedic and Sports Physical Therapy 11: 142–145

Vyse M, Kramer J F 1990 Interaction of concentric and eccentric muscle actions during continuous activation cycles of the elbow flexors. Physiotherapy Canada 42: 123–127

Wilkie D R 1950 The relation between force and velocity in human muscle. Journal of Physiology 110: 249–280

Winter D A, Wells R P, Orr G W 1981 Errors in the use of isokinetic dynamometers. European Journal of Applied Physiology 46: 397–408

Zelig G 1992 Measurement of spasticity in paraplegic patients after washout and during treatment with baclofen. Unpublished thesis, Tel-Aviv University, Tel-Aviv

Hardware, test parameters, and issues in testing

PART 1
HARDWARE

All isokinetic systems are based on the principle that the lever-arm moves at a preset angular velocity (PAV) however great the turning force, or moment, applied by the user. If the user pushes harder, i.e. the muscle-generated moment is increased, tending to increase the angular velocity, the machine increases its resistance correspondingly and maintains movement within very narrow margins about the PAV. The width of these margins is one of the

performance characteristics of each system. It must be stressed that the moment generated by the muscle need not be maximal. On the contrary, using the advanced options available in some systems, users may induce perfectly smooth isokinetic motion without taxing the muscles to their utmost contractile capacity.

Each of the systems on the market has its own individual features, but all have the same basic feature, namely a rotating lever-arm which moves in a single plane. This does not necessarily mean that the motion of the joint/s must be confined to a single anatomical plane. For instance, diagonal movements at the shoulder may be tested using isokinetic dynamometers. The general layout of a typical modern isokinetic system is illustrated in Fig. 2.1.

The basic elements of the system are as follows:

1. *The force acceptance unit* is the interface between the subject and the system. It consists of a metallic attachment on the lever-arm, with or without foam padding, which connects to the lever-arm via the 'load cell'. The location of the unit along the lever-arm is individually adjusted.

2. *The load cell* converts the force signal into an electric signal.

3. *The lever-arm* provides the base for the force acceptance unit and moves radially about a fixed axis.

4. *The head assembly* (Fig. 2.2) houses the motor

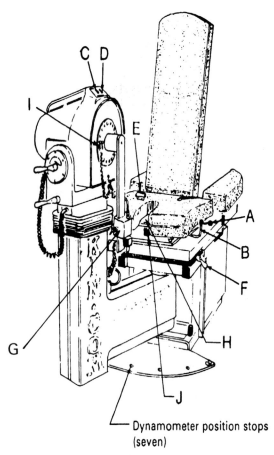

Dynamometer position stops
(seven)

Fig. 2.1 General layout of a modern isokinetic dynamometer: A, rotates seat right and left; B, adjusts seat forward/backward; C, seat up/down control swtich; D, dynamometer head up/down; E, seatbelt; F, forward/backward lock; G, Force acceptance unit and load cell; H, hook to hold thigh straps; I, mechanical stops of lever-arm; J, table extension pad receiving tube.

responsible for the motion of the lever-arm. Its orientation may be adjusted for:

a. tilt, for movement in planes other than the vertical, e.g. rotations of the humerus or subtalar motions.

b. swivelling for applications such as testing of shoulder elevators.

The head may be moved up or down using an electric motor, for the purpose of alignment. Concerning the arrangement of the head assembly and the seat, there are two design approaches. One has a fixed head assembly positioned between two seats, which requires the subject to change seats if, for instance, bilateral knee testing is carried out. The other consists of an adjustable mechanism in which the head assembly is manually moved around the subject. The latter approach, which seems to be

gaining in popularity, is also more convenient for the subjects, besides requiring less space. However, both designs must ensure the stability of the head assembly since this is a crucial factor in the reliability of the system (Herzog 1988).

The incorporation of servomotors in isokinetic systems is now commonplace. These motors move the lever-arm and may do so in either concentric or eccentric modes. In the former, the motor resists a pushing force, whereas in the latter the motor and body segment pull in opposite directions. In some systems the moment which the motor can generate in order to overcome eccentric muscle moment has deliberately been limited, with no appreciable corresponding gain in the maximal angular velocity which may be set. Other designs are characterized by high angular velocities but relatively low active (motor) moment. Consequently neither design can claim to offer genuine eccentric measurement for all joints.

5. *The seat, or plinth* serves to position the subject. The seat must have a stable frame, and independent vertical and horizontal (forward/ backward) alignment options.

6. *The control unit* consists of a personal computer and its associated peripheral equipment. The mode of operation and various other parameters (see below) are fed into the computer using the keyboard. The same computer is also responsible for the real-time data processing.

7. *Specific attachments* are required for the various applications of the isokinetic dynamometer.

PART 2
CONTROL AND PERFORMANCE PARAMETERS

Isokinetic dynamometers are measurement devices, providing clinicians with information about the dynamic, i.e. moving, mechanical performance of muscle groups. It is assumed that the joint spanned by the muscles moves at a constant angular velocity, that is, its motion is isokinetic. This assumption is incorrect even if only because biological joints do not possess a fixed axis of rotation. The extent of the error made in assuming a constant joint angular velocity depends on the joint tested, subject position etc.

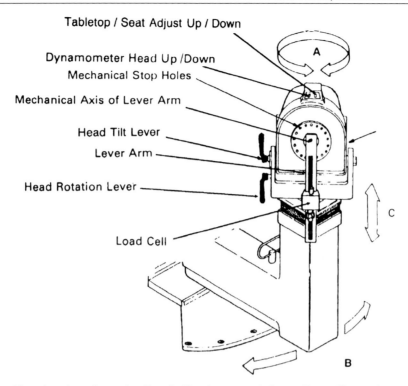

Tabletop / Seat Adjust Up / Down

Dynamometer Head Up /Down

Mechanical Stop Holes

Mechanical Axis of Lever Arm

Head Tilt Lever

Lever Arm

Head Rotation Lever

Load Cell

A

C

B

Fig. 2.2   Head assembly and motions: A, rotation; B, swivelling (seven stops); C – up/down; (tilt, not shown).

It is also possible, using these devices, to measure multijoint motion. In this case, 'isokinetic' refers exclusively to the motion of mechanical elements external to the body, such as the lever arm or handle in angular or linear testing respectively.

Isokinetic dynamometers are also useful for recording static (isometric) performance although this is not their main objective.

In isokinetic dynamometry, the basic measurement record consists of a sequence of numbers which represent the size of the force exerted by the moving distal body segment against the force sensor. In all advanced isokinetic systems, this record is displayed in a graphical form on the computer display.

'Muscle performance' is the collective name for a set of parameters derived from the basic record. These are the 'output' parameters.

Because of the physiological and biomechanical properties of skeletal muscle, which have been discussed in Chapter 1, the magnitudes of the output, or 'performance' parameters, depend, among other variables, on a set of control (input) parameters. These variables, notably the angular velocity, determine the general framework of the test (see Table 2.1). The following sections define and describe the input and output parameters of strength testing, and of fatigue and endurance testing. All parameters are given in SI (metric) units.

CONTROL PARAMETERS OF STRENGTH TESTING

Strength testing is normally understood to consist of a minimal number of maximal effort contractions.

Table 2.1   Control (input) and performance (output) parameters in isokinetic testing

Control	Performance
Joint-dependent	Moment
Range of motion (ROM)	Peak
Angular velocity(ies)	Angle-based
Subject/patient positioning	Angle of peak moment
Stabilization	Average
Alignment of the axes of the	Contractional work
dynamometer and the joint	Contractional power
Contraction mode	Contractional impulse
Joint-independent	
Damp setting	
Isometric preactivation	
Feedback	

This number may vary with different testing protocols (see Chapter 4). The objective is to produce a representative moment–angular position (MAP) curve, from which various performance parameters are derived. The control, or input, parameters which must be specified in advance, fall into two groups, the joint-dependent and joint-independent parameters.

JOINT-DEPENDENT INPUT

The joint-dependent parameters (Table 2.1) vary according to which joint is being tested. These are discussed individually in Chapters 5–9. However, general descriptions of range of motion and angular velocity are given here.

Range of motion

The range of motion (ROM) is the most basic parameter, and describes the allowable angular displacement of the lever arm. It is measured in degrees. This ROM should not be confused with the motion taking place in the biological joint, an error compounded by misalignment of the biological and mechanical axes.

The isokinetic range of motion (IROM)

The specified ROM is not the angular sector in which the distal segment motion is isokinetic. The latter, the isokinetic ROM (IROM) is always smaller than the ROM, as each contraction cycle starts and terminates at a static position. In order to reach a given velocity within the specified ROM, the mobile segment has to be accelerated from 0°/s along a nonisokinetic arc. A certain angular distance must be covered until the segment velocity catches up with the preset velocity. The same rule applies during deceleration. An inverse relationship normally exists between the test velocity and the IROM: an increase in the preset velocity implies a smaller IROM.

Magnitude of the ROM

There is evidence that the size of the ROM has a direct effect on the isokinetic performance, specifically relating to knee extensors in concentric contractions. In a study by Narici et al (1991), two test ROMs, 90° and 120°, were compared under otherwise identical conditions. There was a significant increase, of approximately 9%, in the peak moment, which was attributed to the longer time available for tension development as well as a greater neural activation. Hence although it is a joint-dependent parameter, it may be speculated that in general a greater ROM would have a positive effect on some performance parameters.

Angular velocity

The second input parameter is the test angular velocity (ω), measured in degrees per second (°/s). In some journals another unit, the radian per second (rad/s), is used. As 1 rad is equal to approximately 57.3°, one can hardly see the benefit of abandoning the common and convenient units.

It should be restated that the test angular velocity is that of the lever arm not that of the distal segment. Moreover, the preset velocity does not bear any simple relationship to muscle linear contraction velocity, as indicated by Hinson et al (1979), and this relationship itself would be different for each muscle because of differing anatomical configurations.

As noted above, the preset angular velocity is attained only after a certain sector of motion has been covered, and the greater the preset value, the longer it takes to attain it. In fact, it is possible that such a high angular velocity is prescribed that the patient is not able to perform isokinetically. Examiners should therefore inspect the velocity trace (if one exists) on the screen to ascertain that isokinetic motion indeed took place. Some new attachments/ systems allow linear rather than angular patterns to be tested such as occur in lifting or leg press. In this case the unit of measurement is the centimetre per second (cm/s) or inch per second (in/s).

JOINT-INDEPENDENT CONTROL PARAMETERS

Damp setting

The damp setting controls the acceleration and deceleration of the lever arm and segment combination. The angular sectors occupied by the acceleration and deceleration phases, the so-called 'moment signal transients', are directly proportional to

HIP ADDUCTION

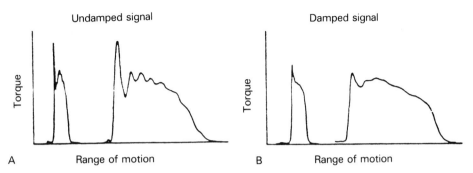

Fig. 2.3 Damp settings and moment overshoot phenomena: **A**, undamped signal; **B**, damped signal. (From Sapega et al 1982 The nature of torque 'overshoot' in Cybex isokinetic dynamometry. Medicine and Science in Sports and Exercise 14: 368–375.)

the angular velocity. For instance, it has been shown that in the concentric mode, these sectors were equal to 1 and 28° at 30 and 210°/s respectively, whereas the corresponding values in the eccentric mode were 2 and 34° (Farrell & Richards 1986).

The effect of damping is demonstrated by the two MAP curves depicted in Fig. 2.3. These curves are based on two consecutive concentric contractions of the quadriceps under conditions identical except for damp settings. A and B refer to undamped and maximally damped contractions. It is evident that the conspicuous spike which occurs at the beginning of the contraction in Fig. 2.3A (undamped) is significantly attenuated Fig. 2.3B (maximally damped).

This spike has been termed the 'impact artifact' (Winter et al 1981), the 'torque overshoot' (Sapega et al 1982) or the 'impact torque' (Sale et al 1987). The term used in this book is 'moment overshoot' or simply 'overshoot'. This phenomenon results from the interaction between the lever arm and the mechanism responsible for arresting its accelerated motion. It is regarded as an obstacle particularly in high velocity testing where, as explained before, the sector of isokinetic motion is significantly reduced (Osternig 1986). Moreover, it does not reflect muscle performance at the preset velocity as it occurs long before isokinetic conditions are reached.

Some modern isokinetic dynamometers overcome the overshoot phenomenon using 'ramping', which allows acceleration of the segment to the preset velocity (Farrell & Richards 1986). The role of this computer-controlled acceleration is to pro-

vide an 'absorber' for the excess force. The resulting movement is hence an overshoot-free, smooth transition from 0°/s to the preset velocity.

It should be emphasized that though the overshoot is an artifact from the point of view of isokinetic testing, physiologically it is very meaningful. First, it has been shown that the factors affecting overshoot are different from those affecting common performance parameters under isokinetic conditions (Sale et al 1987). The magnitude of the overshoot reflects the capacity to recruit the neuromuscular apparatus and generate a moment. In this respect it is reminiscent of the isometric rate of force development. The peak moment, however reflects another facet of strength, that of generating moment under loading. Thus the two are very significant. In addition, one should bear in mind that the magnitude of the overshoot is also a function of the damping technology used in a particular dynamometer and hence should not be compared among different makes.

Variation of the damp setting

The effect on the peak and average moment (see below) of knee extensors, of varying the damp setting has been examined (Rathfon et al 1991). The authors used three damp settings, low, medium and high, which corresponded to a long, medium and short delay in reaching the PAV, which in this study consisted of 90°/s. Both concentric and eccentric modes were tested. The findings indicated that the choice of the damp setting did not appear to have a clinically significant effect on either the peak or average moments. This conclusion can reasonably be extended to lower velocities but its validity for higher velocities cannot be known at present.

Isometric preactivation

Isometric preactivation (IPA) refers to static tension which is generated in the tested muscle/s before motion of the lever-arm and segment ('preloading'). The use of isometric preactivation (IPA) was first reported by Gransberg & Knutsson (1983) who indicated that it had a restraining effect on the initial moment oscillations. Later studies failed to reach a clear answer concerning its effect, probably because of different protocols. Table 2.2 outlines the basic experimental designs and the findings.

As evident from Table 2.2 there are three approaches to setting the IPA: absolute force, absolute moment and relative %MVIC (Maximal Voluntary Isometric Contraction) values. The latter approach conforms to the practice of normalizing muscle performance, and should be preferred. It is also clear that an IPA of 25 %MVIC induces only marginal variations and hence higher values may be used. These have a positive effect on the average moment but do not seem to result in higher peak moment, as there is an increase in the initial moment but not in the mid-range moment. However, this is less characteristic in eccentric exertions. Kramer et al (1991) highlight the point that IPA eccentric knee flexion (quadriceps activity) demands a higher initial contractile moment since, at the usual initial horizontal position, gravity adds about 9 N m. A relevant comparison of the differential effect of IPA on concentric and eccentric contractions would be possible through, for instance, setting of equivalent demands using different IPAs. In addition it would naturally be erroneous to compare muscle performances which are not based on the same IPA.

Lower isometric bias and upper moment limit

Another form of demand on isokinetically contracting muscle/s is the imposition of a lower isometric bias (LIB). The LIB is by definition the minimal magnitude of moment that has to be maintained in order to ensure a smooth progression of isokinetic motion. It thus serves as a complement to IPA.

In addition to the latter, an upper moment limit (UML) may be incorporated for the purpose of ensuring the safety of potentially vulnerable structure. The use of LIB together with UML may be beneficial in nonmaximal efforts (e.g. post-ACL reconstruction), or for the purpose of fine motor performance analysis.

Feedback

Isokinetic performance may be influenced by the provision of feedback to the subject. Feedback may be described in terms of form, amount, delay (Peacock et al 1981) and content (see Box 2.1).

Box 2.1 Characteristics of feedback

- Form: auditory (verbal), visual, or a combination
- Amount: how much information is given to the subject
- Delay: the period of time between the performance and the provision of the information, or between the presentation of the information and the next response
- Content: the elements of performance to which the feedback refers, for instance peak or average moment

---

Table 2.2 Isometric preactivation (IPA): control parameters and effects*

Source	Velocity (°/s)	IPA	Effect
Gransberg & Knutsson (1983)	30, 120, 240	5, 140 N m	Increase in initial moment, damping of oscillations
Piette et al (1986)	30, 180	50, 100%MVIC	Increase in initial moment
Gravel et al (1988)	30	0 100%MVIC	Decrease in mid-ROM moment
Jensen et al (1991)[†]	90	50 N, 75 %MVIC	Increase in average moment, shift in peak moment angle
Narici et al (1991)	180, 240, 300	25 %MVIC	Damping of oscillations, shift of angle-based moment, marginal increase in moment
Kramer et al (1991)[†]	45, 135	20, 50, 100 N	Increase in average moment, increase in mid-ROM eccentric moment, initial proportional increase in moment

* Except for Gravel et al (1988) all studies refer to knee extension.
[†] Contractions performed concentrically and eccentrically.
 MVIC: Maximal Voluntary Isometric Contraction.

In one of the first uses of an isokinetic system for analysing the effect of feedback, it was revealed that isometric quadriceps performance was significantly improved (by about 10%) by combined visual and auditory feedback but not by either of them separately (Peacock et al 1981).

Isokinetic performance with and without visual feedback was examined in a study by Figoni & Morris (1984). The performance criteria were strength (peak moment) and fatigue of knee flexors and extensors, at slow and fast test velocities of 15 and 300 °/s, respectively. The major finding was an improvement of performance at the slow but not at the high velocity, which amounted to about 12% in strength and 24–30% more fatigue (strength decrement) in both muscle groups. The selectivity of the effect was explained by the much longer period of time available for processing the feedback information in the slow test. Also, since the visual feedback consisted of the moment trace and not its numerical value, it was more regular in the slow velocity as opposed to more oscillatory in the fast velocity test. The increase in fatigue was related to higher initial strength values. The general extent of improvement in isokinetic performance and its dependence on the test angular velocity was later confirmed in studies by Hald & Bottjen (1987) and Baltzopoulos et al (1991). Consequently the use of visual feedback may be limited to strength testing at low angular velocities.

Auditory feedback in the form of verbal encouragement, is far more difficult to standardize, which is probably the reason for a lack of information concerning it. It has however been found by Wilk et al (1991) that aggressive verbal commands and encouragement resulted in earlier occurrence of fatigue. It was their recommendation that if encouragement was given, it should be consistent and moderate in intensity.

PERFORMANCE PARAMETERS OF STRENGTH TESTING

Moment

A typical moment-angular position (MAP) curve is depicted in Fig. 2.4. Though it is the force, expressed in newtons (N), which is the most basic mechanical parameter, all isokinetic findings relate to its rotational effect, namely the moment (see below). The latter serves in turn as the basis from which all other performance parameters are derived.

Calculation of the moment

In systems based on a resistance pad and load sensor assembly, whose position on the lever-arm is adjustable, the moment (M) is obtained using the following formula:

$$M = \text{Lever-arm length} \times \text{Force}$$

where the term lever-arm length refers to the distance between the axis of rotation of the lever-arm and the location of the load sensor. In some systems the load sensor is located differently but the calculation is the same.

Moment and torque

The practice of using the term 'torque' rather than moment must be traced to the early days of isokinetic testing. Though torque like moment is associated with a force which acts at a distance from an axis, the mechanical connotation of the two is different. When a torque acts on a body it exerts torsional stresses and may in addition impart axial rotation (winding). When a moment acts on a body it exerts bending stresses and may in addition impart rotation. The difference is therefore in the axes about which the force acts. In this respect, major joint motion along the common anatomical planes are interpretable in terms of *moment* (flexor moment, abductor moment etc.) whereas those relating to internal and external rotations would more correctly be described in terms of *torque*. One of the purposes of proper alignment of the joint axis with that of the dynamometer head is to minimize the effect of torque in tests of muscle performance taking place along the major planes (Oberg et al 1987). The opposite is also true when the purpose of the test is measurement of axial rotations. As a greater proportion of isokinetic testing is devoted to moment-related measurements, the term 'moment' is used in this book e.g. peak or average moment. This will apply for both major planes and axial

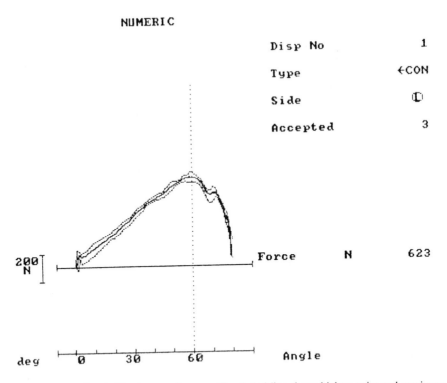

Fig. 2.4 Peak moment (force) of an isokinetic strength curve. The dotted line shows highest point and maximum force value on the MAP curve (623 N). Multiplication of this force value by the length of the lever arm give the peak moment.

rotations (though in the latter, the term torque would have been even more appropriate).

Unit of measurement

The unit of measurement of moment is the newton-meter (N m). Some sources prefer a different notation, N·m which might be misleading. Furthermore, the unit N m should be reserved for moment (see below) whereas the joule, which may also be expressed as newton-meters, should specifically relate to work. Providing gravity is accounted for, the value of the moment at any point on the curve (Fig. 2.4) represents the strength of the tested muscles at that point.

Peak moment

The maximal value of the MAP curve is termed the peak moment (PM). In this book the terms peak moment and maximal strength are synonymous.

The peak moment does not involve specifying its location. For instance, based on the MAP curve depicted in Fig. 2.4, the strength of the muscle is 199 N m, (based on a lever arm of 32 cm and a peak force of 623 N).

The identification of the peak moment is not always straightforward. This is particularly apparent in two instances:

1. Eccentric contractions sometimes involve oscillations of varying amplitude in the moment-angular position curve. In pain-free tests, repeated trials and averaging normally serves to smooth out the curve, yet in certain instances the difficulty persists.

2. If the sampling rate of the data processing unit is fixed at 100 Hz (100 readings per second, the isokinetic industry standard) curves based on very high test velocities appear as dotted rather than solid lines. In this case the accuracy of determining the peak moment may be compromised. Higher sampling rates solve this problem.

Angle-based moment

This is an alternative method of presentation, relating to the value of the moment at a predetermined angular position. It has been used in several studies. Since time and angular position are directly related to each other, except during the transient acceleration periods, the angle-based moment (ABM) is also a time-based value and it may be used for comparing moment generation capacity. Its reproducibility as a performance parameter of the knee extensors has been examined by Kramer et al (1991). Findings revealed that the reproducibility of ABM at 15° of knee flexion was consistently smaller than the corresponding value at 50° of knee flexion at two velocities and three different IPAs. This difference probably derives from the fact that the MAP curve had not settled by 15° of knee flexion. The ABM is less commonly used than the PM and the two are almost never coincident. On the other hand, the ABM allows a more standardized method of comparison, as it relates to the same muscle length. Hence the angle-based form of strength was indicated for multiple velocity measurements (Perrine & Edgerton 1978). It was also used in a recent study of an optimal isokinetic test protocol (Kues et al 1992). However, the decision concerning the specific angle to which reference should be made is basically arbitrary, and on retesting one has to assume absolute reproducibility of the alignment. Such an assumption is not realistic particularly with respect to joint systems such as the shoulder. The potential benefit of using angle-based vs. moment-based strength was studied in a group of patients suffering from chronic insufficiency of the anterior cruciate ligament (Kannus et al 1991). It was indicated that the angle-based method offered little additional information on thigh muscle performance compared with that obtained by the moment-based method. In view of this, and the points already mentioned the use of peak moment is strongly indicated.

Angle of peak moment

The angle at which the peak moment occurs (60° in Fig. 2.4) is called the angle of peak moment (APM). The APM is known to vary as a function of the test velocity (Rothstein 1987). A higher test velocity results in a delay in reaching the peak

moment and hence a greater APM. In addition, the APM varies widely among subjects, particularly in the case of the shoulder (Ivey 1985). Therefore its value as a basis for clinical judgement, at least as far as the shoulder is concerned, is very questionable.

Average moment

Very often strength is expressed in terms of the average moment (AM), also expressed as newton-meters, rather than the peak moment. Clearly the average moment is measured over the isokinetic range of movement (IROM). The use of average moment as an alternative strength parameter demonstrates the controversy over the definition of the theoretical construct 'strength': should strength be represented by a single moment value, i.e. the peak moment, or by the totality of all moment values which produce a single contraction? Since at present there is no unequivocal definition of strength (Rothstein 1987) average moment is no less a legitimate descriptor of strength than peak moment.

Some insight concerning this issue is provided by a recent study of trunk flexors' strength (Wessel et al 1992). The peak concentric moment of the flexors bore a *positive* relationship to the test angular velocity, contrary to the well established moment angular velocity MAV relationship. However, when the average concentric moment was considered the same trend was not apparent, although the expected relationship was only very weakly inverse. Furthermore, compared to their eccentric peak moment the average moment of the trunk flexors increased significantly less with the increase in velocity (30, 60 and 90 °/s). The authors suggested that the relatively high mass of the trunk was responsible for the unevenness of the moment curve and thus created an artifact which was the cause of this effect. It followed that the avereage moment was less affected than the peak moment. Since similar problems could potentially be encountered during testing of muscles operating on other heavy segments (e.g. hip region muscles), the use of average rather than peak moment is strongly recommended.

It is, however, suggested that a possible way to examine the appropriateness of peak or average moment parameter would be to determine the coefficient of variation (CV) associated with each, based on a fixed number of contractions. Since a smaller coefficient of variation indicates a more consistent measure, it could help resolve this issue.

Calculation of the average moment

The average moment is obtained from summing the moment values at each sampling point in the relevant IROM and dividing the result by the number of points (Fig. 2.5). Consider a test performed at an angular velocity of 90 °/s, along a ROM of 90°, with a sampling rate of 100 Hz. In theory, this test will last 1 s and hence if the required average moment is based on the full ROM, the database would consist of 100 moment values. The average moment ($M_{average}$) is therefore:

$$M_{avereage} = (M_1 + M_2 + \ldots + M_{100}/100$$

where M_1, $M_2 \ldots M_{100}$ denote the moment values at each sampling point.

If the number of moment values is n, the average moment value is given by:

$$M_{average} = (M_1 + M_2 + \ldots + M_n)/n$$

or more concisely:

$$M_{average} = \frac{1}{n} \sum_{x=1}^{x=n} M_x$$

To eliminate the transients (moment overshoot, initial oscillations), as already mentioned the average moment is normally based on a sector of, rather than the full ROM. There are no rules concerning the extent of this sector; for instance in knee testing where the common test ROM is 90° the accepted practice is to ignore the first and last 10°. Obviously with a smaller ROM or high test velocities this practice becomes problematic and use of the peak moment is indicated. Also, limiting the average moment to a smaller sector, as described here means that it approximates to the peak moment.

Relationship of peak and average moments

The relationship between average and peak moments has been reported in a few studies (Morrissey 1987, Kramer & MacDermid 1989, Dvir et al 1989, Bandy & Lovelack-Chandler 1991). It was indicated

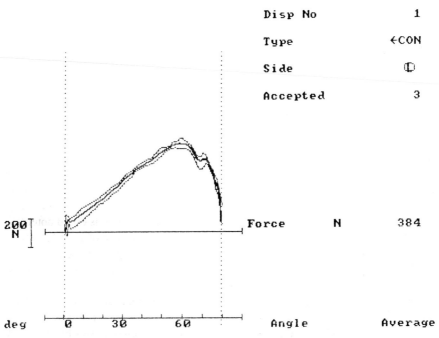

Fig. 2.5 Average moment (force) of an isokinetic strength curve identical to the one depicted in Figure 2.4. Note the approximately 40% difference between the numerical values of the peak force and the average force (384 N).

that the two parameters were strongly correlated, in concentric and eccentric contractions alike, with correlation coefficients (Pearson's r) generally greater than 0.9. Since the peak moment represents, by definition, the greatest moment value, and the average moment is a linear combination incorporation the peak moment, the very high correlation coefficients are not surprising.

Kramer & MacDermid (1989) reported an interesting relationship between the test angular velocity (45, 90, 135 and 180 °/s) and the peak-to-average moment ratio (PM:AM) in concentric and eccentric contractions. For concentric contractions there was an inverse relationship, for eccentric contractions it was direct. Specifically the ratio varied from 1.3 to 1.21, at 45 and 180 °/s respectively, in concentric mode, and in eccentric mode the variation was from 1.3 to 1.36. Although not discussed by the authors, it seems from the findings that the concentric peak moments declined more rapidly than the corresponding average moments whereas this was not the case in eccentric contractions. In other words, the shape of the moment–angular velocity curve was different for peak moment and average moment. Consequently, although correlation coefficients of between 0.94 and 0.96 were found, in both modes of contraction, for a given velocity this degree of correspondence may not hold for comparisons at different velocities. This leads to the conclusion that average and peak moments cannot be used interchangeably because of their different magnitudes, and their probably different relationships to angular velocity.

Both the peak and average moments are commonly quoted in N m units. In quite a number of papers, the preferred unit was m/kilogram of body-weight (N m/kgbw) or ft-lb/lb, namely the absolute strength values were 'normalized' according to the subject's weight. Though weight does seem to be a factor in strength production, the current approach seems to be against the practice of normalization (see, for instance, DeLitto et al 1991, Newton et al 1993). Therefore users are advised to quote the average or peak moment in N m (or ft-lb).

Contractional work

A parameter which is closely associated with average moment is the contractional work (CW), whose unit of measurement is the joule (J). It is a measure of the work done, or energy expended, by the muscle/s under test. It is equal to the area under the MAP curve or alternatively to the average moment times the angular displacement (A) (Fig. 2.3). In mathematical form, where work is represented by W:

$$W = M_{average} \times A$$

A normally refers to the angular displacement in the truly isokinetic sector of the MAP curve, as with the calculation of the average moment, described earlier.

Since contractional work is derived from the average moment through multiplication by a constant (the angular sector) their correlation coefficient is $r = 1.0$. Like average moment, contractional work eliminates the intricacies of the MAP curve.

Contractional power

Contractional power (CP), which is measured in watts, is an important performance parameter which relates to the average time rate of work namely:

$$Power = \frac{Work\ done}{Time\ taken}$$

or, if T is the total time for the movement through the angular sector (A):

$$P = \frac{W}{T}$$

This can be expressed:

$$P = \frac{M_{average} \times A}{T}$$

Hence:

$$P = M_{average} \times \omega$$

where ω is the test angular velocity.

The importance of this parameter derives from the fact that it reflects aspects other than strength although it bears a close relationship to the latter (Rothstein et al 1983, Bandy & Lovelace-Chandler 1991). For instance, although the concentric peak moment is inversely related to the test velocities (moment–angular velocity relationship), contractional power may be positively related to the latter as has been indicated with respect to the ankle plantarflexors (Gerdle et al 1985). This phenomenon results from the nonlinear (decelerated) decay in the moment–velocity curve. Although it is theoretically valid to relate to an instantaneous P, (the power based on a small angular sector), it probably has no value for the purpose of interpreting test findings based on normal or patient populations.

Contractional impulse

The performance parameter contractional impulse (CI) is the product of the moment multiplied by the time for which it acts namely where I is the value of the impulse namely:

$$I = M_{average} \times T$$

Impulse is measured in N m s. Studies of athletes and patients have shown that impulse has a special significance. Sale (1991) analysed the performance of sprinters versus cross-country skiers, using knee extension performance. The contractional impulse at 180 °/s was the best discriminator between the two groups, while the peak moment at 30 °/s revealed no differences. In another study in patients suffering from patellofemoral pain syndrome, the contractional impulse was highly correlated with the subjective pain ratings whereas the average moment was not (Dvir et al 1991a). Both studies

have suggested the wider application of this parameter.

Suggested convention for specification of parameters

Used correctly, all of the above parameters must be used with reference to test angular velocity and mode of contraction. Since it is the concentric strength that is most commonly referred to, the latter should be used as a default. The following is suggested as a convenient way of quoting isokinetic parameters: parameter, angular velocity, contraction mode (only if eccentric). Examples are PM-120, AM-30 or CI-60E (PM, peak moment; AM, average moment; CI, contractional impulse).

Table 2.3 outlines the performance parameters of strength testing, their acronyms, measurement metric units, conversion factors and mechanical relationships.

FATIGUE AND ENDURANCE TESTING

Isokinetic testing of fatigue and endurance (F & E) is based on a series of repetitive contractions,

Table 2.3 Performance and related parameters: units, conversion formulae and mechanical relationships

Parameter	Abbreviation	Symbol	Unit	Conversion	Relation to other parameters
Force		F	newton (N)	1 N = 0.2248 lb = 0.102 kgf	$F = M/r$ (r = lever length)
Moment		M	newton-meter (N m)	1 N m = 0.738 ft lb = 0.102 kg m 1 ft lb = 1.356 N m 1 kg m = 9.81 N m	$M = rF$
Peak	PM	M_{peak}	N m		$M = rF_{peak}$
Average	AM	$M_{average}$	N m		
Angle-based moment	ABM		N m		
Angle of peak moment	APM		degree (°) radian (rad)	1 ° = 0.0174 rad 1 rad = 57.3°	
Contractional work	CW	W	joule (J)	1 J = 1 N m = 0.737 ft lb 1 ft lb = 1.356 J	$W = M_{average}A$ (A = angular displacement) $W = \int_{o}^{a} Mda$
Angular velocity		ω	degree per second (°/s) radian per second (rad/s)	1 °/s = 0.0174 rad/s 1 rad/s = 57.3 °/s	$v = r\omega$ (v = linear velocity)
Contractional power	CP	P	watt (W)	1 W = 1 J/s = 0 00134 hp	$P = W/T$ (T = contraction time) $P = M_{average}\omega$
Contractional impulse	CI	I	newton-meter-second (N m s)		$T = M_{average}T$ $I = M_{average}T$ $I = \int_{o}^{t} Mdt$

performed at preset angular velocity and contraction modes. A number of additional/alternative criteria are involved.

CONTROL PARAMETERS IN F & E TESTING

Number of repetitions

There is no rule governing the number of contractions (NOC) required in a fully fledged F & E test although some guidelines have been formulated. The reported NOC in a single testing session ranges typically from 10 (Barnes 1981) to 150 (Elert & Gerdle 1989, Gerdle et al 1989).

In the latter studies the authors examined the relationship: PM, (CW,CP) vs. NOC, in the mechanical output of the shoulder flexors. They identified two phases. The first, termed the 'fatigue' phase, was characterized by a steep decrease in the mechanical output. The second, or 'endurance' phase showed a steady state performance. It follows from this dichotomy, which may apply only when a relatively high NOC is involved, that the NOC determines the quality of the phenomenon one is measuring. Obviously, where the NOC is maximal, one does not attain the endurance phase without first passing through the fatigue phase. Thus the isokinetic 'endurance' test of the elbow flexors and extensors in a study by Motzkin et al (1991) probably related to fatigue.

Contraction time (CT)

This parameter refers to the ratio between the time actually spent in contractional activity and the total testing time (Mathiassen 1989). Contraction time (CT) which is expressed as a percentage reflects therefore the relationship between the activity and pause time.

PERFORMANCE PARAMETERS IN F & E TESTING

The same set of performance parameters which applies in strength analysis is generally valid for F & E. However, instead of considering the performance within the framework of a single contraction, the basis is an ensemble of contractions. The following performance parameters have been used in analysing fatigue and endurance in isokinetic situations.

Reductions in peak moment (PM) contractional work (CW) and contractional power (CP)

Reduction in peak moment (PM) is probably the most commonly used performance measure. It is based on the percentage ratio, of the last and first contractions. There are some variations. Thorstensson & Karlsson (1976), for instance, compared the average peak moment of the first five contractions with that of the last five, whereas Gray & Chandler (1989) selected the three highest peak moment values from the five initial and five final contractions.

Reductions in contractional work and contractional power are used as performance measures in a way comparable to peak moment (Elert & Gerdle 1989, Gerdle et al 1989). Mathiassen (1989) used a variant of contractional work reduction in F & E analysis of the quadriceps. Instead of dividing the final by the initial work output, the initial work output was replaced by a contractional work value based on a strength test.

Time to 50% of peak moment

This performance parameter refers to the period of time in which a subject can maintain a repetitive peak moment level of 50% or above the peak moment obtained at the initial contraction (Motzkin et al 1991). It is therefore a time-based rather than an NOC-based indicator. One disadvantage associated with this parameter is the inability to predict the exact number of contractions. Moreover, whether or not a single contraction with a peak moment value of 50% that of the initial peak moment should be sufficient to terminate the test is as yet unresolved.

PART 3
ISSUES IN ISOKINETIC MEASUREMENT AND REHABILITATION

SOURCES OF ERROR

It is possibly the most basic assumption of isokinetic dynamometry that the moment recorded by the system is the resultant joint moment and hence may be used for deriving the performance parameters. Analysing the relation between the measured and the actual moment exerted by the quadriceps during knee extension, Herzog (1988) identified three areas of error that could undermine this assumption:

1. Acceleration effects have to be factored in or 'trimmed' in order to obtain a meaningful record (Sapega et al 1982).
2. Failure to account for the effect of gravity can result in very large errors (Winter et al 1981).
3. Optimal biological–mechanical alignment and firm stabilization have to be ensured, otherwise the motion pattern of the joint does not bear an interpretable relation to the movement of the lever-arm (Herzog 1988).

As previously discussed modern isokinetic systems offer a partial solution to the first problem by using the damp setting. Furthermore, as both ends of the tested ROM are ignored, the basis for interpretation is the middle sector, IROM. The second problem is largely being overcome by the use of gravity correction procedures.

The third source of error is probably the most problematic and so far, unless one is dealing with the knee at specific IROMs, there is a good chance of involving components that do not reflect the true performance of the joint. In the shoulder, for example, this is responsible for the generally poor reproducibility of test findings (Magnusson 1990). This source of error is therefore discussed in detail in the chapters dedicated to the individual joint systems.

THE MEASUREMENT SCALE AND ISOKINETIC RATIOS

The classification of isokinetic measurements as consisting of interval and not ratio scales has been advocated in a review article by Rothstein et al (1987). It was stated that:

. .isokinetic torque measurements must be considered to be interval scaled; that is, the zero level on the torque curve does not represent a true absence of muscularly generated torque. The torque curve actually represents the resistive torque generated by the machine to keep a limb segment from accelerating. The torque generated by the muscle to move the limb segment up to the

machine speed is not registered. Ratios, or percentages, thus cannot be formed from interval-scaled data.

Although from the strictly mathematical viewpoint this remark is correct, in practice zero moment levels (which in this case are equivalent to grade 3 in manual muscle testing) are never compared. Therefore, the question whether, for instance, a muscle which generates a PM of 80 N m is twice as strong as another muscle which generates 40 N m must be answered affirmatively. The relevance of these ratios is discussed in the chapters on the isokinetics of the trunk (extension/flexion), the knee (extension/flexion) and the shoulder (internal/external rotation).

SHAPE OF THE MAP CURVE

This is one of the most interesting and controversial issues associated with isokinetic measurements. The advent of active dynamometers, capable of measuring eccentric performance led to the production of even more complex curves. These led to correspondingly higher expectations that the shape of the MAP curves could furnish information that went beyond the performance parameters. To what extent have these expectations been fulfilled?

Problems of interpretation

There are a number of difficulties that must first be addressed. First, it would be of prime importance to know the extent to which simple visual analysis can reveal the same idiosyncrasies to different observers. Although human perception lacks the mathematical probing power of the computer, it is capable of good pattern recognition. It was suggested in a few studies that the shape of the curve could be instrumental in identifying various knee pathologies (Blackburn et al, Hoke et al 1983, Grace et al 1984, Grace 1985). However, none of these studies attempted to investigate this using an inter-observer analysis.

Second, it would indeed be necessary to use processing techniques that so far have not been applied in this field. An original attempt has been reported by Afzali et al (1992) who found a mathematical expression which described quadriceps MAP curves. As pointed out by Mayhew (1992) the study suffered some weaknesses notably a lack of reproducibility. From another point of view a major drawback was that the curves analysed were derived from normal subjects or from the uninvolved side of patients with knee problems. Thus the curves could be described as 'simple' or 'regular' with the characteristic inverted U shape. However most problematic of all seemed to be the use of averaged MAP curves rather than original curves as the database. Hence the applicability of the findings, which did not deal with outstanding curves, is questionable.

There is a third difficulty concerning the issue of the MAP curve shape: reiterating Mayhew's criticism, unless 'reproducibility of shape' can be confirmed, the question is pointless. In fact, when performing an isokinetic test, examiners are looking for a 'representative' or 'the same' curve but this convergence is not always achieved, and is estimated using visual inspection only. The real obstacle is, however, consistency from one session to another. Whereas parameters like peak moment or contractional work may manifest acceptable reproducibility, this may not necessarily be the case with respect to shape.

Specificity in MAP curves

On the positive side it should be recognized that not all isokinetic curves have the same typical inverted U shape. Consequently there is a certain degree of specificity associated with these curves. A typical example is the difference between the quadriceps and hamstring concentric MAP curves, obtained upon testing the muscles in the sitting position. Whereas the quadriceps curve starts and normally ends at near zero moment, the hamstring is characterized by a monotonously increasing curve which peaks near or at the end of the ROM.

Another example is the phenomenon of 'break' or 'dip' in the curve, which has been associated with pain in the knee joint (Nordgren et al 1983, Dvir et al 1991b) (see detailed discussion in Chapter 6). These breaks disappeared following surgical intervention (Nordgren et al 1983), a finding which correlated well with the alleviation of pain in the joint. On the other hand the reproducibility of this phenomenon in terms of both magnitude and location has not been confirmed. Paradoxically it does not mean that this is an invalid criterion as the

source of pain, e.g. tissue stretching, may vary its responsivity even within the same testing session. Nevertheless the shape may vary quite considerably and thus few inferences may be drawn from it.

Clearly these issues must be investigated before the incorporation of shape analysis into clinical decision making can be considered.

INDICATIONS AND CONTRAINDICATIONS FOR ISOKINETIC PROCEDURES

Indications

These have been finely elaborated by Timm (1992), regarding the special case of the trunk. They may be generalized, with the appropriate limitations, to other joint systems, and include:

1. Trunk deconditioning syndrome (Mayer & Gatchel 1987) or general muscle weakness. With respect to the trunk, the syndrome refers to a general decline in muscle and cardiovascular performance which results from chronic low back dysfunction without a definite spinal pathology. General muscle weakness, in other joint systems, may result from long periods of significantly reduced activity such as those following cast immobilization. However, there is a definite pathology associated with the immobilization and the status of the injured tissues must carefully be considered (see contraindications).

2. Testing and correction of muscle imbalance which is often closely related to muscle weakness, may be reduced through the use of isokinetics. However, the precise extent of the imbalance must be assessed and confirmed. For instance, one views with alarm the common practice of determining the balance between trunk flexor and extensor performance without regard to the gravitational effect. Imbalance may be revealed between various muscle groups, like the glenohumeral rotators, and its rectification, as a therapeutic means, had been indicated (Glousman et al 1988).

3. Provision of additional data when the patient's available information cannot be satisfactorily interpreted, or where symptoms do not diminish using other therapeutic approaches. In this instance also, attention must be paid to any existing contraindications.

4. An alternative source of information may be provided by isokinetic testing when reporting the results of new forms of treatment (Sapega 1990).

Contraindications

The use of preset moment and force levels, an option which is available in modern systems, has drastically reduced the risk associated with isokinetic exertions. These levels work two ways: they ensure the generation of muscular tension greater than a certain threshold yet protect the involved structures from a potentially damaging stress. Moreover, as previously stated, an isokinetic motion pattern can be produced even without maximal contraction. Consequently the 'relative' versus 'absolute' classification of contraindications, suggested by Davies (1992), may be modified to consist of a spectrum (Box 2.2). The clinical status appearing

---

Box 2.2 Contraindications spectrum (based on Davies 1992)

1. Severely limited ROM ...... limited ROM
2. Severe pain .... pain
3. Severe effusion .... effusion or synovitis
4. Acute sprain .... chronic third degree sprain
5. Acute strain .... subacute strain of the musculotendinous unit
6. Soft tissue healing constraints
7. Unstable bone fracture or joint

---

on the left hand side of Box 2.2 signifies the 'no testing permitted zone' whereas that on the right shows those clinical situations in which the decision to test is left to the clinician, while exercising maximal caution.

In addition, isokinetic testing of maximal muscle performance is *absolutely contraindicated in patients suffering from heart disease.*

REFERENCES

Afzali L, Kuwabara F, Zachazewski J, Browne P, Robinson B 1992 A new method for the determination of the characteristic shape of an isokinetic quadriceps femoris muscle torque curve. Physical Therapy 72: 585–595

Amundsen L R 1990 Measurement of skeletal muscle strength: an overview of instrumented and non-instrumented systems. In: Amundsen L R (ed) Muscle strength testing: instrumented and non-instrumented systems. Churchill Livingstone, New York, pp 1–24

Baltzopoulos V, Williams J G, Brodie D E 1991 Sources of error in isokinetic dynamometry: effects of visual feedback on maximum torque measurements. Journal of Orthopaedic and Sports Physical Therapy 13: 138–142

Bandy W D, Lovelack-Chandler V 1991 Relationship of peak torque to peak work and peak power of the quadriceps and hamstring muscles in a normal sample using an accommodating resistance measurement device. Isokinetics and Exercise Science 1: 87–91

Barnes W S 1981 Isokinetic fatigue curves at different contractile velocities. Archives of Physical Medicine and Rehabilitation 62: 66–69

Blackburn T, Eiland W, Bandy W 1982 An introduction to the plica. Journal of Orthopaedic and Sports Physical Therapy 3: 171–177

Davies G J 1992 Isokinetic testing. In: Davies G J (ed) A compendium of isokinetics in clinical usage. S & S Publishers, Onalaska, Wisconsin, p 37

Delitto A, Rose S J, Crandell C C, Strube M J 1991 Reliability of isokinetic measurements of trunk muscle performance. Spine 16: 800–803

Dvir Z, Eger G, Halperin N, Shklar A 1989 Thigh muscles activity and anterior cruciate ligament insufficiency. Clinical Biomechanics 4: 87–91

Dvir Z, Halperin N, Shklar A, Robinson D (1991a) Quadriceps function and patellofemoral pain syndrome. Part I: pain provocation during concentric and eccentric isokinetic activity. Isokinetics and Exercise Science 1: 26–30

Dvir Z, Halperin N, Robinson D, Shklar A (1991b) Quadriceps function with patellofemoral pain syndrome. Part II: the break phenomenon during eccentric activity. Isokinetics and Exercise Science 1: 31–35

Elert J, Gerdle B 1989 The relationship between contraction and relaxation during fatiguing isokinetic shoulder flexions. An electromyographic study. European Journal of Applied Physiology 59: 303–309

Farrell M, Richards J E 1986 Analysis of the reliability and validity of the kinetic communicator exercise device. Medicine and Science in Sports and Exercise 18: 44–49

Figoni S F, Morris A F 1984 Effects of knowledge of results on reciprocal isokinetic strength and fatigue. Journal of Orthopaedic and Sports Physical Therapy 6: 190–197

Gerdle B, Fugl-Meyer A R 1985 Mechanical output and iEMG of isokinetic plantarflexion in 40–64 years old subjects. Acta Physiologica Scandinavica 124: 210–211

Gerdle B, Elert J, Hendriksson-Larsen K 1989 Muscular fatigue during repeated isokinetic shoulder forward flexions in young females. European Journal of Applied Physiology 59: 666–673

Glousman R, Jobe F, Tibone J, Moynes D, Antonelli D, Perry J 1988 Dynamic electromyographic analysis of the throwing shoulder with glenohumeral instability. Journal of Bone and Joint Surgery 70A: 220–226

Grace T G 1985 Muscle imbalance and extremity injury: a perplexing relationship. Sports Medicine 2: 77–82

Grace T G, Sweetser E, Nelson M, Skipper B J 1984 Isokinetic muscle imbalance and knee joint injuries. Journal of Bone and Joint Surgery 66A: 734–740

Gransberg L, Knutsson E 1983 Determination of dynamic muscle strength in man with acceleration controlled isokinetic movements. Acta Physiologica Scandinavica 119: 317–320

Gravel D, Richards C L, Filion M 1988 Influence of contractile tension development on dynamic strength measurements of the plantarflexors in man. Journal of Biomechanics 21: 89–96

Gray J C, Chandler J M 1989 Percent decline in peak torque production during repeated concentric and eccentric contractions of the quadriceps femoris muscle. Journal of Orthopaedic and Sports Physical Therapy 10: 309–313

Hald R D, Bottjen E J 1987 Effect of visual feedback on maximal and submaximal isokinetic test measurements of normal quadriceps and hamstrings. Journal of Orthopaedic and Sports Physical Therapy 9: 86–93

Herzog W 1988 The relation between the resultant moments at a joint and the moments measured by an isokinetic dynamometer. Journal of Biomechanics 21: 5–12

Hinson M N, Smith S C, Funk S 1979 Isokinetics: a clarification. Research Quarterly 50: 30–35

Hoke B, Howell D, Stack M 1983 The relationship between isokinetic testing and dynamic patellofemoral compression. Journal of Orthopaedic and Sports Physical Therapy 4: 150–153

Ivey F M, Calhoun J H, Rusche K, Bierschenk J 1985 Isokinetic testing of shoulder strength: normal values. Archives of Physical Medicine and Rehabilitation 66: 384–386

Jensen R C, Warren B, Laursen C, Morrissey M C 1991 Static pre-load effect on knee extensor isokinetic concentric and eccentric performance. Medicine and Science in Sports and Exercise 23: 10–14

Kannus P, Jarvinen M, Lehto M 1991 Maximal peak torque as a predictor of angle-specific torques of hamstring and quadriceps muscles in man. European Journal of Applied Physiology 63: 112–118

Kramer J F, MacDermid J 1989 Isokinetic measures during concentric–eccentric cycles of the knee extensors. Physiotherapy Canada 35: 9–14

Kramer J F, Vaz M D, Hakansson D 1991 Effect of activation force on knee extensor torques. Medicine and Science in Sports and Exercise 23: 231–237

Kues J M, Rothstein J M, Lamb R L 1992 Obtaining reliable measurements of knee extensor torque produced during maximal voluntary contractions: an experimental investigation. Physical Therapy 72: 492–504

Magnusson S P, Gleim G W, Nicholas J A 1990 Subject variability of shoulder abduction strength testing. American Journal of Sports Medicine 18: 349–353

Mathiassen S E 1989 Influence of angular velocity and movement frequency on development of fatigue in repeated isokinetic knee extensions. European Journal of Applied Physiology 59: 80–88

Mayer T G, Gatchel R 1987 A prospective two-year study of functional restoration in industrial low back injury. Journal of the American Medical Association 258: 1763–1767

Mayhem T P 1992 Commentary. Physical Therapy 72: 593–594

Mayhem T P, Rothstein J M 1985 Measurement of muscle performance with instruments. In: Rothstein J M (ed) Measurement in physical therapy. Churchill Livingstone, Edinburgh, pp 73–91

Morrissey M C 1987 The relationship between peak torque and work of the quadriceps and hamstring after meniscectomy. Journal of Orthopaedics and Sports Physical Therapy 8: 405–408

Motzkin N, Cahalan T D, Morrey B F, An K-N, Chao E Y S 1991 Isometric and isokinetic endurance testing of the forearm complex. American Journal of Sports Medicine 19: 107–111

Narici M V, Sirtori M D, Mastore P, Mognoni P 1991 The effect of range of motion and isometric preactivation on isokinetic torques. European Journal of Applied Physiology 62: 216–220

Newton M, Thow M, Somerville D, Henderson I, Waddell G 1993 Trunk strength testing with isomachines part II: experimental evaluation of the Cybex II back resting system in normal subjects and patients with chronic low back pain.

Spine 18: 812–824

Nordgren B, Nordesjo L, Rauschning W 1983 Isokinetic knee extension strength and pain before and after advanced osteotomy of the tibial tuberosity. Archives of Orthopaedic and Traumatic Surgery 192: 95–101

Oberg B, Bergman T, Tropp H 1987 Testing of isokinetic muscle strength in the ankle. Medicine and Science in Sports and Exercise 19: 318–322

Osternig L R 1986 Isokinetic dynamometry: implications for muscle testing and rehabilitation. Exercise and Sports Science Reviews 14: 45–80

Peacock B, Westers S, Walsh S, Nicholson K 1981 Feedback and maximum voluntary contraction. Ergonomics 24: 223–228

Perrine J, Edgerton V R 1978 Muscle force–velocity and power–velocity relationships under isokinetic loading. Medicine and Science in Sports 10: 159–166

Piette V, Richards C, Milton F 1986 Use of static preloading in estimation of dynamic strength with the KinCom dynamometer. In: Proceedings of the North American Congress on Biomechanics, Montreal, pp 261–262

Rathfon J A, Matthews K M, Yang A N, Levangie P K, Morrissey M C 1991 Effects of different acceleration and deceleration rates on isokinetic performance of the knee extensors. Journal of Orthopaedic and Sports Physical Therapy 14: 161–168

Reid D C, Saboe L A, Burnham R 1991 Common shoulder problems in the athlete. In: Donatelli R (ed) Physical therapy of the shoulder, 2nd ed. Churchill Livingstone, Edinburgh

Rothstein J M, Delitto A, Sinacore D R, Rose S J 1983 Electromyographic, peak torque and power relationships during isokinetic movements. Physical Therapy 63: 926–933

Rothstein J M, Lamb R L, Mayhew T P 1987 Clinical uses of isokinetic measurements: critical issues. Physical Therapy 67: 1840–1844

Sale D G 1991 Testing strength and power. In: MacDougall J D, Wenger H A, Green H J (eds) Physiological testing of the high performance athlete, 2nd edn. Human Kinetics Books, Champaign, Illinois

Sale D G, MacDougall J D, Alway S E, Sutton J R 1987 Voluntary strength and muscle characteristics in untrained men and women and male bodybuilders. Journal of Applied Physiology 62: 1786–1793

Sapega A A 1990 Muscle performance evaluation in orthpaedic practice. Journal of Bone and Joint Surgery 72A: 1562–1574

Sapega A A, Nicholas J A, Sokolow D, Saraniti A 1982 The nature of torque 'overshoot' in Cybex isokinetic dynamometry. Medicine and Science in Sports and Exercise 14: 368–375

Thorstensson A, Karlsson J 1976 Fatiguability and fibre composition of human skeletal muscle. Acta Physiologica Scandinvavica 98: 318–322

Timm K E 1992 Lumbar spine testing and rehabilitation. In: Davies G J (ed) A compendium of isokinetics in clinical usage. S & S Publishers, Onalaska, Wisconsin, pp 497–532

Wessel J, Ford D, Van Driesum D 1992 Measurement of torque of trunk flexors at different velocities. Scandinavian Journal of Rehabilitation Medicine 24: 175–180

Westing S H, Seger J Y, Thorstensson A 1991 Isoacceleration: a new concept of resistive exercise. Medicine and Science in Sports and Exercise 23: 631–635

Wilk K E, Arrigo C A, Andrews J R 1991 Standardized isokinetic testing protocol for the throwing shoulder: the throwers' series. Isokinetics and Exercise Science 1: 63–71

Winter D A, Wells R P, Orr G W 1981 Errors in the use of isokinetic dynamometers. European Journal of Applied Physiology 46: 397–408

Reproducibility, validity and related topics

It is now close to a decade since the publication of Mayhew & Rothstein's (1985) excellent work on measurement of muscle performance with instruments. Here, as elsewhere in the same book (Rothstein 1985) special emphasis was given to the issues of reproducibility and validity of isokinetic test findings, and the major problems associated with these two mainstays of measurement theory and practice. Some of those problems remain unsolved and thus the rigor with which test findings can be interpreted is still compromised.

On the other hand, the development of isokinetic technology, especially during the last decade, did solve some problems and rendered others obsolete. First and foremost these developments accompanied the advent of computer-controlled active dynamometers, computer processing and presentation of the data, and more advanced engineering components. Some of the current systems are far more versatile, and allow the measurement of performance such as eccentric activity, which was previously almost impossible to measure accurately. Secondly, procedures like gravity correction, whose absence in the first models of the Cybex system largely accounted for the misuse of strength ratios, are now incorporated as a matter of course in most modern dynamometers. There also exist options for manipulating (smoothing) of data, and derivation of quantities other than strength which were not available at the beginning of the 1980s.

Above all, however, the clinical community has become far more aware of the crucial significance of reproducibility and validity in using and interpreting isokinetic test findings. This awareness is not only expressed at the formal, academic levels, such as journal papers or scientific conference presentations, but mostly at the informal level. Here, one of the first questions asked by users of isokinetic systems concerns the ability to reproduce findings under similar conditions, and the legitimacy of interpreting the findings. This, I would respectfully submit, is the greatest contribution of Dr Rothstein and his colleagues.

Analyses of the reproducibility of isokinetic findings relating to ankle, hip, shoulder and trunk muscles appear in the appropriate chapters. The analysis of knee muscle testing is presented largely within this chapter, since knee testing has served (and still does) as the most common model for studying the reproducibility and validity of the isokinetic method.

PART 1
REPRODUCIBILITY

Reproducibility, validity and sensitivity are the three requirements which must be satisfied in order for a measurement to be meaningful and interpretable. Since modern isokinetic systems offer high sensitivity this requirement is fully satisfied. Consideration of the other two qualities indicates that while reproducibility is somewhat easier to prove, the question of validity is irrelevant if an acceptable level of reproducibility is not ensured. Consequently the establishment of reproducibility is even more vital to the admissibility of isokinetics, although the method is ultimately useless without proven validity.

'Reproducibility' refers to the consistence of the measurement: if test results are described as reproducible, this implies that under the same test (experimental) conditions the measured entities will be assigned the same values. Furthermore, in the present context, reproducibility refers to the measurement of human performance and not of the effect of an externally applied load (see below). The present author has chosen to use the term 'reproducibility' rather than the more common 'reliability' since the latter conveys the impression that one can rely on the findings. This, at least partly,

implies a validity which may not obtain.

Whatever mathematical method is used to derive its numerical value, the reproducibility of test findings is affected by the following potential sources of error:

1. Machine-linked inconsistences, e.g. lack of calibration
2. Subject/patient-linked variations, e.g. motivation
3. Testing procedure-linked errors, e.g. poor stabilization
4. Protocol-linked variations, e.g. different intercontraction pauses
5. Examiner-linked variations, e.g. differences between examiners
6. Data processing-linked factors, e.g. smoothing.

Of course these elements affect reproducibility of findings for both the individual tester (intra-tester) and from tester to tester ('inter-tester'). The following sections deal with the problems associated with the first four abovementioned sources of errors, especially protocol. In some instances the reader is referred to other parts of this volume, where a more detailed treatment is given.

MACHINE-LINKED VARIATIONS

Isokinetic test results may vary between the different models or systems, between individual machines of the same model type, and even between tests on the same machine during normal operation.

Reproducibility during normal operation: calibration

Isokinetic dynamometers are based on a large number of interconnected components, and a fault in any of these may interfere with the normal operation of the system. Such faults may sometimes be detected by the system itself using dedicated hardware or software. However, the main demand, accurate calibration, is the responsibility of the operator.

Calibration is the process by which the system-measured quantities are compared with a standard, and, if necessary corrected. Correction may be carried out either through physical intervention, such as adjustment of amplification, sensitivity etc. or by the use of correction formulae.

Calibration is the essential condition for reproducibility, albeit not sufficient of itself.

It should in principle be applied for all parameters measurable by the system. This includes the force (moment) exerted on the dynamometer's arm as recorded by the sensors, as well as the angular position and velocity of the arm. To these, calibration of the damp setting should be added. In fact, a full calibration would even extend to components further along the processing chain, such as the amplifiers and analogue-to-digital converters, but these are rarely necessary.

Calibration should be conducted in static and dynamic conditions. A relatively detailed description of measuring the performance of an isokinetic dynamometer was given by Farrell & Richards (1986) and by Bemben et al (1988). Some elements in these studies can be applied to calibration of isokinetic systems.

A system which is not calibrated often may yield different values for the same standard. On-site calibration is indeed a relatively straightforward process involving the use of a set of exact weights. It is also quite simple to measure angular velocity, providing an elementary optical sensor and pulse counter and an electronic timer are available. However, the present author is not aware that any manufacturer of isokinetic systems provides users with all the necessary tools for calibration. Similarly, it is not always apparent how often either the moment- or the velocity-measuring modules should be calibrated. Moreover, not all manufacturers point out the differing extents to which the various sensors change over time.

Level of accuracy

How great an error must be to compromise interpretation is a difficult question. However, consider the case where the criterion for discharge calls for a 10% improvement in a given muscle's peak strength. Suppose also that an unrectified drift in the measuring circuits caused an offset of 3% in the moment. Thus if the drift leads to overestimation, the patient may be discharged too soon, and vice versa. Errors with even harsher consequences, such as those encountered in personal injury claims, may be the result of poor reproducibility because of

failure to calibrate. Hence the rule is always aim at the most accurate calibration.

Frequency of calibration

The issue of how often calibration should be carried out has been examined by Olds et al (1981), with respect to the Cybex II system, using nine different angular velocities. Olds and colleagues concluded that it was necessary to calibrate the moment-measuring module of this system, every testing day and at every test velocity. This recommendation did not take damping into account, but as shown by Sinacore et al (1983) this parameter must also be calibrated.

To what extent modern systems require the same frequency of calibration is difficult to tell. However, it would seem that omitting to calibrate at least once a week, particularly in a heavily used system, jeopardizes the reproducibility of findings based on the system.

Stability of measurement

Calibration is intimately related to the stability of the measurement. Whereas calibration is based on comparison of measurements with an external standard, stability refers to the machine's own consistency from measurement to measurement. The length of the period between measurements is obviously a critical factor as the drift in the measurements is likely to increase with a longer period. The proper way to assess stability is to retest the system performance without first calibrating it. The differences in the recorded measurements between the test (calibrated) and retest (uncalibrated) indicate the stability.

A recent comparison of several isokinetic systems indicated that a proper level of moment-measurement stability was maintained throughout the test session (Timm et al 1992). As indicated by the authors, the systems were recalibrated before the second test session and therefore stability was not the measured parameter. What the study did demonstrate however was high skill in calibrating the systems (an important issue on its own) rather than reliability of the system. On the other hand, excellent reproducibility (as defined above) was indicated, for strength in particular and, depending on the system used, excellent to acceptable reproducibility for average power and total work.

'Intra-model' reproducibility

This factor refers to findings based on the same model but using different machines operated by different examiners. It is of particular significance for the establishment of norms for specific pathologies. Such norms are likely to be generated using multicenter studies and hence intra-model reproducibility, using different examiners, must first be established. In addition, patients may receive treatment and assessment in different facilities (e.g. hospital first and then a clinic) and therefore 'intra-model' reproducibility is essential.

Molczyk et al (1991) examined this issue using Cybex II dynamometers at two clinical facilities. The examiners applied identical protocols for testing strength and endurance of the knee flexors and extensors. The inter-tester (intra-model) reliability ranges were 0.86–0.95 and 0.69–0.95, for extension and flexion respectively. Muscle endurance, based on total work values, showed ranges of 0.80–0.85 and 0.81–0.89 for extension and flexion respectively. It was suggested that comparable strength and endurance values could be obtained with different testers using this particular dynamometer.

In another study Byl et al (1991) used a similar design and Cybex 340 systems. It was found that with the measurement of knee flexor and extensor performance, there were no significant differences betweed the two examiners regarding strength (at 90, 120 and 180 °/s) and endurance (120 °/s). There was however a significant difference in the work done in extension. The authors concluded that:

physical therapists from different sites could collaborate to pool data for developing norms for isokinetic knee flexion and extension torque as long as the same test protocol was followed. However, the large variation in retest measurements and the coefficient of variation suggest that when a therapist wants to determine if a patient has made a significant gain in strength, the remeasurement should be taken by the same examiner at the same site.

Consequently, although intra-model reproducibility for normal subjects exists, at least with respect to the abovementioned systems, retesting should replicate testing conditions.

Byl & Sadowski (1993) have recently extended their analysis of inter-site reproducibility by measuring trunk muscle performance in 10 individuals at three different centers. The performance was assessed during flexion and extension (FE), rotation (R) and lifting (L). No statistically significant differences in peak and average moment, average power, total work (in L) or best work (in FE or R) were found. Intraclass correlation coefficients ranged from 0.91 to 0.98, 0.88 to 0.93 and 0.94 to 0.98 for L, FE and R respectively. It was hence concluded that, with respect to these activities, normative values could be established based on data collected at different sites.

'Inter-model' reproducibility

Because of differences in engineering components, data manipulation, positioning, stabilization and attachments, there is a reasonable likelihood of disagreement between isokinetic models/systems. Presumably at the heart of this issue is the question: which system measures best? The present author does not believe a judgement can be made while no acceptable standard exists. It has been suggested that the Cybex system should fulfil this role as almost all studies up to the mid-1980s used it exclusively for measurement. This argument can no longer be voiced, given an interest in ensuring instrument accuracy and reliability. This point was brought out very clearly and strongly in the concluding remarks of a paper by Bemben et al (1988):

. . the instrument [Cybex II] is suitable for clinical work and research where there is an interest in peak torque and lever arm angle at peak torque but only when used at lower velocities and higher damping setting. The velocity should not exceed the velocity specified by the manufactuer, 120 °/s. Possibly it would be feasible to use the instrument under other conditions if calibration curves are developed which can be used to correct for the errors in recorded torque and angle.

Every instrument is unique; therefore, it is recommended that anyone planning to use a Cybex II isokinetic system for research or in clinical practice where precision of measurement is important, thoroughly analyse and become fully acquainted with the measurement characteristics of the particular instrument to be used.

Therefore, since even intra-model reproducibility cannot always be guaranteed due to the abovementioned uniqueness of every system, it is obvious that the far more complex inter-model reproducibility cannot be obtained. (It is indeed surprising that so much effort has been put into this subject.) This has been proven in a number of papers comparing test findings with the same subjects, based on Cybex II and Lido 2.0 (Francis & Hoobler 1987); Cybex II and Kin-Com (Reitz et al 1988); Cybex II and Biodex 2000 (Thompson et al 1989, Gross 1991), and Cybex 340 and Merac (Timm 1990). Consequently it may be stated that findings obtained using one system (model) cannot serve as a baseline for or compared with those obtained by another system.

SUBJECT/PATIENT-LINKED VARIATIONS

It can be stated that any factor which is liable to influence subject performance is a potential source of difference when the first and the second (or beyond) tests are compared. Consequently, control of such a factor, however difficult, is essential in order to ensure reproducibility.

Among the factors most commonly operating are:

1. pain and its intensity post- vs. pretesting
2. fatigue and/or an underlying problem of inconsistent pattern
3. level of motivation and cooperation.

Admittedly, these factors are often difficult to assess quantitatively, and hence interpreting their effects is notoriously problematic. Nevertheless each of these factors ought to be considered before initiating the test. When they have been assessed, it is up to the clinician whether to proceed with the test.

Generally, the presence of pain contraindicates testing. However, in certain instances moderate or weak pain does not preclude testing and indeed its effect on performance is precisely what one is looking for (see isokinetic evaluation of patellofemoral pain in Ch. 6). On the other hand, pain may subside, and hence on retesting reproducibility would be low.

The relevance of fatigue in measurement of performance is self-evident, though at times this factor may not become apparent unless one is testing endurance. It is easily controllable and requires that the subject/patient be asked about activities before commencement of the test. Clearly, fatigue should not be confused with the preparatory phase ('warm-up') essential for appropriate testing.

Lack of motivation or cooperation may often be deduced directly or indirectly. The response of the patient to verbal encouragement, a factor which has

already been discussed in Chapter 2, is central to this issue. Additionally, autonomous and psychological responses may indicate to what extent effort is indeed optimal. Finally, the within-test reproducibility is often an excellent indicator of these factors (see detailed discussion in Ch. 8). An acceptable and compatible level of motivation and cooperation is essential, both at very short and long retesting intervals, for reproducibility.

TESTING PROCEDURE ERRORS

The significance of this cluster of factors which includes test range of motion (ROM), positioning, stabilization, biological-mechanical axes alignment and test angular velocities is discussed in detail in each of the chapters dedicated to joint testing. To achieve reproducibility these factors must be kept exactly the same on retesting. Consider, for instance, nonequal ROMs on two testing occasions. Though the peak moment may not differ, there is a good chance that angular work would, as the generated force is allowed to move a longer distance. This would automatically compromise test reproducibility.

PROTOCOL AND REPRODUCIBILITY

INTRODUCTION

The test protocol is undoubtedly the most complex and least understood of the issues concerning reproducibility, and of the most central significance once subjective factors are controlled. Maintaining the consistency of the system is largely a technical matter which is achievable. Deciding which testing procedures should be applied may not be as mechanical, but at least a number of procedures may be described as common practice (e.g. knee ROM). There is however no doubt that the testing procedures are intimately related to the protocol factors, most notably the question of test angular velocities.

The correct identification, selection and application of protocol factors requires considerable knowledge and understanding of the testing process. For instance, although most strength testing protocols advocate the use of the mean (or of the maximal score) of 3–5 maximal contractions as the basis for interpretation, it is common experience to come across a patient who requires more trials to reach an optimal level of performance. Likewise, whether endurance is more correctly measured by a fixed number of contractions, by a percentage decline in performance or by the greatest number of contractions exerted during a given time, is a problem of protocol and physiology combined.

Protocol factors are not those which are inherent to the technical set-up of the test nor those which must be keyed in order to initiate testing. The test protocol leads ultimately to a specific interpretation and therefore ensuring the reproducibility of the findings based on it is of the most profound significance. Protocol factors include amongst others:

1. the choice of a unidirectional vs. a bidirectional movement, e.g. extension only or extension followed by flexion ('reciprocal')
2. the choice of contraction mode, e.g. concentric contraction/s only, or concentric–eccentric sequence
3. inter-contraction pause (if any and how long)
4. number of contraction cycles/set
5. inter-set pause
6. test-retest interval.

All of these factors may be applied in different ways with respect to different joints and the clinical status. It is self-evident that there is an infinite number of potential protocols, and the core problem is therefore the selection of the optimal one. The subject of protocol design has occupied many scholars and it is extremely difficult to review the literature on this subject. Given that in every study a protocol of some sort is employed, this task is even more daunting.

Time span

The time span of a protocol is highly relevant to reproducibility. For instance, reproducibility may be defined as the level of agreement between measured individual contractions or reciprocal contractions, within the same test session, with a gap of a few seconds between measures. Alternatively it may refer to the same relationship but in terms of inter-session agreement, and here the time span is days, weeks or even years (Fugl-Meyer et al 1985). Since there are no rules about the shortest relevant

period for reproducibility, it may be defined as one chooses.

Given that sequential (repeated) contractions yield close scores (Stratford et al 1990, Stratford 1991), it is usually inter-session reproducibility which requires most attention. (However in certain instances it is definitely the intra-session reproducibility which becomes the object of interest. For instance in the medico-legal area, inconsistency of performance within the same test session indicates lack of effort.) Hence in the following exposition, inter-session reproducibility studies are emphasized. The more relevant studies, i.e. those in which the authors were expressly investigating the relationship between protocol design and reproducibility are considered. This review is not conclusive and there may well be other sources, but it outlines the major principles of the topic.

Experimental and statistical rigor

Recent years have seen the publication of a few excellent studies on this topic. There is not only a commendable degree of experimental sophistication, but rigorous statistical analyses of data. The former is characterized by more demanding experimental procedures, with the object of defining what might be called an 'acceptable protocol domain.' The latter incorporate modern correlational techniques to the extent that a background in statistics is needed to appreciate the full scope of the findings.

NORMAL SUBJECTS

An early study

A study by Johnson & Siegel (1978) was one of the first attempts to examine reproducibility, and it is still a valuable source which is frequently referred to. A group of 40 normal women, 17–50 years of age, took part and were tested on 6 consecutive days. The performance examined was the strength of the knee extensors using a Cybex II system. The protocol was based on unidirectional movement only, (extension) tested at 180 °/s. The subjects were asked to submaximally contract the quadriceps three times and then attempt six maximal contractions with an inter-contraction pause of 20 sec. Due to a significant ascending linear trend in strength values, the criterion was defined as the average value of the last three contractions.

Reproducibility which was determined using intra-class correlation coefficients (ICCs) varied between 0.93 for the first day and 0.99 for the fifth days.

Variation depending on day of testing

The variability in ICCs values as a function of the testing day was recently reexamined by Kues et al (1992). The complex protocol involved measurement of isometric, concentric and eccentric performance using a spectrum of velocities.

It was indicated that subjects reached their greatest peak moment, which served as the performance criterion, on the second and third day. Within each velocity, the fourth repetition was associated with the highest peak moment. The ICC ranges were 0.94–0.98 and 0.87–0.96 for concentric and eccentric strengths respectively. This protocol did not however incorporate practice repetitions and hence testing on the first day may have fulfilled this function.

Variations over a 6-week period

Mawdsley & Knapik (1982) studied reproducibility with a longer time span, three tests 2 weeks apart, using the same dynamometer. The experimental group consisted of 16 normal women and men, aged 20–50 years. Knee extensor strength was examined at a velocity of 30 °/s, using a series of six maximal contractions separated by 1 min pauses. In the absence of significant variations the authors concluded that the strength measurements were stable over the 6-week period. No correlational analysis was presented.

Reciprocal protocols

Protocols involving alternating extension and flexion movements are known as reciprocal protocols.

Intermittent reciprocal protocol

The reproducibility of a protocol for testing of intermittent reciprocal extension and flexion contractions in the knee, was studied by Harding et al (1989). Testing took place during two sessions on different days. Only one test velocity, 60 °/s, was examined. Following warm-up, subjects were instructed to perform six maximal alternating (reciprocal) extension and flexion movements with a 5 s pause between extension and flexion followed by a 30 sec pause until the next extension. The maximal strength and the angle at which it occurred were the criterion parameters. Reproducibility was expressed in terms of ICCs and standard error of the mean (SEM).

High ICCs, 0.936–0.952, were reported for the strength of both muscle groups, whereas lower figures were obtained for the angle of peak moment. The SEMs were 5.46 and 2.4 N m for the strength of the extensors and flexors respectively. This meant that for an extensor peak moment of 135 N m, the 95% confidence interval was 10.7 N m; for a flexor peak moment of 57 N m, the 95% confidence limit was 4.7% N m. These are relatively narrow intervals indicating good reproducibility for this protocol. The protocol was also associated with extremely low repetition and session variance which indicated minimal bias (systematic error due to either test session or repetition).

Subject–session interaction was greater than that of subject–repetition. The authors suggested therefore that a reproducibility analysis based on multiple observations taken on a single occasion, could probably underestimate the errors derived from the device, the subject and their mutual interaction and 'as a result, the clinician will be more likely to declare a future measurement (taken following an intervention) as indicating a change when in fact no true change has occurred'. This means that, another series of test repetitions has to be taken to ensure correct interpretation.

Continuous-reciprocal protocols

Developing the reciprocal protocol, Stratford et al (1990) have shown that eliminating the long pause between extensions resulted in even higher ICCs. This continuous reciprocal protocol resulted however in a significant linear decline in strength, probably due to fatigue.

A further step was taken by Montgomery et al (1989) in an in-depth reproducibility study of knee extensor and flexor strength and endurance.

Measurements consisted of three test sessions, 2–4 days apart. A spectrum of velocities which was eventually reduced to five, 90, 150, 210, 270 and 330 °/s, served for the strength analysis. At each test velocity, subjects were instructed to complete five maximal continuous reciprocal contractions. There was a pause of 1 min between tests. The criterion parameter was the single maximal strength attained during the test. Endurance was rated according to the number of contractions performed at 180 °/s during 45 s, and endurance parameters included work and power.

Findings revealed no significant differences in mean extension or flexion strength across test days at any velocity. The across-all-velocities ICCs relating to strength were 0.88 and 0.79 for extension and flexion respectively with a tendency to be higher at the two lower velocities and better in extension than in flexion. The lower velocities were also associated with lower coefficients of variation (CV). For the endurance test, the two reproducible measures were total work performed and average power, both with an ICC of 0.92.

The authors concluded therefore that this protocol was appropriate for intervention studies because it demonstrated 'minimal within-subject and inherent variation due to repeated testing'. This statement could not be made so definitively regarding other aspects of endurance.

This protocol however has two disadvantages:

1. Its applicability has never been tested in patients.
2. It involves the exposure of the relevant dysfunctional muscle/joint complex to a relatively large number of maximal contractions. Hence it may not be applicable in certain conditions.

Nevertheless, this is one of the most advanced and carefully designed protocols and as such deserves considerable attention.

It also coincides with the recent tendency to use a range of velocities, demonstrating different physiological facets of the muscle.

The main findings of the above reciprocal protocol studies have generally been supported by other studies notably Levene et al (1991).

Eccentric contractions

The incorporation of eccentric contractions sig-
nalled the opening of a new research topic related to protocol. In one of the first studies Wessel et al (1989) examined the reproducibility of concentric and eccentric work measurement based on isokinetic testing of knee extensors. The test–retest period was 1 week. The protocol was three submaximal and six maximal intermittent reciprocal cycles at 60 and 180 °/s with a 1 min inter-cycle pause. The criterion was the maximum of four trials. The ICCs for each combination of contraction mode, test session and angular velocity were all greater than 0.85. The coefficients were generally higher for the second week (pointing to some learning effect), the slower velocity and the concentric contraction. The findings for slower velocity and concentric mode are now well established.

Kramer (1990) designed another protocol which consisted of continuous reciprocal concentric and eccentric flexion and extension cycles at the velocities of 45 and 90 °/s. A group of normal subjects were tested three times in 10 days. The testing involved three submaximal and one maximal concentric–eccentric practice cycles, followed by a 2 min pause and three test cycles. Using the peak moment as the criterion, the single-session-based ICCs ranges were 0.82–0.91 and 0.79–0.88 for concentric and eccentric strength respectively. It was claimed that these figures could be much improved if ICCs calculations included two or more testing sessions. It is not clear why this additional analysis had not been performed. The ICCs were generally higher in extension than in flexion. There were apparently no differences in reproducibility as a function of the test velocity. This finding may be explained by the fact that both velocities belong to the lower end of the spectrum. The author emphasized patient compliance and indicated that this protocol offered acceptable reproducibility.

Order of test velocities

Quite apart from the issue of the order and spacing of contractions, the order of test velocities has been shown to have an effect on test reproducibility. In a study by Wilhite et al (1992) three angular velocities, 60, 120 and 180 °/s were used within a testing session. Testing involved concentric and eccentric contractions of the knee extensors. The basic design of the protocol was intermittent reciprocal with a 5 s pause between each contraction and four contraction cycles (concentric–eccentric) per velocity. The average of the peak moment of the second, third and fourth repetitions served as the criterion.

The inter-session ICCs, combined across the testing order were in the range 0.75–0.96 and were highly significant. However, when testing order was analysed, it was indicated that the reproducibility of measurements of subjects who began testing at 180 °/s was much lower compared to when this velocity was second or third in the order. Consequently when this protocol is applied, subjects should first be tested at the slower velocities.

Isometric preactivation

The incorporation of isometric preactivation (IPA) in intermittent reciprocal (concentric–eccentric) testing of the knee extensors has been examined by Kramer et al (1991). The authors used three IPA levels, 20, 50 and 100 N for determination of the peak moment, average moment and angle-based moment. High reproducibility (ICC>0.75) was indicated for all IPAs and for each of the above performance parameters. Since IPA tended to have a more pronounced effect on average moment, it is suggested that if average moment is the preferred performance criterion, IPA may be incorporated without compromising the test reproducibility.

Factors associated with reproducibility

Which of the above protocols is optimal is not a question that can be answered conclusively. Nevertheless there are a number of factors, common to these and other studies, which seem to be associated with acceptable reproducibility:

1. Three to six submaximal practice repetitions followed by one or two maximal repetitions enhance reproducibility.
2. Four to six test repetitions are sufficient to yield a representative performance parameter.
3. A continuous reciprocal protocol is appropriate for both concentric and eccentric performance.
4. Reproducibility may be higher for lower velocities, i.e. 30–120 °/s.
5. The criterion par excellence in non-endurance testing is strength, which may be equal either to the highest peak moment reached during any single movement or to the average of the peak

moments of the second half of the sequence.
6. Work may serve a parallel function in endurance testing.

PATIENTS

The issue of protocol reproducibility becomes even more complex when the subjects are afflicted with some disorder/dysfunction. For instance, variables such as pain may not be 'stable'; during the course of even a short period of time they may vary in a significant fashion. Hence, almost by definition it may not be possible to ascertain the repeatability of a given performance criterion.

However, reproducibility is a necessary condition, particularly for demonstrating changes brought about by a therapeutic intervention. A relevant performance criterion must be shown to be reproducible over a specified period of time. Only then, and under appropriate conditions, may it be claimed that an intervention was responsible for a specific change.

This statement assumes that the isokinetically-based criterion under consideration is a valid one for a given clinical group (see section on validity).

There are several orthopaedic and neurological dysfunctions in which isokinetic testing, follow-up and conditioning is indicated, especially where a conspicuous (neuro)muscular component is involved. Such cases include patellofemoral pain syndrome, low back dysfunction, surgical repair of the rotator cuff, or reconstruction of the anterior cruciate ligament. Equally relevant are measurements of muscle performance in patients with central nervous system (CNS) lesions such as multiple sclerosis or cerebrovascular accident (CVA).

The reproducibility of isokinetically-derived parameters in these cases has hardly been ever tested. Thus although there exists an acceptable body of evidence with respect to normal subjects it should not be taken for granted that a similar situation prevails for the clinical groups.

Complexity of clinical studies

The complexities associated with clinical studies were well demonstrated by Giles et al (1990) who compared the reproducibility of knee flexion and extension and hip flexion strength in groups of normal and arthritic subjects. Tests were administered five times at fortnightly intervals. The protocol consisted of continuous reciprocal flexion–extension contractions at the velocities of 60, 120 and 180 °/s for the knee and 45, 90 and 135 °/s for the hip. Hip testing was performed in the supine position. Gravity correction was not incorporated for either joint. It is suggested that this omission, as well as the unconventional hip testing position, could be one of the reasons for the qualified reproducibility which was obtained, using coefficients of variation.

A peak moment of 54 N m was determined as being critical. For both control and arthritic subjects, and irrespective of the muscle group, the average coefficient of variation, in the case of a mean strength greater or lower than 54 N m was 10% ± 5.8 or 19.8% ± 12.1 respectively. It was concluded that:

1. In untrained subjects reproducibility could not be demonstrated based on a biweekly interval (using a Cybex II dynamometer).
2. For subjects whose average strength was above a given level (54 N m) the first test could serve as an acceptable baseline, otherwise the second test was more representative.
3. Reproducibility could be established only in those instances where the average strength was above a given level (54 N m).

The numerical values quoted apply, of course, to this study only. The authors offered some reasons for the high variability (low reproducibility) of their test findings. The activity level of the normal subjects was a central issue; it was claimed that untrained subjects were less likely to reproduce their performance compared with subjects who were involved in regular physical activity. For the patients with rheumatoid arthritis, the instability in performance was derived from considerable fluctuations in symptoms and activity, even over brief periods of time. Their strength values were, as expected, not only smaller than those of their counterparts but the associated variability was much higher. Consequently, Giles et al stated, appropriately:

'while a variation of around 5% may be satisfactory in the analysis of groups of subjects tested over brief periods of time, the data suggest that in most clinical situations,

particularly where individuals have disease or disability, reliance on such narrow ranges may be misleading'.

As demonstrated by Montgomery et al (1989) the threshold for proving an experimental effect, using the coefficient of variation as the criterion, and a range of velocities, is an increase (decrease) of 7% or more in the performance index (based on 20 subjects or more). Bearing in mind that the performance of current isokinetic systems is probably better than the system used by Giles et al and applying more rational protocols, one could reduce the suggested 20% margin of variability in patients with rheumatoid arthritis. It would be entirely speculative to suggest a figure though a margin of between 10–15% does not seem overly liberal.

Neurological involvement

Studies of patients with neurological involvement have appeared in recent years.

Perhaps the first was by Armstrong et al (1983) which dealt with the muscular performance of three ambulatory patients with multiple sclerosis. Test–retest reproducibility of strength was determined 6 and 11 weeks after the original test session. An intermittent reciprocal protocol with a wide spectrum of velocities was used. Because of the large fluctuations observed in the peak moment, it was concluded that strength was not a reproducible parameter over such periods. Changes in clinical condition and a learning effect were potential sources of error. It should be mentioned that intra-session stability was excellent (0.99, Pearson's r) which incidentally proves the point that the agreement among trials within the same testing session may not necessarily serve as a valid clinical index for reproducibility .

Spastic hemiparesis

An excellent degree of test–retest reproducibility of knee flexion and extension strength, in patients suffering from spastic hemiparesis, was demonstrated in a study by Tripp & Harris (1991). The patients who participated in this study, all victims of CVA or traumatic brain injury, met a strict list of criteria hence ensuring the homogeneity of the group. Both knees were tested, 2–4 days apart, using velocities of 60 and 120 °/s. A continuous reciprocal protocol consisting of five maximal flexion–extension contractions with 5 min inter-velocity and inter-limb pauses was used. Peak and average moment served as the performance indices.

The ICCs of the test–retest scores had ranges of 0.91–0.98 and 0.92–0.97 for the involved and uninvolved extremities respectively. No difference was indicated between the extremities. Though in two isolated patients there were large differences in the above indices on retesting, the group as a whole performed very consistently. The authors have attributed these findings to the specific inclusion criteria and the high motivation among all participants. It was concluded that under similar circumstances, one could reliably test hemiparetic patients.

Future development of clinical studies

It is obvious that before isokinetic dynamometry can be legitimately used as a basis for inference, more clinical studies are needed. The technology is sufficiently established in terms of patient safety and comfort, reasonable testing protocols and sensitive and sophisticated systems, to allow the consistent pursuit of this issue. In this context the following recommendations concerning reproducibility standards are appropriate (Johnstone et al 1992):

1. Reports of measurements in rehabilitation should be accompanied by numerical estimates of reliability, the population(s) used, and the method of determining the reliability of the scores.
2. Developers of measurements have the primary responsibility for establishing initial reliability estimates for the population to which the measurement is to be applied.

PART 2
VALIDITY

The validity of inferences based on isokinetic measurements is probably the single most important issue which users of this technology face today. As shown in the preceding sections, the requirement for reproducibility has in some instances been met, notably with regard to specific parameters of normal muscle performance.

Such is not the case vis-à-vis clinical conditions where reproducibility has yet to be established in most cases. Since reproducibility is a prerequisite for validity, inference based on isokinetic testing must hence be limited to the above parameters, and to the specific group of dysfunctions for which reproducibility has been shown. Validity, as with reproducibility, is therefore group- and purpose-specific.

Assuming that for a given dysfunction, testing procedure and protocol, reproducibility of the test findings has indeed been proven, the interrelated types of validity (see Box 3.1) have to be examined

Box 3.1 Validity of isokinetic testing: does it measure what it is expected to measure?	
Content validity	Are the parameters measured relevant to muscle performance?
Construct validity	Does isokinetic testing measure strength?
Convergent	Do isokinetic findings display expected patterns, e.g. of changes with age?
Discriminant/divergent	Are tests good at distinguishing muscle performance from confounding factors, e.g. pain?
Criterion-referenced validity	Do isokinetic test results correlate well with external criteria or outcomes?
Concurrent	Do findings match existing situations, e.g. functional capacity, such as walking?
Predictive	Can isokinetic testing predict future outcomes, e.g. injury or progress?

in the light of established principles of muscle performance.

CONTENT VALIDITY

This type of validity has been defined by Johnstone et al (1992) as:

... the extent to which measures represent functions or items of relevance given the purpose and matter at issue. If items in a measure sample representative or outstanding items in a domain, the measure at least has content validity.

Isokinetic method belongs to the domain of

muscle performance. Peak moment, work, power and impulse are all 'items' which are relevant to and in some respects representative of the performance.

There are strong interrelationships between these items, but this does not disprove the basic argument, and these items still reflect independent functions. For instance, whereas the force generated by a muscle (as derived from the moment–velocity curve) decreases with an increase in the velocity, the power developed by the same muscle increases, at least up to a certain point (Fugl-Meyer et al 1982).

The fact that for the ankle plantarflexors, maximum isokinetically-derived power is reached at the functional velocity of 'toe-off' during walking is an excellent example of an item connecting the general domain to a subset, functional muscle performance. Thus isokinetic dynamometry has content validity with respect to specific aspects of muscle performance.

CONSTRUCT VALIDITY

This type of validity concerns the extent to which an instrument measures the theoretical construct it was designed to measure. Strength, the basic theoretical construction at the core of isokinetic findings, is commonly derived from the moment–angular velocity relationship. Strength, and its relevant mechanical counterparts, work, power and impulse, are not directly observable. However the construct validity of inferences based on these variables may be tested by:

1. Observing whether findings display the pattern of converging or predictive relationships one would expect (convergent validity).
2. Distinguishing the construct from confounding factors (divergent or discriminant validity) (Johnstone et al 1992).

In other words what one is looking for in this context is a 'network of relationships' with other well established factors. A number of such factors are discussed below.

Convergent validity

Gender differences

A number of isokinetic studies have shown that men are significantly and consistently stronger than women (see Tables in Chapters 6–9). This is compatible with one of the most obvious observations concerning gender differences.

Effect of age

Children and adolescents A study relating to dorsiflexor strength and contractional work (Backman & Oberg 1989) has demonstrated a consistent increase in strength through the ages of 6, 9 and 12 years in girls. Strength did not differ in girls between the ages of 12 and 15 years. In boys the corresponding increase persisted through the oldest age group namely 15 years, with the most intense rise in strength occurring between 12 and 15 years of age. These variations are in very good agreement with puberty processes, both for girls and boys. Furthermore there were no gender variations until early puberty.

Adults Strength normally reaches its peak at the third decade and thereafter declines very moderately with aging. A steeper decline may occur at the seventh/eighth decade. A good demonstration of the isokinetic correlates of these variations may be found in Timm (1988) and Borges (1989), concerning isokinetic norms for trunk lifting and knee muscle performances respectively.

Activity level

Individuals who maintain a physically active lifestyle are likely to have a better developed muscular system. The study by Fugl-Meyer (1981), of ankle plantar and dorsiflexors in age-matched trained versus sedentary subjects, underscores this point.

Body weight

Since in normal individuals muslce mass rises proportionately with body weight, heavier subjects generally produce higher isokinetic moments. This relationship which is not linear, constitutes the main reason for 'normalizing' strength with respect to body weight, using the unit N m/kgbw (newton-meter per kilogram bodyweight).

Muscle characteristics

Stiffness As shown by Backman & Oberg (1989) the slope of the moment–angular velocity curve changes with age, indicating that strength, especially in the adolescent groups, was mostly greater at slow velocities. This phenomenon is compatible with the observation that children cannot utilize stretch–shortening cycles to the same extent as can adults (Bosco & Komi 1980), possibly due to 'softer' (more 'flexible') muscles.

Fiber types Some evidence exists concerning the association between isokinetic strength and the histological composition of the quadriceps. Thorstensson et al (1976) examined muscle performance of active individuals, as expressed by maximal contraction speed and the ability to generate force. It was indicated that performance at 180 °/s was correlated with the percentage and relative area of fast twitch fibers. This relationship was not substantiated in another study (Fugl-Meyer et al 1989). One of the possible reasons for the difference was that the latter study used non-active subjects.

Static (isometric) moment Numerous studies have compared the static and dynamic strength of various groups of muscles. Even though static strength itself is rather vaguely defined, the aggregate of the two helps in cross-validation. Generally, most studies indicate a significant correlation between the two measures.

Discriminant validity

Association with pain

Injection of local anesthetic into the knee joint resulted in normalization of the otherwise depressed moment curve in patients with patellofemoral chondromalacia and osteoarthrosis, prior to advancement osteotomy of the tibial tuberosity (Nordgren et al 1983). This is probably one of the most direct proofs of the validity of strength measurement in the light of its relation to pain, which is a significant confounding factor.

CRITERION-REFERENCED VALIDITY

This type of validity concerns the extent to which a measure is related to some outcome or external criterion (Johnstone et al 1992). Criterion-referenced validity consists of two main forms: concurrent and predictive. Concurrent validity relates to whether an inference is justifiable at the time of measurement. Predictive validity refers to the extent to which a measure is able to forecast some future event. In accord with the principle of specificity mentioned earlier, these forms of validity may be associated with specific dysfunctions but may not be generalized to others. The followings describe instances where criterion-referenced validity has been indicated.

Concurrent validity

Isokinetic endurance and walking capacity

There is some evidence that isokinetic endurance tests may be helpful in estimating function in patients suffering from peripheral arterial insufficiency with intermittent claudication (Gerdle et al 1986). In this study (see Ch. 7) the authors have indicated that the contractional (total) work performed during repeated plantarflexion contractions was 'well correlated with the maximum functional walking'.

Moreover, isokinetic endurance was a preferable testing modality in patients with arteriosclerosis and cardiac insufficiency, as these disorders could create difficulties in tests, such as measurement of walking distance, which required general exertions. Hence if a patient has a low score on this specific endurance test, it may be inferred that her/his walking capacity is correspondingly limited.

Angular velocity and patellofemoral pain

The magnitude of pain sensation during knee testing, as reported by patients suffering from patellofemoral pain syndrome, has also been linked to isokinetic findings. Pain was found to be closely associated with the test angular velocity during isokinetic contractions. In other words, the longer the joint was exposed (lower angular velocity) the higher was the pain (Nordgren et al 1983, Lankhorst et al 1985, Lysholm 1987, Dvir et al 1991, see Ch. 6).

If after therapeutic intervention, slower tests were associated with less pain, the present author believes that this finding could be regarded as a significant, but not the only, measure of a successful outcome.

Isokinetic findings in osteoarthritis

In contrast, for patients with osteoarthritis of the knee, Lankhorst et al (1985) found that isokinetically derived strength did not provide a valid indicator of functional capacity. The correlations between pain and strength were low at all test velocities. In addition, isokinetic measures reflected only a fraction, 23–35%, of the variations in functional capacity, pain and walking. This method of analysis should be compared with that of Dvir et al (1991) where the load (impulse), rather than strength, was the criterion parameter. It is possible that if load had been used as the criterion, a different conclusion might have been reached.

Functional ability in anterior crucitate ligament deficiency

The functional ability, knee laxity and a number of isokinetic variables were tested in 47 atheletes with anterior cruciate ligament (ACL) deficiency (Shelbourne et al 1987). Out of 56 isokinetic variables, 37 were significantly correlated with knee score. On the other hand, laxity, running, cutting and hamstring/quadriceps ratio did not correlate with functional ability, suggesting that knee strength testing was the only objective means of determining functional ability in ACL-deficient patients. Thus some isokinetic findings may be valid for estimating functional ability in these patients.

Predictive validity

The predictive validity of isokinetic testing is a matter of great debate. Two categories may be discussed:

1. the power to predict dysfunction/injury from prior testing
2. the power to predict progress in rehabilitation based on repeated postinjury testing.

Prediction of injury

There are two major and conflicting sources concerning the predictive validity of isokinetic testing regarding injury. In the first and often-quoted study, Grace et al (1984) examined a group of 174 athletes preseasonally and compared the isokinetic performance findings of those who were injured in-season with those who were not. The performance measures included a large number of variables.

The findings indicated that across all parameters the differences between these two subgroups were insignificant. Therefore the authors failed to substantiate a claimed predictive validity.

This conclusion was later supported in a prospective study of ice-hockey injuries (Eriksson 1991). No relationship was indicated between the concentric and eccentric knee flexor and extensor strength, pre- or postseason, to the in-season rate of injury.

In a later study which made no reference to Grace et al, Knapik et al (1991) examined preseasonal strength and flexibility in a group of 138 women collegiate athletes. In-season injuries were evaluated and recorded, but apparently no attention was given to the mechanism of injury. Concentric knee extensor and flexor strength tests, uncorrected for gravity, were conducted at 30 and 180 °/s. It was indicated that athletes experienced more lower extremity injury if they had:

1. right knee flexor 15% stronger than the left knee flexor at 180 °/s,
2. a knee flexor/extensor (H/Q) ratio of 75% or less at this velocity, and
3. a right hip extensor 15% or more flexible than its left counterpart.

The fact that the risk factors were better associated with the high velocity tests is in itself of significance for validation. Moreover, hamstring involvement in all three factors is, speculatively, indicative of knee decelerator deficiency which could contribute to a higher sprain rate. This possibility was not elaborated by the authors.

It is nevertheless questionable whether the conclusions drawn may be generalized to male athletes: the claimed predictive validity should be reserved to the specific group tested. In view of this, the existence of predictive validity seems somewhat unlikely.

Prediction of progress

Prediction of progress is an entirely different issue. It is likely that repeated tests during a rehabilitation process could generally provide a valid forecast, based on trend analysis. What is the optimal follow-up rate, how many tests have to be performed and for how long such a prediction would be effective, are all questions which, to the best of the present author's knowledge, have not been examined in a systematic way. Therefore for the time being, isokinetic test findings seem to lack predictive validity for any particular dysfunction.

SPECIFIC VALIDITY OF ISOKINETIC TESTING

To summarize, isokinetic test findings are valid for a number of specific dysfunctions. In other words they furnish a reasonable basis for inference relevant to these dysfunctions only. The field of isokinetic testing clearly and urgently needs more validity-oriented research regarding other dysfunctions. This objective is certainly attainable but unless it is achieved, legitimate clinical inferences are bound to be limited in number and scope.

PART 3
PRINCIPLES OF INTERPRETATION

The interpretation of isokinetic findings with respect to each of the major joint systems is discussed in Chapters 5–9. Irrespective of the muscle systems involved, there are principles which form a basis for interpretation. These have been discussed in a large number of studies, outlined in an excellent paper by Sapega (1990), and are as follows:

1. In the case of unilateral involvement, the contralateral, sound side, constitutes the basis for comparison. This assumption is reasonable for symmetrical use of the body segments. In athletes who use their extremities, particularly the upper, in a non-symmetrical manner this assumption may not be valid. Thus referring to normal individuals:
   a. imbalance of strength (normally peak moment) of up to 10% can be considered normal
   b. imbalance of between 10 and 20% is possibly abnormal
   c. imbalance greater than 20% is probably abnormal.
2. If one extremity is expected to be weaker due to a previous injury or disuse:
   a. imbalance of between 10 and 20% is probably abnormal

   b. imbalance greater than 20% is almost certainly abnormal.
3. As a criterion for resumption of sports activity or strenuous physical exertion, a maximum deficit of the involved extremity is 20% for individual muscle groups and 10% for total limb strength, namely the combined strength of all the muscle groups of the limb. No corresponding figures were suggested for resumption of light activities but 30% for individual muscle groups and 20% for total limb strength seem reasonable.
4. In the case of bilateral or trunk involvement norms should be used. The norms must be gender-, age- and activity level-specific.
5. Imbalance of muscle performance ratios, for instance the bilateral difference in the ratios of the peak moments of external and internal shoulder rotators, may be employed in a similar fashion to the absolute peak moments. However it is advisable to consider using ratios in a physiologically meaningful way, namely the concentric performance of the agonist relative to the eccentric performance of the antagonist.
6. The use of bodyweight-normalized parameters is advisable.

PART 4
MEDICOLEGAL USES OF ISOKINETICS

From its advent, isokinetic dynamometry was an attractive tool in legal proceedings involving certain cases of musculoskeletally-based injury, impairment and/or disability. The possibility of objectively measuring some muscle functions which were previously assessed manually and subjectively was in many ways a revelation, if not a revolution. This, coupled with the immense financial consequences of personal injury litigation, particularly in the US, helped to secure for isokinetic findings an important niche among the various types of evidence. In some promotional literature the manufacturers have even quoted legal cases in which isokinetic test findings were used.

The two main issues concerning the medicolegal use of isokinetic findings are: veracity or sincerity of claim and, where impairment or disability are concerned, comparison with a standard.

SINCERITY OF CLAIM

APPROACHES TO SOC

Curve reproducibility

The issue of SOC has received considerable attention among users of isokinetic systems, but its scientific foundations have not been commensurately established. Rather than facing the difficulties of a verifying a claim in a broad context, the 'perfect' reproducibility of the MAP curves became the exclusive test of the claimant's sincerity. The problem in applying this test in the legal arena is that isokinetic findings do not necessarily lead to the type of yes/no answer obtained when testing nonvolitional parameters, such as the muscle's histological composition. Since a certain variance will always be present, given even optimal control of test parameters, the application of perfect curve reproducibility as an *exclusive* legal test is very restrictive, scientifically unjustifiable and, hence, should be strongly discouraged.

Use of an aggregate of factors

An alternative approach to the problem of veracity of claim is decidedly more global; it examines the extent to which a subject is capable of presenting a coherent neuromuscular performance in terms of established physiological and/or clinical criteria. In other words, instead of referring to a single parameter (curve variance) the general motor behavior of the subject as manifested by her/his isokinetic performance is examined. The importance of using an aggregate of factors in verifying the claim cannot be overstated, and even then there may be cases where error must be seriously considered.

Some general principles

In attempting to prove or disprove the veracity of a claim, emphasis is commonly put on a behavioral construct known as sincerity of effort (SOE). This construct refers to the question of whether the severity of the manifested muscle deficiency is on a par with the clinically diagnosed motor dysfunction. A typical example is sometimes seen in patients with low back dysfunction, but this instance is by no means exclusive. Therefore, when a claim for muscle (strength) deficiency is presented, the veracity of the claim and/or SOE may be tested in the

light of the following:

- Consistency of the strength curves within an isolated testing session
- Compatibility of the findings with physiological principles
- Symmetry in terms of bilateral performance
- Specificity of the deficiency in terms of the involved muscles.

This conceptual system, which for reasons of facility will be termed CCSS, will now be explored in more detail.

With respect to the element of consistency, the following principles have been established:

1. There exists an individual level of maximal performance which cannot vary during a single test session. This level depends on physiological and motivational factors.

2. Though consecutive maximal efforts (contractions) are supposed to overlap in terms of their strength curves, lack of overlapping does not necessarily indicate submaximal effort. The extent of overlapping may be determined using different mathematical/statistical operations, but no unanimity regarding the most appropriate one currently exists (see also below).

3. The ability and, indeed, legitimacy of dissociating maximal from submaximal effort curves is highly controversial, reflected by the positive approach of Hazard et al (1988) against the negative approach taken by Newton & Waddel (1993). It is, however, suggested that this controversy relates specifically to the case of trunk muscle testing. This dissociation may prove to be easier when simpler joint systems (in terms of the number of operating muscles) are considered.

With respect to the element of compatibility, the following describe muscle behavior under a wide spectrum of test conditions:

a. In concentric testing, the strength peak moment is inversely proportional to the test velocity.

b. Eccentric strength is normally expected to be greater than concentric strength.

The element of symmetry refers to the specific case where there is no side preference in terms of muscular deficiency, namely in the case of a general pathological condition or a disease.

Finally, the element of specificity relates to the location of the muscular deficiency and its relationship to other deficiencies.

Endurance testing can point out specific deficiencies and hence can serve as accessory evidence.

This list is by no means final: other parameters may, in view of circumstances, be legitimately considered. Furthermore, all elements should not be included in every case.

The application of these principles creates a web of indications that taken together support or deny the claim. Support or denial is not always absolute and should be judged according to individual merits and the prevailing circumstances. The latter statement is particularly significant in those cases where an element of conflict among the different sources is apparent. The following describe the application of the CCSS system.

Consistency of maximal and submaximal performance

Concerning the consistency of maximal voluntary contractions (MVCs), as mentioned in point 1. above, it has been suggested that only MVCs can be faithfully reproduced through multiple trials (Mayer & Gatchel 1988, Reid et al 1991). Moreover, even in tasks such as lifting which involve a significant number of joints and muscles, the variability in the MVC output was less than 10%.

On the other hand, the ability to reproduce the same submaximal strength output by a specific muscle group is poor (Carlsoo 1986). Although the type of contraction studied by Carlsoo was isometric, the further findings by Hazard et al (1988) do not deny the applicability of the former's results. It follows that if a subject is consciously exerting a submaximal (suboptimal) effort which she or he has been asked to repeat as accurately as possible, the likelihood of doing so to within ± 10% of the previous score is low. This normally refers to the third to sixth contractions during a carefully conducted test protocol (see 'Protocol' section above). If performance is not reproducible, it is advisable to retest the subject following a rest period of about 15–30 min. One group of individuals who may show particularly low consistency are claimants who have been clinically diagnosed as suffering from post-traumatic neurosis or depression. This observation is based on as yet unpublished findings

drawn from the author's personal experience with a small group of such patients. In over one half of the cases, no truly representative strength curve could be established.

If one exerts a maximal effort this margin of reproducibility is very reasonable.

The coefficient of variation is much in use as a measure of variability. It relates the standard deviation of the scores to the average. The coefficient of variation is a single number which is based on one performance parameter, normally the peak moment. The selection of the criterion for reproducibility is of critical significance to the trustworthiness of any decision regarding SOE. Clearly, more research is needed to substantiate the use of such a criterion.

Examples of the use of multiple elements

An example of utilization of a number of elements was given by Martensson (1991), who attempted to verify the diagnosis in the case of hysterical paresis. Knee flexor and extensor strength at three velocities were tested in 25 patients. Three characteristics were demonstrated that are not usually associated with organic paresis, that is, caused by CNS or peripheral lesions:

1. Variability in peak moment, based on successive contractions, exceeded 20% in 22 of the patients (element of *consistency*).
2. The moment–angular velocity curve was atypical, showing higher strength at relatively higher velocities in 8 patients (element of *compatibility*).
3. Flexor moment was less than expected from the weight of the shank and lever-arm due to quadriceps antagonistic activity, but in the absence of spasticity in 12 patients (element of *compatibility*).

The following case, drawn from the author's own (unpublished) experience, is an example of incorporating the elements of *specificity* and *symmetry*. The case involved a bilateral frostbite injury to both legs, which was particularly severe from the mid-shank level down. The main complaints were total loss of sensation in the foot and ankle regions, combined with a virtual paralysis of the ankle and foot muscles and a severe weakness of the knee region muscles.

Bilateral isokinetic tests of the plantar and dorsi-flexors and knee extensors revealed:

1. No strength output from either the plantar or dorsiflexors
2. Measurable but low strength output from the knee extensors which were tested at 30 °/s, in both concentric and eccentric contractions.

Findings (1) and (2) embody the element of specificity.

Other knee extensors findings:

1. Consistency was very good as judged by a maximal deviation of 7% in the average moment (AVM) among individual repetitions and in all tests (element of consistency).
2. Concentric AVM strength was 16 N m in the right and left muscles; the bilateral concentric AVM ratio was therefore 1.0 (element of symmetry).
3. Eccentric AVM was 20 and 22 N m in the right and left muscles respectively; the bilateral eccentric AVM ratio was 1.1 (element of symmetry).
4. The eccentric/concentric AVM ratio was 1.25 and 1.38 for the right and left muscles respectively, well within the expected values for this ratio (element of compatibility).

In view of the isokinetic findings, the impairment rating of this claimant was doubled, compared to the initial decision.

Another example of the incorporation of the element of specificity is the case of a woman who had suffered an injury to the shoulder. The victim claimed loss of 'power' in shoulder elevation and elbow flexion, which the insurers refused to accept as genuine. Six years after the accident, bilateral isokinetic testing, conducted at 30–60 °/s, revealed a reduction of 57% in abduction; 32% in adduction; 62% in internal and 66% in external rotation; 38% in elbow flexion; 16% in elbow extension; 40% in supination; 7% in pronation, and completely symmetrical hand grip strengths as measured by the JAMAR isometric dynamometer. Eccentric tests were consistent and revealed in all cases a higher strength than the concentric at a ratio of between 1.16 and 1.54. In addition the curves indicated a reasonable degree of reproducibility. Taken together, these circumstances, locality of deficiency, eccentric/concentric ratios and overlapping, served to conclusively justify the patient's claim.

Lower back dysfunction and SOE

Finally, it should be borne in mind that most of the arguments for and against using isokinetics for SOE settling were centered on trunk analysis in the context of lower back dysfunction. Given the enormity of the problem, any attempt to determine veracity of low back dysfunction claims is seen with appropriate suspicion. In the author's opinion the trunk is far from being an ideal area for isokinetic SOE testing because of a number of problems, substantive as well as technical. This is not, however, to decry the specific power this technology has to unravel SOE-related cases which center on other joints, notably those of the extremities.

PAIN AND SOE

Effect of pain

Pain is an important confounding factor in muscle performance testing, and may significantly affect the SOE findings. Pain can, and often does, inhibit muscle function but not always in a predictable fashion. For example, MAP curves sometimes demonstrate serious irregularities on one repetition which subside on the next. As another example, though the peak moments of the curves in Figure 3.1 are sufficiently close, the breaks in two of them are significantly different in magnitude.

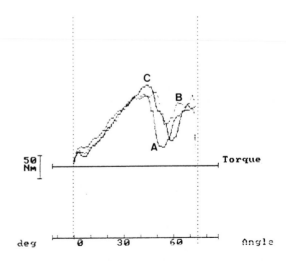

Fig. 3.1 Consecutive isokinetic eccentric moment–angular position (MAP) curves in a patient with patellar pain. The peak moments of the individual curves, A, B and C were 149 N m (at 43°), 157 N m (46°) and 173 N m (44°) respectively. The lowest within-break moment values were 40 N m (53°), 91 N m (56°) and 54 N m (58°) respectively, i.e. with a 128% difference between curves A and B.

It may not be impossible to present reproducible test findings, even in the presence of pain, but there is a high probability that they will be significantly attenuated. In such a case the examiner may mistakenly believe that a genuine muscular insufficiency exists, when the examination actually relates to the degree of pain intolerance. Clearly the test is invalid. Therefore the presence of pain, which contraindicates isokinetic testing in general, should preclude the use of isokinetic data in SOE cases, unless the MAP curves consistently overlap in terms of the angle of peak moment, peak moment, the extent of the break and the angle at which it occurs. Such a rare example is illustrated in Figure 3.2.

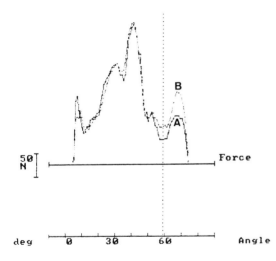

Fig. 3.2 Consecutive isokinetic eccentric peak moments MAP curves, A and B in a patient suffering from peripheral neuropathy. Peak moments were almost identical for both curves, 94 N m and 95 N m respectively, both at 41°. The lowest within-break moment values were 53 N m and 82 N m at the same angle of 59°, with a 54% difference.

'Proving' existence and magnitude of pain

However, 'proving' the existence of pain may be the aim of the test. Generally, the extent of impairment and disability arising primarily from pain, especially chronic pain, is controversial (American Medical Association 1991). This situation results mostly from the impossibility of measuring pain objectively. Furthermore, if pain is assumed to be present, its effect on function is no less difficult to judge.

Concerning the existence of pain, it is suggested that if its source can be traced to muscle or joint involvement, then in some instances it may be possible to objectively confirm its presence using isokinetics.

As detailed in Chapter 6, a few studies have indicated that the magnitude of pain, as subjectively rated by the subject, was inversely proportional to the concentric test angular velocity. In other words, a longer exposure to load resulted in a more intense pain. Therefore, if a protocol with a wide range of velocities is used, there is reason to believe that in specific cases of myogenic or arthrogenic pain, this relationship will prevail. The protocol should be conventional and a random order of velocities should be used. Tests must be repeated at least twice. If the patient's pain ratings conform to the inverse relationship, her/his claim concerning the existence of pain is further supported. Moreover, the demands, in terms of the loads developed during the tests, may be compared with those typical of habitual activities and hence the extent of disability could be decided more accurately. The present author has used this approach successfully with three patients presenting with severe pain, due to a rare combination of chronic viral infection and Charcot–Marie–Tooth disease. On the other hand, since the research concerning this issue is still at a very early stage, the absence of such a relationship should not be viewed as necessarily discrediting the claim.

FATIGUE AND ANXIETY

It should be emphasized that fatigue, which may impair normal motor control (Parnianpour et al 1988), may also interfere with a proper SOE assessment. Consequently testing should not be performed when subjects complain of exhaustion or fatigue. From the point of view of motivation, it should be borne in mind that as subjects are generally aware of the test objectives, a certain level of anxiety is almost inevitable. It is therefore crucial that the test should be carried out in as relaxed an atmosphere as possible. Also, subjects should not be allowed to view the computer screen for obvious reasons, nor should any verbal encouragement be offered.

COMPARISON WITH A STANDARD

EVALUATION OF IMPAIRMENT

Sincerity of effort: this must positively be demonstrated in those cases where the extent of impairment, if any, is not clear cut.

Limitations of existing systems

The American Medical Association's Guide to the evaluation of permanent impairment (1991) states:

Muscle testing, including tests for *strength, duration and repetition of contraction and function*, helps evaluate the motor function of specific nerves. Muscle testing is based on the principle of gravity and resistance, that is, *the ability to raise a part of the body through its range of motion against gravity and to hold that part at the end of its range of motion against resistance*. In interpreting muscle testing, *comparable muscle function on both sides of the body should be considered*. A grading scheme and procedure for determining impairment of the upper (lower) extremity due to loss of *power*... (present author's italics)

The phrases in italics show some of the inconsistencies, and the confusion inherent in defining the muscle performance component in impairment evaluation. Strength, duration and repetition of contraction are never quoted in operative terms. For instance, concentric performance (raising a limb against gravity) is not related to the angular velocity, duration and the number and nature of contractions are not defined. The crucial eccentric performance component is not mentioned at all. Muscle function explicity appears but its meaning is vague. Furthermore, although substitutions are mentioned (in a previous paragraph) their signficance in interpreting function is again left to the discretion of the examiner. Examiners are also encouraged to perform a bilateral test but how a bilateral involvement should be interpreted, or what should happen if the other limb is not available for comparison, is not at all clear. Finally loss of power, which strictly speaking is a reduction in the rate of work output, here refers probably to a general decline in performance.

Crudity of grading system

Experienced users of isokinetic systems will immediately realize the scope of the problems associated with the above approach. It should, in all fairness, be mentioned that the American system is not different from, and is often even superior to, its counterparts in other western countries. However, isokinetics introduces a new dimension to motor loss analysis, which many physicians still find difficult to assimilate. This applies even more emphatically to the law, which is normally impervious to changes. Therefore very often one has to downgrade the isokinetic findings in order to render them compatible with the prevailing regulations.

This is particularly marked with regard to grade 4 of the American system: the ability of a patient to demonstrate 'complete ROM against gravity and some resistance'. The 'some resistance' factor is especially vague, since it spans the entire strength (moment) continuum, starting with the minimal (against gravity only), and terminating at the maximal strength.

As mentioned in Chapter 2, if muscle moment is to be measured during the performance of an antigravity motion, the essential condition for measurability is that the moment exerted by the muscle exceeds the gravitational moment of the distal segment. Thus if a muscle is judged to have a 'grade 3 strength' the resulting moment record will be zero. In other words, grade 3 is tantamount to a complete palsy of this muscle/muscle group. The consequence of this is that the full 'in excess of gravity' potential of any muscle is covered by grades 4 and 5 only, a situation which greatly impedes the expression of precise isokinetic findings in terms of the manual muscle testing grades, which are still binding in most books of impairment regulations.

For example, consider a male patient, with a unilateral 'strength loss' in a shoulder flexor which is judged to be at grade 3, and whose upper extremity weighs 70 N. Assuming a center of gravity location at 30 cm distal to the joint, the highest isometric moment expected to be generated by his involved flexors at an elevation of 90° is 21 N m. A comparison is then made with the uninvolved side. If the flexors of the uninvolved side of this patient are completely normal, Table 9.7 (see Ch. 9) indicates that he would reasonably be expected to generate a peak moment of the uninvolved flexors of 49–75 N m (mean, standard deviation – 62, 13 N m) at 60 °/s. These values are 150 to almost 300% greater than the calculated isometric strength in the most demanding position, without additional resistance, a considerable margin by any standard. What is then the corresponding meaning of 'some' resistance? Put quantitatively, does it correspond to a peak moment of 30, 40 or 50 N m?

Adapting isokinetic data

Thus, instead of increased precision, one has to

redefine the meaning of the findings to fit the crude categories of the impairment rating.

In other rating systems, the severity of impairment may relate to specific muscles or muscle groups and the categories are defined in terms of light (10%), medium (20%) and severe (30%) impairment to the limb. In this case the decision on how to categorize performance may be more difficult. One possible solution is to use the gravity-corrected peak moment of the uninvolved side as a criterion and use its value to obtain three ranges. Consider again the example mentioned earlier, and assume that the peak moment of the uninvolved flexors is 57 N m. Dividing by three gives sub-ranges as follows: 0–19, 20–38 and 39–57 N m. To differentiate between light and no impairment, the third category is divided into two: 39–48 and 49–57 N m respectively. If the involved side flexor peak moment is, for instance, 29 N m this figure would correspond to medium impairment. If on the other hand the result is 50 N m, no impairment is indicated.

The impairment figure is subsequently multiplied by the relative weight of the flexors compared to the other muscles of the shoulder and again by the limb factor to obtain the impairment to the whole person.

Bilateral comparisons

Use of the absolute values of the uninvolved limb as the standard for comparison has been supported in a recent paper by Motzkin et al (1991), and is generally accepted.

However, the major source in this regard are the guidelines recommended by Sapega (1990):

1. When presumably normal individuals are evaluated (such as when screening athletic teams), imbalances of strength in an individual muscle group of less than 10% can be considered normal; differences of 10–20% as possibly abnormal; those greater than 20% as probably abnormal.
2. When one extremity is clearly expected to be weaker, on the basis of a previous injury or disease, differences of 10–20% can be considered probably abnormal and those of more than 20% as almost certainly abnormal. (p. 1569 in the paper)

Precise bilateral comparison is probably one of the most distinguishing facets of isokinetic dynamometry, and has a specific medicolegal role. This derives mainly from the sensitivity of the apparatus, which is far superior to human ability.

Consider for instance the following case of a male patient, 54 years old, whose elbow rotational strength was impaired following an attempt to lift a very heavy object (Fig. 3.3). Eight months after the injury he was diagnosed by two orthopaedic surgeons as having a complete recovery of both supination and pronation strength. Therefore the muscle strength rating stood at 5 according to the manual scale. His persistent complaint, a clear weakness in turning his elbow, proved to be well substantiated in the light of the isokinetic findings: a 57 and 54% reduction in supination and pronation strength respectively. What had probably led both surgeons to decide that this patient had completely recovered was his ability to exert a reasonable counterresistance with his involved upper extremity. That this ability was more than 50% less than that of the uninvolved extremity was not detected because of the insensitivity of the human force sensing mechanism, particularly when relatively high forces are involved.

Population norms

Representative isokinetic performance values (RIPVs) are not yet in general use as a standard for comparison. However, they are acutely needed where the patient is afflicted with bilateral damage or some disease state so that no 'sound side' is available. Typical examples, respectively, are bilateral osteoarthritis of the knee with severe deterioration of involved muscles and a neurological disease such as Charcot-Marie-Tooth. RIPVs should normally consist of the elements of gender, age and activity level, but the latter hardly exists. Therefore, it is suggested that, except in extreme situations, the element of activity level is waived and the comparison is based on the elements of gender and age only. Some relevant RIPVs are outlined in this book.

DISABILITY RATING

The incorporation of isokinetic findings into disability ratings is even more problematic, although

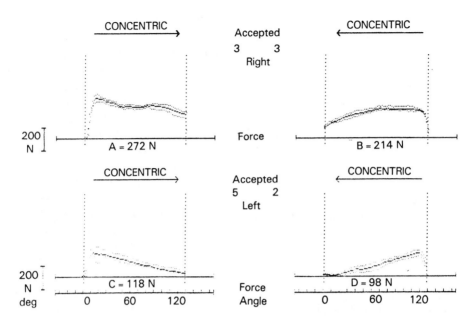

Fig. 3.3 Concentric strength differences in forearm pronators (upper and lower right-hand traces) and supinators (left-hand traces), in a 54-year-old male patient following injury to the elbow. Upper traces: the uninvolved extremity, lower traces: the involved extremity. Tests performed at 30 °/s and medium damping.

not without promise. Disability has been defined as a limitation in the amount or the kind of gainful work that can be performed because of a chronic condition or impairment (Snook & Webster 1987), or limitation in the performance of the individual when compared to a fit person of the same age and sex (Waddell 1987). Both definitions refer explicity to performance. However, parameters based on a single test, like peak moment or contractional work can hardly be extrapolated to this kind of performance. Rather, fatigue or endurance testing are more appropriate.

With the rapid increase in automatization of manual tasks, the demands put on the human body by strenuous jobs is decreasing, but some occupations, such as firefighting or agricultural work, still need a certain level of cardiopulmonary and musculoskeletal fitness. Impairment of key components in these systems might render individuals incapable of continuing with their occupations, and/or to loss of earning capacity. Isokinetic testing can provide vital information regarding the musculoskeletal component. Together with cardiopulmonary testing, a comprehensive quantitative picture may be obtained.

However, loss of function is far more difficult to define as it involves so many more components (see below) and consequently isokinetic testing has hardly been used in this context. It is possible, however, that the development of multijoint testing (see for instance Chapter 8) and of representative databases will open the way for assessment of disability as well as of impairment.

PART 5
ISOKINETIC MUSCLE PERFORMANCE AND FUNCTIONAL ACTIVITY

ISOKINETICS AND FUNCTIONAL TESTING

'Functional measurement' refers to a situation where the tested muscle/s perform a certain habitual function in an uninterrupted fashion. Habitual human motion very seldom occurs in an isokinetic manner, which is one of the main reservations concerning the wider use of isokinetics in muscle performance analysis.

Moreover, even where an isokinetic-like movement takes place, for instance arm motion in swimming, isokinetic tests have failed to reveal specificity. Thus Reid et al (1991) found that isokinetically measured shoulder muscle strength in swimmers did not differ from that measured in other athletes. This contrasts with the expectaction that the swimmers would have significantly stronger shoulder muscles and ostensibly casts doubts on the validity of isokinetic testing.

Can isokinetic testing be of value?

Given the reservation about the nonisokineticity of human motion, the first question is therefore whether a so-called nonfunctional testing method can have any value in indicating functional capacity. As discussed earlier, in certain instances isokinetic findings are of significant value in assessing functional capacity. In fact, according to a recent review of muscle performance measurement (Sapega 1990) 'Results of isokinetic tests have considerable inferential value with regard to human manual or locomotor functional capacity'. Thus, prima facie, the application of isokinetic technology cannot be ignored simply because of its specific mode of operation.

Difficulty of testing functional capacity

However there are other salient issues concerning the measurement of functional capacity, by whatever means. Certain assumptions may be made:

1. Although normal muscle performance is one of the prerequisites for normal functioning (Amundsen 1990) other factors, such as coordination, are essential for correct movement patterns.
2. Objective and accurate measurements have to be made in order to determine the extent to which the relevant muscle performance is within accepted standards (Sapega 1990).
3. Such measurements can seldom be performed in an completely functional setting.

Consider the case of a patient in whom quadriceps performance has been observed to decline. Functional measurement of knee extension performance may be carried out in the following way. In the absence of reactive forces, such as in the swing phase of gait, it would be possible, using optical instruments and the laws of dynamics, to calculate the moment developed. In this instance, the process of measurement is completely external to the movement and consequently the measurement would 'functional'. It would however require the use of a very expensive set-up.

Once external loads were introduced, such as during foot–ground contact in stair ascent and descent, kinematic measurement would not suffice and force measurement devices would have to be used. If 'functionality' was to be preserved, these devices would take the form of sophisticated force platforms, fully synchronized with optical equipment via a computer. Such systems would become prohibitively expensive and require a laboratory set-up which could be afforded only by large institutions.

Moreover, at times the patient is not capable of walking, or the function/s may not be amendable for quantitative assessment. For instance in this particular case, one may be interested in assessing the moments generated by the quadriceps during assisted seat rise, which in turn would necessitate an even more complex set of devices. Consequently the full scope of muscle performance analysis in the context of functional activity may remain elusive.

Functionally oriented isokinetic testing

The logical alternative is therefore to employ instruments which may not allow total 'functionality' yet permit the making of reasonable inferences. Isometric tests yield 'peak moment' findings only and are heavily dependent on the skill of the examiner. Although the isometric 'peak moments' generally correlate well with those obtained from isokinetic tests, the advantage of the latter technique, whenever it is applicable, over the former is unquestionable. The same, or even more forceful, arguments are valid as far as the so-called isotonic measurement technique is concerned. Other methods such as the isoinertial or isoacceleration techniques (Westing et al 1990) have, so far, not improved the current understanding of muscle performance in any significant way.

Isokinetic testing may, however, be performed in a more functionally oriented way. Consider for instance Figure 3.4. This shows the findings of a bilateral isokinetic test of the quadriceps in a woman who suffered from unilateral polio. This woman complained of a progessive weakness of the quadri-

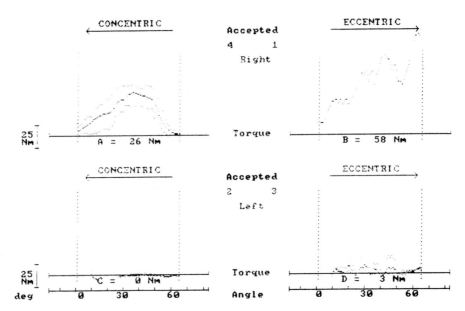

Fig. 3.4 Knee extensor concentric and eccentric strength in a postpolio female patient. Upper traces, uninvolved lower extremity; lower traces, involved lower extremity. Note the zero strength of the involved extremity, in both contraction modes, in the single-joint-testing configuration.

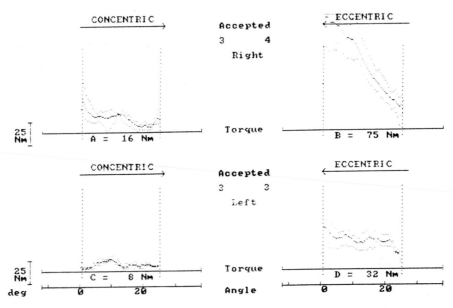

Fig. 3.5 Same patient as in Figure 3.4, in leg press test. Note considerable improvement in closed kinetic chain configuration in both contraction modes. Upper traces uninvolved lower extremity; lower traces, involved lower extremity.

ceps with pelvic muscle involvement, which was particularly problematic on stair ascending. The external manifestation of her situation, however, was a very slight limp and some heaviness in gait.

The initial test consisted of concentric/eccentric quadriceps testing, performed sitting with a ROM of about 60°. Compared with the uninvolved side, there was an almost total loss of muscle strength to the extent that she was unable to extend the knee. The loss, approximately 96% relative to the sound limb, was expressed in both the concentric and eccentric tests which were deliberately conducted at the very low velocity of 10 °/s. This velocity was chosen in order to compare the performance in this single joint testing (open kinetic chain) configuration with the performance in the leg press test which followed. It also contributed to the large dispersion which is very conspicuous in the findings.

This patient was subsequently asked to perform a multiple-joint isokinetic leg press test in the supine position. Starting with the hip and knee in the 90° position, the patient pressed her foot as forcefully as possible, effecting concentric contractions in the hip and knee extensors. This motion corresponded to about 25° in each joint. The return motion involved eccentric contractions of the same muscle groups. Stabilization of the trunk and the foot was ensured using special attachments. Figure 3.5 illustrates the findings.

Although the involved side still demonstrated marked weakness, 40 and 50% in the concentric and eccentric contractions respectively, the extent was markedly limited compared with that in the single muscle. A significant contribution from the hip extensors together, probably, with altered nervous input and knee joint motion could account for this dramatic variation. These findings agree with the clinical picture, in that only a limited moment has to be generated by the quadriceps during free gait. Indeed 'quadriceps gait' is a well known clinical entity which does not present a totally disrupted gait cycle. On the other hand, performance of a more taxing, closed kinetic chain activity, like that simulated by the leg press, calls for a significantly higher quadriceps moment and hence the difficulty in climbing stairs.

MUSCLE CONDITION

As far as muscle conditioning is concerned, the ability to preset the control parameters affords an extraordinary degree of flexibility in preparing the muscle/s to resume certain activities. It should be emphasized that muscle performance spans a continuum across all of the control parameters. Functionally means that the nervous system can freely operate within the available ranges of these parameters. The present author believes, therefore, that even though every functional element is not simulated, used correctly, isokinetics allows maximization of muscle performance. It lays the ground for optimal utilization of the relevant muscles in a fashion which is probably unsurpassed by other techniques.

REFERENCES

American Medical Association 1991 Guides to evaluation of permanent impairment, 3rd edn. American Medical Association, Milwaukee, Wisconsin

Amundsen L R 1990 Measurement of skeletal muscle strength: an overview of instrumented and non-instrumented systems. In:Amundsen L R (ed) Muscle strength testing: instrumented and non-instrumented systems, Churchill Livingstone, New York, pp 1–24

Armstrong L E, Winat D M, Swasey P R, Seidle M E, Carter A L, Gehlsen G 1983 Using isokinetic dynamometry to test ambulatory patients with multiple sclerosis. Physical Therapy 63: 1274–1279

Backman E, Oberg B 1989 Isokinetic torque in the dorsiflexors of the ankle in children 6–15 years of age. Scandinavian Journal of Rehabilitation Medicine 21: 97–103

Bemben M G, Grump K J, Massey B H 1989 Assessment of technical accuracy of the Cybex II isokinetic dynamometer and analog recording system. Journal of Orthopaedic and Sports Physical Therapy 10: 12–17

Bennett G J, Stauber W T 1986 Evaluation and treatment of anterior knee pain using eccentric exercise. Medicine and Science in Sports and Exercise 18: 526–530

Borges O 1989 Isometric and isokinetic knee extension and flexion torque in men and women aged 20–70. Scandinavian Journal of Rehabilitation Medicine 21: 45–53

Bosco C, Komi P V 1980 Influence of aging on the mechanical behavior of leg extensor muscle. European Journal of Applied Physiology 45: 209–219

Byl N N, Sadowski S H 1993 Intersite reliability of repeated isokinetic measurements: Cybex back systems including trunk rotation, trunk extension-flexion and Liftask. Isokinetics and Exercise Science 3: 139–147

Byl N N, Wells L, Grady D, Friedlander A, Sadowski S 1991 Consistency of repeated isokinetic testing: effect of different examiners, sites and protocol. Isokinetic and Exercise Science 1: 122–130

Carlsoo S 1986 With what degree of precision can voluntary muscle force be repeated? Scandinavian Journal of Rehabilitation Medicine 18: 1–3

Dvir Z, Halperin N, Shklar A, Robinson D 1991 Quadriceps function and patellofemoral pain syndrome. Part I: pain provocation during concentric and eccentric isokinetic contractions. Isokinetics and Exercise Science 1: 26–30

Engleberg A L 1988 Guide to the evaluation of permanent impairment, 4th edn. American Medical Association, Chicago, pp 40–45

Eriksson E 1991 The use of isokinetic dynamometers in sports orthopaedic research. In: Eriksson E, Grimby G, Knutsson E, Thorstensson A (eds) Dynamic dynamometry in research and clinical work. (Seminar proceedings), Karolinska Institute, Stockholm

Farrell M, Richards J G 1986 Analysis of the reliability and validity of the kinetic communicator exercise device. Medicine and Science in Sports and Exercise 18: 44–49

Francis K, Hoobler T 1987 Comparison of peak torque values of the knee flexor and extensor muscle groups using the Cybex II and Lido 2.0 isokinetic dynamometers. Journal of Orthopaedic and Sports Physical Therapy 8: 480–484

Fugl-Meyer AR 1981 Maximum ankle plantar and dorsiflexor torque in trained subjects. European Journal of Applied Physiology 47: 393–404

Fugl-Meyer AR, Sjöstrom M, Wahlby L 1979 Human plantar flexion strength and structure. Acta Physiologica Scandinavica 107: 47–56

Fugl-Meyer A R, Mild K H, Hornsten J 1982 Output of skeletal muscle contractions:a study of isokinetic plantar flexion in athletes. Acta Physiologica Scandinavica 115: 193–199

Fugl-Meyer A R, Gerdle B, Eriksson B E, Jonsson B 1985 Isokinetic plantar flexion endurance: reliability and validity of output/excitation measurements. Scandinavian Journal of Rehabilitation Medicine 17: 47–52

Gerdle B, Hedberg B, Angquist K-A, Fugl-Meyer A R 1986 Isokinetic strength and endurance in peripheral arterial insufficiency with intermittent claudication. Scandinavian Journal of Rehabilitation Medicine 18: 9–15

Giles B, Henke P, Edmonds J, McNeil D 1990 Reproducibility of isokinetic muscle strength measurements in normal and arthritic individuals. Scandinavian Journal of Rehabilitation Medicine 22: 93–99

Grace TG, Sweetser E R, Nelson M A, Ydens L R, Skipper B J 1984 Isokinetic muscle imbalance and knee joint injury. Journal of Bone and Joint Surgery 66A: 734–740

Gross M 1991 Intra-machine and inter-machine reliability of the Biodex and Cybex II for knee flexion and extension peak torque and angular work. Journal of Orthopaedic and Sports Physical Therapy 13: 329–330

Harding B, Black T, Bruulsema A, Maxwell B, Stratford P 1988 Reliability of a reciprocal test protocol performed on the Kinetic Communicator: an isokinetic test of knee extensor and flexor strength. Journal of Orthopaedic and Sports Physical Therapy 10: 218–223

Hazard R G, Reid S, Fenwick J, Reeves V 1988 Isokinetic trunk and lifting strength measurements: variability as an indicator of effort. Spine 13: 54–57

Johnson J, Siegel D 1978 Reliability of an isokinetic movement of the knee extensors. Research Quarterely 49: 88–98

Johnstone M V, Keith R A, Hinderer S R 1992 Measurement standards for interdisciplinary medical rehabilitation. Archives of Physical Medicine and Rehabilitation 73: S3–S23

Knapik J J, Bauman C L, Jones B H, Harris J McA, Vaughan L 1991 Preseason strength and flexibility imbalances associated with athletic injuries in female collegiate athletes. Medicine and Science in Sports and Exercise 19: 76–81

Kramer J F 1990 Reliability of knee extensor and flexor torques during continuous concentric-eccentric cycles. Archives of Physical Medicine and Rehabilitation 71: 460–464

Kramer J F, Vaz M D, Hakansson D 1991 Effect of activation force on knee extensor torques. Medicine and Science in Sports and Exercise 23: 231–237

Kues J, Rothstein J M, Lamb R L 1992 Obtaining reliable measurements of knee extensor torque produced during maximal voluntary contractions: an experimental investigation. Physical Therapy 72: 492–504

Lankhorst G J, Van de Stadt R J, Van de Korst J K 1985 The relationship of functional capacity pain and isometric and isokinetic torque in osteoarthritis of the knee. Scandinavian Journal of Rehabilitation Medicine 17: 167–172

Levene J A, Hart B A, Seeds R A, Fuhrman G A 1991 Reliability of reciprocal isokinetic testing of the knee extensors and flexors. Journal of Orthopaedic and Sports Physical Therapy 14: 121–127

Lysholm J 1987 The relationship between pain and torque in an isokinetic strength test of knee extension. Arthroscopy 3: 182–184

Martensson A 1991 Isokinetic dynamometry in hysterical paresis. In: Eriksson E, Grimby G, Knutsson E, Thorstensson A (eds) Dynamic dynamometry in research and clinical work. (Seminar proceedings, Karolinska Institute, Stockholm)

Mawdsley R H, Knapik J J 1982 Comparison of isokinetic measurements with test repetitions. Physical Therapy 62: 169–172

Mayhew T P, Rothstein J M 1985 Measurement of muscle performance with instruments. In: Rothstein J M (ed) Measurement in physical therapy. Churchill Livingstone, Edinburgh

Molczyk L, Thigpen L K, Eickhoff J, Coldgar D, Gallagher J C 1991 Reliability of testing the knee extensors and flexors in healthy adult women using a Cybex II isokinetic dynamometer. Journal of Orthopaedic and Sports Physical Therapy 14: 37–41

Montgomery L C, Douglass L W, Deuster P A 1989 Reliability of an isokinetic test of muscle strength and endurance. Journal of Orthopaedic and Sports Physical Therapy 11: 315–322

Motzkin N, Cahalan T D, Morrey B F, An K-N, Chao E Y S 1991 Isometric and isokinetic endurance testing of the forearm complex. American Journal of Sports Medicine 19: 107–111

Newton M, Waddell G 1993 Trunk strength testing with iso-machines Part I: review of a decade of scientific evidence. Spine 18: 801–811

Nordgren B, Nordesjo L-O, Rauschning W 1983 Isokinetic knee extension strength and pain before and after advancement osteotomy of the tibial tuberosity. Archives of Orthopaedic and Traumatic Surgery 102: 95–101

Olds K, Godfrey C, Rosenrot P 1981 Computer assisted isokinetic dynamometry: a calibration study. In: Fourth annual conference on rehabilitation engineering, Washington DC

Parnianpour M, Nordin M, Kahanovitz N, Frankel V 1988 The triaxial coupling of torque generation of the trunk muscles during isometric exertions and the effect of fatiguing isoinertial movements on the motor output and movement patterns. Spine 9: 982–992

Reid D C, Saboe L A, Burnham R 1991 Common shoulder problems in the athlete. In: Donatelli R (ed) Physical therapy of the shoulder, 2nd edn. Churchill Livingstone, Edinburgh

Reitz C, Rowinski M, Davies G J 1988 Comparison of Cybex II and Kin-Com reliability on the measures of peak torque, work and power at three speeds. Physical Therapy 68: 782

Sapega A A 1990 Muscle performance evaluation in orthopaedic practice. Journal of Bone and Joint Surgery 72A: 1562–1574

Shelbourne K D, Rettig AC, McCarroll J R, Vogel A, Kuhn D, Bisesi M A 1987 Functional ability in athletes with an anterior ligament deficient knee. American Journal of Sports Medicine 16: 628

Sinacore D R, Rothstein J M, Delitto A, Rose S J 1983 Effect of damp on isokinetic measurements. Physical Therapy 63: 1248–1253

Snook S H, Webster B S 1987 The cost of disability. Clinical Orthopaedics and Related Research 221: 77–84

Stratford P 1991 Reliability of a peak knee extensor and flexor torque protocol: a study of post ACL reconstructed knees. Physiotherapy Canada 43: 27–30

Stratford P, Bruulsema A, Maxwell B, Black T, Harding B 1990 The effect of inter-trial rest interval on the assessment of thigh muscle torque. Journal of Orthopaedic and Sports Physical Therapy 11: 362–366

Thompson M C, Shingleton G, Kegerreis S T 1989 Comparison of values generated in testing of the knee using the Cybex II and Biodex B-2000. Journal of Orthopaedic and Sports Physical Therapy 10: 108–112

Thorstensson A, Grimby G, Karlsson J 1976 Force-velocity relations and fiber composition in human knee extensor muscles. Journal of Applied Physiology 40: 12–16

Timm K 1988 Isokinetic lifting simulation: a normative data study. Journal of Orthopaedic and Sports Physical Therapy 9: 156–166

Timm K 1990 Reliability of the Cybex 340 and Merac isokinetic measures of peak torque, total work and average power at five test speeds. Physical Therapy 69: 389

Timm K E, Gennrich P, Burns R, Fyke D 1992 The mechanical and physiological performance reliability of selected isokinetic dynamometers. Isokinetics and Exercise Science 2: 182–190

Tripp E J, Harris S R 1991 Test-retest reliability of isokinetic knee extension and flexion torque measurements in persons with spastic hemiparesis. Physical Therapy 71: 390–396

Waddell G 1987 Clinical assessment of lumbar impairment. Clinical Orthopaedic and Related Research 221: 110–120

Wessel J, Gray G, Luongo F, Isherwood L 1989 Reliability of work measurements recorded during concentric and eccentric contractions of the knee extensors in healthy subjects. Physiotherapy Canada 41: 250–253

Westing S H, Seger J Y, Thorstensson A 1991 Isoacceleration: a new concept of resistive exercise. Medicine and Science in Sports and Exercise 23: 631–635

Wilhite M R, Cohen E S, Wilhite S C 1992 Reliability of concentric and eccentric measurement of quadriceps performance using the Kin-Com dynamometer: the effect of testing order for three different speeds. Journal of Orthopaedic and Sports Physical Therapy 15: 175–182

CHAPTER 4

Application of isokinetics to muscle conditioning and rehabilitation

PART 1
INTRODUCTION

Compared with the use of isokinetics in testing, where there are relatively well-established rules and procedures, its clinical role in the conditioning of muscle performance is far less researched and understood. A number of difficulties seriously undermine and sometimes even preclude the estab-

lishment of pathology- or intervention-specific protocols. These difficulties result from a range of factors which may be divided into two groups: methodological and patient-linked on one hand, and the predominantly logistic on the other.

From the methodological viewpoint, there are complex interactions between factors ranging from the type of injury or pathology to the patient's motivation. This is reflected in a paper by Zarins et al (1985), discussing rehabilitation after the relatively straightforward meniscectomy procedure:

Thus a large amount of variability exists in rehabilitation patterns following meniscectomy. Patient-to-patient differences dictate that each recovery program be tailored to meet the individual needs.

For instance for surgical cases the following factors must be taken into account when designing the rehabilitation protocol (Zarins et al 1985, Wilk & Andrews 1992):

1. surgical approach, e.g. arthrotomy vs. arthroscopy
2. amount of periarticular soft tissue dissection
3. type of tissue used (in reconstruction)
4. grafting factors
5. coexisting lesions and concomitant surgery
6. preoperative status
7. patient compliance and expectations.

Protocol problems

Muscle conditioning protocols are another critical methodological component. The difficulties in managing effectively isokinetic testing variables are described in Chapter 3. The complexity associated with rational implementation of conditioning protocols is considerably greater. Problems arise in various quarters, for instance, the impact on tissues other than muscle. During isokinetic conditioning significant loads may be exerted on structures such as the articular surfaces, capsule or ligaments. The cumulative effect of this, which is notoriously hard to determine, must be considered.

The question of submaximal versus maximal exertions has to be answered with regard to healing stage, pain and the potential of the muscles and/or other involved tissues. The issues of protocol structure, mainly the conditioning dose and which performance criteria should be optimized, have never been settled in a systematic manner. Clinicians have therefore to rely either on a very limited number of studies and/or on their own experience which may be even more restricted.

Logistic limitations

The logistic problems, though not necessarily limited to isokinetic conditioning are no less daunting. The time frame for significant improvements in muscle performance, is measured in weeks rather than minutes. Moreover, within this period, subjects have to attend all sessions, typically at least three per week. Hence, even a 'minimal size' study consisting of 20 patients, who exercise at this rate for a period of 6 weeks, necessitates 360 sessions, an undertaking which can be met only by large and well-equipped centers.

This obstacle is associated with the difficulty of obtaining a large homogeneous sample for a given symptom and/or interventions. Small clinics and some medical centers rarely treat more than a handful of patients afflicted with the same pathology during a limited time period. Consequently, the likelihood of generating original conditioning (rather than testing) protocols and more significantly, their objective assessment, is very low. For instance, the body of knowledge relating to the isokinetic testing of thigh muscles in chronic deficiency of, or reconstruction of, the anterior cruciate

ligament (ACL) is disproportionately larger than that relating to isokinetic-based rehabilitation.

Moreover, the success rate reported by one center may not apply to others in spite of the same conditioning philosophy being used. This may, for example, be the case with the 'accelerated rehabilitation' approach for patients with reconstructed ACL (Shelbourne & Nitz 1990); surgical skills accumulated after many hundreds, perhaps thousands, of reconstructions at a particular center, are bound to be reflected in the immediate postoperative status of the patient. Although this issue is common to all conditioning methods, its effects are more pronounced with isokinetic rehabilitation in view of the large range of options inherent in this technology.

Limitations of knowledge base

Finally, the studies which form the conceptual background of this chapter were based almost exclusively on young and healthy individuals, and practically all studies were based on a single muscle system, that of the thigh. It should also be noted that whereas the quadriceps and hamstring muscle groups frequently operate within the framework of a closed isokinetic chain, these muscles have usually been isokinetically conditioned in the open kinetic chain configuration. Consequently, though the results may be valid for other major muscle groups, the specific joint and dysfunction would dictate the individual approach.

Issues in therapeutic use of isokinetics

These difficulties (and probably others) contribute to a situation in which professionals, who are well-known in the practice of muscle performance rehabilitation, advocate the use of specific methods without the backing of solid research and its later recognition in peer-reviewed literature. For example, in a recently published book, one author quoted certain protocols which allegedly were implemented in the rehabilitation of more than 1000 patients. These patients were reported to have significantly benefited from these protocols. The present author believes that since, in the present context, muscle conditioning refers to the therapeutic use of isokinetics, it must be considered with the utmost care. Consequently, one may rely only on those studies which systematically pursued relevant issues such as the principle of physiological overflow or the comparison of resistance training methods.

The purpose of this chapter is to review a number of issues which are relevant to the therapeutic use of isokinetic dynamometry. These issues include:

1. Physiological interactions in the course of muscle conditioning
2. Specificity of muscle performance conditioning
3. Principles of isokinetic conditioning programs in clinical rehabilitation.

PART 2
PHYSIOLOGICAL INTERACTIONS IN MUSCLE CONDITIONING

This subject has received considerable attention and hundreds of papers have been published, representing the scientific output of the fields of exercise physiology, physical therapy, rehabilitation medicine, athletic training, kinesiology, biomechanics and motor behavior. The following is a short exposition of relevant topics, based on the excellent reviews of Komi (1986), Enoka (1988) and Sale (1988). These reviews deal particularly with the development of muscle strength, mostly in healthy individuals, often athletes. However, in the clinical context, patients are not aiming at a 'stronger body' or improved athletic prowess, but simply to reach performance levels which enable the resumption of activity. This requirement is generally met by bringing muscle performance in the dysfunctional segment to a level comparable with that of the uninvolved side.

Overloading

The process of strength development is reflected in adaptive processes, both in the muscle tissue itself and in the neural apparatus associated with motor activity. These processes can be realized by 'almost any method provided that the frequency of the exercises and the loading intensities sufficiently

exceed those of normal activation of an individual muscle' (Komi 1986). This statement defines the principle of overloading. Isokinetic is one of the methods that can be employed very effectively for this purpose.

NEURAL ADAPTATIONS AND MUSCLE TISSUE CHANGES

Although the maximal force that a muscle can develop is related directly to its area of cross-section, the correlation between increases in muscle moment and in size is generally poor (Luthi et al 1986). This is particularly typical in naive subjects and patients. The lack of correlation exists because, at least during the initial stage of conditioning, increase in muscle moment is due to neural adaptations and possibly improved force transmission from individual sarcomeres to the skeletal apparatus (Enoka 1988).

The size changes, which characterize the later stage of strength conditioning, are brought about mainly by the increase in size of individual muscle fibers, and probably by some proliferation of the latter (hypertrophy and hyperplasia respectively). Moreover, there is a greater increase in the area of fast twitch (type II) compared with slow twitch (type I) fibers (Tesch 1988).

Neural activity and conditioning

Electromyographic changes highlight the interaction between the conditioning process and the neural adaptations. In studies of changes in motor unit activation following strength conditioning, it has been suggested that these adaptations consisted of an enhanced activation of prime movers and synergic patterns (agonist–antagonist). This conclusion was based on findings from a number of conditioning methods, including the isokinetic, (Komi & Burskirk 1972). An example of these effects is shown in Figure 4.1, which illustrates facilitation of the gastrocnemius during a drop jump in a trained subject, compared with an inhibition of the same muscle in an untrained subject.

Increased neural activation during strength conditioning has been attributed to an increase in the number of active motor units and/or their rate of firing. The source of this enhanced activity may

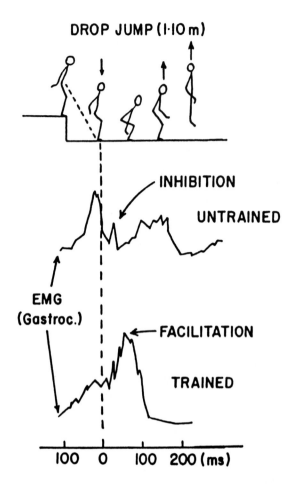

DROP JUMP (1·10 m)

INHIBITION

UNTRAINED

EMG
(Gastroc.)

FACILITATION

TRAINED

100   0   100   200 (ms)

Fig. 4.1 EMG recordings from the gastrocnemius muscle during drop jumps in an untrained subject (top) and in a trained jumper (bottom). During the eccentric phase of high stretch load (to immediate right of vertical dashed line at time 0) the untrained subject responded with a period of inhibition whereas the trained jumper responded with a period of facilitation. (From Komi 1986 Training of muscle strength and power. International Journal of Sports Medicine 7(suppl): 10–15.)

reside at the spinal and/or supraspinal levels. The role of motor unit synchronization is less clear. According to the theory proposed by Milner-Brown et al (1974) synchronization results either from increased input from the sensory fibers, which in turn operate on the alpha motor neurons, or from increased activity from higher centers. On the other hand, synchronization activity would actually be detrimental to force potentiation at submaximal firing frequencies (Sale 1988).

However, the recruitment of additional motor units and/or the increased rate of discharge may also serve as a stimulus for the second important stage of adaptation: hypertrophy.

Morphological changes

The time course of neural and morphological adaptations in the context of isokinetic conditioning, using the commonly employed regimens, is not immediately obvious. Earlier studies have shown no adaptive hypertrophy within the first weeks of conditioning at slow or medium velocities (Costill et al 1979, Caiozzo et al 1981, Coyle et al 1981), but did indicate a significant increase for type II fibers at the high conditioning velocity of 300 °/s (Coyle et al 1981). Komi (1986) suggested a period of 8 weeks before hypertrophy is apparent, though not with particular reference to isokinetics. However, recent papers present opposite views with respect to this issue.

Cote et al (1988)

In one study, 23 sedentary individuals (Cote et al 1988) trained for 5 days per week, for 10 weeks. During each session 30 maximal concentric contractions of the quadriceps and hamstring were performed. Seven subjects then participated in the latter part of the study which consisted of 50 days without training, and then retraining according to the same protocol as before. Biopsies were performed on the vastus lateralis for histological and biochemical analyses.

While the strength of the quadriceps increased by 54%, no overall increase in the fiber area was observed. However the percentage of type IIa fibers did increase significantly in number and area. For the 7 subjects who underwent retraining, the pre- and posttraining quadriceps strength scores in the first conditioning period were 89 and 133 N m. For the second conditioning period the scores were 117 and 123 N m.

In other words, retraining after a 50-day detraining period did not result in any significant variation, either in strength or fiber area. It was concluded that although isokinetic conditioning could increase the functional capacity of skeletal muscle, it did not appear to induce hypertrophy.

Ewing et al (1990)

Isokinetic and biopsy studies of muscle performance and adaptation following conditioning were also undertaken by Ewing et al (1990) and Esselman et al (1991). In the former study subjects trained for 10 weeks using maximal concentric quadriceps and hamstring contractions. Relatively modest increases in performance criteria (peak moment and contractional power) were recorded. Although there were no significant increases in the percentage of any fiber type (I, IIa or IIb) the area of type I and IIa fibers increased significantly, contrasting with the findings of Cote et al.

Esselman et al (1991)

The sophisticated protocol of Esselman et al (1991) consisted of a 12-week period of quadriceps conditioning with a different input for the opposite lower extremity of each subject. Twenty men were randomized into four groups. Subjects in group I trained at 36 °/s (low velocity) with 20 or 60 repetitions (reps), group II did 20 reps at 36 °/s with one limb and 60 reps at 108 °/s (medium velocity) contralaterally, and group III trained at 108 °/s with 20 or 60 reps. Group IV (control) did not train. The significant increases in strength, especially in the low velocity conditioning group, following this relatively long period of conditioning, were not correlated with muscle hypertrophy, as no signifi-

cant changes in type I and II fiber area were indicated. On the other hand, there was a significant increase in glycolytic and mitochondrial enzyme activity, in line with the findings of Cote et al (1988).

Figure 4.2 shows the times course of strength variations in the study of Esselman et al. Whereas the low-velocity group showed consistent gains up to the eighth week of conditioning, strength improvement in the medium/low velocity group leveled off after only 4 weeks. The authors suggested that these variations were consistent with neural adaptation and concluded that, in view of the absence of hypertrophy, the muscle adaptation had a smaller role in the overall strength gains.

The studies of Petersen et al

In a series of three studies, (Petersen et al 1989, 1990, 1991) the cross-sectional area (CSA) of muscle (quadriceps, hamstring or both) was shown to increase significantly following different protocols of concentric conditioning, lasting 6 and 12 weeks respectively (see section on specifity of conditioning for description of the regimen used).

In the first study, various hydraulic strength

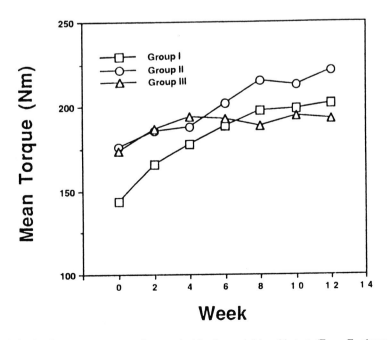

Fig. 4.2 Mean strength in the three groups across all test velocities for each biweekly test. (From Esselman et al 1991.)

conditioning devices were used to overload the lower limb. In the second, maximal knee extension was used as the overloading stimulus, whereas in the third study, conditioning was based on a combination of loading patterns for the lower limb, some of which were identical to those used in the first study. The authors used computed tomography (CT) for the calculation of thigh muscle cross-sectional area.

In all the studies significant hypertrophy was indicated, but the effect was not uniform; whereas quadriceps area increased during the first 6 weeks, a significant change in hamstring area occurred only after 12 weeks. The latter finding should be compared with a significant increase in hamstring strength, half way into the program, which could be explained by neural adaptation.

The weekly variations in strength found in the 1990 study of Petersen et al are shown in Figure 4.3. The accelerating gain in strength shown in this study contrasts notably with the decelerating gain shown in that of Esselman et al (1991). This discrepancy, doubtless the result of the different protocols used by the investigators, serves to emphasize the complexities associated with interpretation of conditioning outcome.

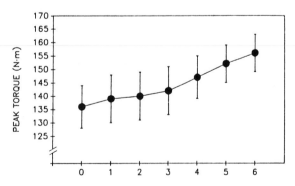

Fig. 4.3 Peak concentric extension moment (mean ± SE) observed during the final training session of each week at 60 °/s. (From Petersen et al 1990.)

Incompatibility of findings

Another plausible explanation for the incompatible findings lies in the different techniques employed to analyse the morphological data. There is a clear

dichotomy between the more conservative findings, which relied on biopsy-based histology, and those based on CT, which indicated significant changes. In the latter case the inclusion of connective tissue elements of noncontractile nature, which are known to increase in size during training (Sale 1988), might possibly account for the difference. Sometimes also, the initial phase of rehabilitation uses conditioning methods other than isokinetic, and it is reasonable to assume that morphological and neural adaptations are already in progress by the time isokinetic conditioning is initiated.

PART 3
SPECIFICITY OF MUSCLE PERFORMANCE CONDITIONING

As mentioned earlier conditioning of muscle performance can be effected using the overloading principle in various contraction modes: isometric, concentric, eccentric, plyometric or combinations. For instance, for the purpose of conditioning of knee extensor performance, one may use single or multiple isometrics; concentric (nonisokinetic) resisted extension in an open kinetic chain mode; concentric isokinetic leg press (closed kinetic chain mode); resisted eccentric isokinetic in an open kinetic chain mode, drop jumps from different heights (plyometrics), or combinations.

If a well-designed conditioning program is based on a single system of performance improvement, postconditioning testing using the same system that was used for conditioning, is likely to reveal significant gains in strength (and/or other performance parameters). However, when testing is performed using other systems, improvement may not necessarily be indicated. This illustrates the principle of specificity of conditioning. Specificity, therefore, concerns the degree to which gains from one system of performance enhancement may be transferred. The degree of specificity is considered mainly with respect to mode of contraction (e.g. concentric versus eccentric), conditioning velocity (high versus low), the nature of the kinetic chain and bilateral effects.

SPECIFICITY OF MODES OF CONTRACTION

Research data

The findings from a few studies which investigated this problem using nonisokinetic conditioning methods did not confirm specificity for any of them (see Petersen et al 1990). With isokinetic performance, the problem has been defined as either one or two-way transfer of gains. Table 4.1 presents a sample of studies which have either measured transfer from eccentric conditioning to concentric performance (Bishop et al 1991), from concentric conditioning to eccentric performance (Petersen et al 1990, Petersen et al 1991) or mutual transfer (Duncan et al 1989, Tomberlin et al 1991). The data from these studies suggest that:

1. On balance, concentric conditioning results in eccentric strength gains and therefore this method is not specific.
2. Eccentric conditioning does not result in concentric strength gains and therefore this method is specific.

Another study, however (Nicely et al 1988), which appeared in abstract form and hence did not provide sufficient protocol data, indicated mode specificity.

Limitations

Since different protocols were employed in these studies the above indications must be viewed with caution; the scope of their interpretation is qualified because:

1. Most findings, notably of Peterson and colleagues, are based on conditioning at the slow velocity of 60 °/s. Although a study of contraction mode specificity as a function of conditioning velocity is not currently available, it is possible that gains from lower velocities might be more effectively transferable. This speculation arises from the principle of physiological overflow (see below); low conditioning velocities are closer to the 'transfer zone' from one contraction mode to the other. The study by Duncan et al (1989) may provide some evidence for this, as at least with regard to eccentric conditioning, the concentric gains were higher at the lower velocity.

2. None of the abovementioned studies was applied in a clinical setting and the extent to which one may generalize from findings from healthy individuals must be qualified.

Clinical implication

If indeed '[isokinetic] resistance training effects are not always as specific to the training mode as has been thought' (Petersen et al 1990), the clinical implication cannot be overlooked. Eccentric contractions are important for the performance of daily activities as well as for the induction of muscle hypertrophy, but can potentially damage muscle fiber (Stauber 1989). In addition, eccentric conditioning would not be desirable in the rehabilitation of previously inactive individuals (Peterson et al 1990). It should also be borne in mind that not every rehabilitation facility has access to an active dynamometer. Hence, it is significant that concentric conditioning can produce an increase in eccentric strength.

The magnitude of this increase is not negligible; it was about 20 and 15% in the studies of Petersen et al (1990, 1991), about 10% in the study of Tomberlin et al (1991) and less than 10% in the findings of Duncan et al (1989). Clearly, though, these transfers may not be sufficient in every case, necessitating either more vigorous exercising or ultimately the use of eccentric conditioning.

SPECIFICITY OF CONDITIONING VELOCITIES

The question of whether gains achieved during conditioning at a given velocity are transferable to other velocities has received much attention. The physiological rationale underlying the possible phenomenon of velocity specificity is the differential recruitment of muscle fibers. It has been suggested (see Ewing et al 1990) that fast twitch fibers could be selectively stressed (and hence 'conditioned') during high velocity conditioning and vice versa.

Practical implication of velocity transfer

In the field of isokinetic dynamometry, the undisputed stimulus to this debate was the option of controlling the angular velocity of the lever-arm.

Table 4.1   Specificity of contraction mode in isokinetic conditioning protocols*

Source and subjects	Protocol		Muscle(s)	Condition contraction mode	Transfer of gains
	Weeks × days × sets (repetitions)	Velocity			
Bishop et al (1991)					
n = 13	8 w × 3 d × 3 sets (6 max)	60 °/s	Quadriceps + hamstring	Eccentric	Specific for quadriceps, not specific for hamstring
n = 15	8 w × 3 d × 3 sets (6 max)	180 °/s	Quadriceps + hamstring	Eccentric	Negligible effect of pain in eccentric mode
Duncan et al (1989)					
n = 16	6 w × 3 d × 1 set (10 max)	120 °/s	Quadriceps	Eccentric	Highly specific
n = 14	6 w × 3 d × 1 set (10 max)	120 °/s	Quadriceps	Concentric	More general Negligible effect of pain in eccentric mode
Petersen et al (1990)					
n = 8	6 w × 3 d × 5 sets (10 max)	60 °/s	Quadriceps	Concentric	Not specific
Petersen et al (1991)					
n = 14	12 w × 3 d × (2–3) sets (8–12 max)	60 °/s	Quadriceps + hamstring and other muscles	Concentric	Not specific
Tomberlin et al					
n = 19	6 w × 3 d × 3 sets (10 max)	100 °/s	Quadriceps	Concentric	Not specific
n = 21	6 w × 3 d × 3 sets (10 max)	100 °/s	Quadriceps	Eccentric	Specific

* All findings refer to gain in peak moment.

The need to assess the extent of velocity specificity is no less practical than theoretical. In isokinetic rehabilitation, the demands for reaching optimal muscle performance must be reconciled with the limited resources of time and equipment.

For instance, consider a unilateral muscular dysfunction and assume that 'optimal' means a bilateral parity in strength along the spectrum of velocities 30–300 °/s. Further assume that this spectrum is represented by 10 velocities 30 °/s apart. The question would then be: is it essential to exercise at each of these discrete velocities or will the use of two 'anchor point' velocities, low and high, be sufficient. The problem is really that of defining the optimal velocity differentials.

Research findings

The findings obtained in a number of representative studies which explored the phenomenon of velocity specificity are outlined in Table 4.2. It would appear that except for one study (Perrin et al 1989) all studies indicated the existence of a so-called 'physiological overflow,' or transfer, which is the reciprocal of specificity. This lack of specificity acted both ways; conditioning at a certain velocity resulted in strength gains at velocities higher and lower than the said velocity.

In these studies, the range of overflow was 30–120 °/s. One study included eccentric conditioning (Duncan et al 1989) where there was an up/down overflow of 60 °/s.

In other studies this phenomenon was analysed in terms of a one-way effect and the data were generally of the same or even higher magnitude.

Using these findings it is not possible to determine whether the lack of specificity has some preferential directionality, i.e. whether the overflow should be associated more with higher or lower velocities. However, a velocity differential of 90 °/s may confidently be used in isokinetic conditioning protocols.

SPECIFICITY OF OPEN AND CLOSED KINETIC CHAIN CONDITIONING

The use of closed kinetic chain-based conditioning (CKCC) has been gathering considerable momentum in recent years (Albert 1991, Davies 1992, see also Chapter 1).The advantages of CKCC are both its more functional nature and, in some instances, a better load distribution within the joints that are spanned by the working muscles. Closed kinetic chain movements can be realized using linear or angular patterns. Though purely linear isokinetic systems are not yet commercially available, the angular versions have long been in use in the form of isokinetic bicycles or exercisers for the upper limb.

Since CKCC typically involves simultaneous action of several muscles for the purpose of executing a given task, it is possible that individual muscles would be denied the full effect of the overloading stimulus such as occurs during open kinetic chain conditioning (OKCC). Hence, a well-balanced regimen should incorporate both CKC and OKC movement patterns. It is however imperative to assess the enhancement of OKC-based performance by CKCC and vice versa, in order to design an optimal combination of the two variants. This, in other words, is a problem of specificity.

Currently, knowledge regarding this issue is almost nonexistent. There is probably only one study where systematic OKCC was applied in order to test its effect on nonisokinetic constant load cycling (Mannion et al 1992). This CKC activity was chosen since it was a functional activity which put considerable demand on the knee extensors, but in a different coordination pattern from the conditioning (OKC) manoeuvre. In this study, two experimental groups underwent bilateral quadriceps conditioning at 60 and 240 °/s respectively, using the regimen, 6 sets, 3 days per week, for 16 weeks, with a maximum of 25 repetitions per set: (16 w × 3 d × 6 sets (25 max)). The performance criteria were isometric knee extensor strength and power output during a 6-second all-out sprint on a bicycle ergometer. Findings indicated significant increases in the peak power output and peak pedal velocity during sprint cycling, with no difference between the two conditioning velocity groups. It was therefore concluded that the gains achieved in the course of isokinetic OKCC could be positively transferred to a nonisokinetic CKC activity.

CROSS-EDUCATION (BILATERAL EFFECTS)

Isometric conditioning

Cross-education refers to the effect which conditioning of one extremity has on the other, where

Table 4.2 Specificity of velocities in isokinetic conditioning protocol*. (↑,↓; upwards, downwards transfer)

Source and subjects	Protocol Weeks × days × sets (repetitions)	Muscle(s)	Velocity	Transfer
Caiozzo et al (1981)				
n = 5	4 w × 3 d × 2 sets (10 max)	Quadriceps	96 °/s	↑ to 240 °/s
n = 5	4 w × 3 d × 2 sets (10 max)	Quadriceps	240 °/s	↓ to 144 °/s
Coyle et al (1981)				
n = 4	6 w × 3 d × 5 sets (6 or 12 max)	Quadriceps	60 °/s	↑ to 180 °/s
n = 4	6 w × 3 d × 5 sets (6 or 12 max)	Quadriceps	300 °/s	↓ to 0 °/s
Duncan et al (1989)				
n = 14	6 w × 3 d × 1 set (10 max)	Quadriceps	120 °/s	↑ to 180 °/s C only
n = 16 (eccentric)	6 w × 3 d × 1 set (10 max)	Quadriceps	120 °/s	↑/↓ in E only: 60 °/s
Esselman et al (1991)				
n = 5	12 w × 5 d × 1 set (20 or 60 max)	Quadriceps	36 °/s	
n = 5	12 w × 5 d × 1 set (20 or 60 max)	Quadriceps	36, 108 °/s	General ↑ and ↓ overflow
n = 5	12 w × 5 d × 1 set (20 or 60 max)	Quadriceps	108 °/s	
Ewing et al (1990)				
n = 10	10 w × 3 d × 3 sets (8–20 max)	Quadriceps	60 °/s	↑ to 180 °/s (peak moment and contractional power)
n = 10	10 w × 3 d × 3 sets (8–20 max)	Quadriceps	240 °/s	↓ to 180 °/s (peak moment and contractional power)
Jenkins et al (1984)				
n = 12	6 w × 3 d × 1 set (15 max)	Quadriceps	60 °/s	↑ to 240 °/s
n = 12	6 w × 3 d × 1 set (15 max)	Quadriceps	240 °/s	↓ to 30 °/s
Lesmes et al (1978)				
n = 5	7 w × 4 d × 2 or 10 sets (30 or 6 s max)	Quadriceps	180 °/s	↓ to 0 °/s ↓ to 60 °/s (contractional work)
	7 w × 4 d × 2 or 10 sets (30 or 6 s max)	Hamstring	180 °/s	120–0 °/s ↓ to 60 °/s (contractional work)
Perrin et al (1989)				
n = 7	7 w × 3 d × 3 sets (25 max)	Quadriceps + hamstring	70 °/s	No ↓ (at 180, 60 °/s)
Petersen et al (1989)				
n = 15	6 w × 3 d × (2–3) sets (20 s max)		180 °/s	↑ and ↓ (+ 60 and –30 °/s)
n = 15	6 w × 3 d × (2–3) sets (20 s max)		60 °/s	↑ to 180 °/s
Timm (1987)				
n = 30	8 w × 3 d × 1 set (to 50% fatigue)		180 °/s	↑ 120 °/s, and ↓ 120 °/s overflow (peak moment and contractional power)

* All findings refer to gains in peak moment, and using concentric contraction mode, except where indicated otherwise.

the latter may or may not be conditioned. If side-specificity prevails, no transfer of strength would be expected. This however is not the case, as has been revealed by a number of studies, relating to isometric conditioning (Enoka 1988). For instance Moritani & DeVries (1979) used the regimen: 8 w × 3 d × 2 s (10 at 67% max) to isometrically condition the elbow flexors of one extremity. Postconditioning strength increased by 36 and 25% in the conditioned and control (unconditioned) muscles. As a result of other studies, an association between conditioning intensity (predominantly isometric) and the magnitude of the cross-education has been proposed (Enoka 1988).

Isokinetic conditioning

Some indications concerning cross-education during isokinetic concentric conditioning appear in the study mentioned earlier (Esselman et al 1991). The experimental design included three subject groups, who trained the knee extensors of both limbs but with differing protocols (Table 4.3). The identical

Table 4.3 Cross-education effect due to isokinetic conditioning. (Based on Esselman et al (1991)

Group	n	Velocity (°/s)	Repetitions	% increase	P
IA	5	36	60	129	<0.05
IB	5	36	20	126	<0.05
IIC	5	36	20	58	<0.05
IID	5	108	60	50	<0.05
IIIE	5	108	60	25	NS*
IIIF	5	108	20	23	NS
Control				16	NS

* Not significant.

protocols of subgroups B and C (36 °/s, 20 repetitions) and D and E (108 °/s, 60 repetitions) enabled the analysis of cross-education.

The findings indicated that the increase in strength made by subgroup B was greater than that made by subgroup C, and those by subgroup D greater by 100% than E. It should be noted that in spite of an identical 'training dose' in both subgroups B and C as well as D and E, the contralateral leg was trained differently, namely A versus D or C versus F respectively. In spite of the fact that direct comparisons cannot be performed (e.g. subgroups A and B did not train with the same number of repetitions), this study indicates that the tendency for the opposite lower extremity to respond simi-

larly to conditioning, could be more important than the number of repetitions. In order to substantiate this speculation, modified designs which also include the effect of eccentric contractions should be applied.

PART 4
PRINCIPLES OF ISOKINETIC CONDITIONING PROGRAMS (ICPS) IN CLINICAL REHABILITATION

In spite of more than 25 years' intensive use of isokinetic dynamometry, the body of clinical knowledge, especially research-based, concerning its use in rehabilitation leaves much to be desired. Some of the reasons for this have already been discussed with regard to conditioning studies in general. On the other hand, promotional material and courses offered by manufacturers, presentations given in user group meetings and, presumably, personal experience and sound clinical common sense, assist practitioners to extend the use of isokinetic systems beyond that of pure testing.

In the area of clinical rehabilitation, the great advantage of isokinetics lies in its capacity to accommodate the moment generated by the contracting muscle/s. Furthermore, it is possible:

1. to adjust the control parameters, particularly the upper limit of the muscular moment which may safely be generated, and
2. to visually display the trace of the strength curve in real time, sometimes for feedback to the subject.

These facilities enable clinicians to ensure that certain muscle/joint load values will not be exceeded. However, to the best of the present author's knowledge, these very values and their progressive modification during the course of rehabilitation, have never been systematically investigated. This is but one of a cluster of issues that makes the therapeutic use of isokinetics, the most complicated of all topics discussed in this book. The final part of this chapter discusses some major problems associated with the therapeutic applications of isokinetics. These include:

1. isokinetics versus other performance conditioning methods

2. the objective of isokinetic conditioning programs (ICPs)
3. the timing of ICP introduction into the general rehabilitation program
4. protocol-related issues
5. selected protocols
6. delayed onset muscle soreness as a result of isokinetic conditioning programs.

ISOKINETICS VERSUS OTHER PERFORMANCE CONDITIONING METHODS

A compelling reason for employing isokinetic dynamometry in rehabilitation is its assumed superiority to other methods such as the isometric or isotonic. Only a handful of studies have tested the veracity of this assumption, and they cannot be compared with one another because of lack of consistency between studies on any variable.

Isokinetics versus weight- or self-training

Clinical evidence of the superiority of isokinetic conditioning comes from the illuminating findings of a study relating to quadriceps function by Grimby et al (1980). All the patients investigated had undergone surgery on the isolated anterior cruciate ligament (ACL), medial collateral ligament or a combination of both. During the postoperative period all were engaged in structured physical therapy programs and the athletes among them even resumed their activity.

Following a period of 14 months, on average, a comparative study of the effect of isokinetic conditioning versus weight training or self-training was undertaken. Preconditioning measurements had indicated a significant strength reduction in the quadriceps of the involved side. Histological findings had failed to indicate any significant bilateral differences.

The general regimen was similar for the weight training and isokinetic methods: 6 w × 3 d × 3 s (10 max) with the latter performed at the low velocity of 42 °/s. The self-training program was somewhat different: 3 w × 6 d (25 × 2–8 kg) + 3 w × 6 d × (50 × 2–8 kg).

The results, based on testing at 0, 30, 42 and 120 °/s are shown in Figure 4.4. A very important finding was that the isokinetic group showed a complete restoration of bilateral symmetry in strength at all velocities. Although all groups increased their quadriceps strength significantly, the highest gains were made by the isokinetic group. These gains were however significant only with respect to an isometric test. This is not very surprising since the conditioning velocity was low. The present author believes Grimby et al were correct in anticipating more significant improvement (over the other methods) had the conditioning velocity been higher. On the other hand, there was a conspicuous overflow effect, which is apparent from the relatively flat shape of the isokinetic curve.

A distinguishing feature of this study was the fact that all participants were pain-free, with a reasonable ROM and already engaged in various athletic activities. This study indicates therefore that:

1. There is a need for a more systematized follow-up of patients with knee injury.
2. Spontaneous activity including athletic training may not suffice to restore muscular function.
3. This insufficiency can be remedied very effectively using ICPs.

An epidemiological study

The most comprehensive study of this issue is epidemiological in nature and summarizes the post-surgical knee rehabilitation findings of more than 5000 patients, with a roughly equal gender division, during a period of 5 years (Timm 1988). The surgery involved a large variety of nonACL procedures. The resumption of required activities without symptom recurrence, during the 5-year postoperative period, was defined as the criterion for success. This criterion was examined with respect to four methods of rehabilitation: no exercise, home exercise, isotonic exercise and isokinetic exercise.

Those patients who used isokinetic methods had a significantly shorter rehabilitation interval, 8.9 ± 3.7 weeks, compared to isotonic-based rehabilitation, 12.3 ± 6.1 weeks or home exercise, 10.0 ± 4.5 weeks. In addition an impressive correlation with success ($r = 0.92$) was recorded for patients comprising the isokinetic group compared with the isotonic and home exercise groups (0.48, and 0.09 respectively). Although these findings cannot be interpreted with the same confidence as

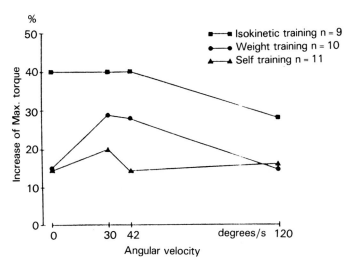

Fig. 4.4 Percentage increase in strength for knee extension for three training groups. (From Grimby et al 1980 Quadriceps function and training after knee ligament surgery. Medicine and Science in Sports Exercise 12: 70–75.)

those of a well controlled prospective study, they may indicate a 'general superiority' of isokinetics over other methods.

Effectiveness of ICPs

Consequently, in the light of the above studies it can legitimately be concluded that among the methods commonly employed for muscle strength enhancement in clinical and normal populations, ICPs are probably more effective, assuming equal resources. However, in the absence of other studies, this conclusion should currently be reserved for knee rehabilitation.

THE OBJECTIVE OF ISOKINETIC CONDITIONING

Progressive over-loading

As with other methods of strength conditioning, isokinetics operates according to the mechanism of progressive overloading of the involved muscles. Muscle tension of the magnitude that is expected to develop during even submaximal isokinetic contractions is bound to have an effect on structures other than the muscle itself, that is the bones comprising the joint, the articular surfaces, the joint capsule and the ligaments. However, the extent to which isokinetic contractions are directly responsible for better proprioception, cartilage nourishment and the repair or growth enhancement of connective tissue is unknown. It is possible to generalize

from other sources which have elucidated the important role which physical activity has in preserving the functional state of the abovementioned structures (Stone 1988). The objective of isokinetic conditioning is considered in this book to be related to the effect isokinetics has on its target organ: the skeletal muscle.

In terms of the control parameters, overloading refers to:

1. Progressively increasing the active range of motion (ROM).
2. Progressively raising the upper limit imposed on the generation of either the peak or average moment; the former parameter is the almost universal criterion.
3. Extending the range of angular velocities, concurrently with 1 and 2.
4. The incorporation of isokinetic eccentric loading.

Optimization of muscle strength

Clearly since, with respect to either concentric or eccentric exertions, the moment levels that can be generated during isokinetic contractions span the full spectrum of muscle strength, the main objective of isokinetic conditioning is to optimize muscle strength through the induction of maximal gains at all angular positions of the available joint ROM and along a predetermined spectrum of angular velocities.

It should be emphasized that:

1. Optimization rather than maximization defines the special advantage of an ICP. In theory it is possible to maximize strength gains through multiple angle isometric contractions. However, such a method demands the consumption of resources far in excess of those used in an ICP.

2. Enhancement of strength, rather than other performance parameters, is explicitly defined although the specificity of velocity studies, mentioned earlier, showed conditioning-based improvements in other performance parameters such as contractional work and power. These parameters, it should be remembered, are very closely correlated with the peak moment, the mechanical 'name' of strength. In addition, strength is the only parameter to which reference has been made in the few clinical studies of conditioning protocols.

3. The decision concerning the spectrum of velocities involved must rely on the patient's performance and functional requirements.

TIMING OF ISOKINETIC CONDITIONING

Leaving aside patient-linked factors such as compliance, the timing of the introduction of isokinetic conditioning into rehabilitation depends on two factors: the nature of the injury or dysfunction including its anatomical location, and the therapeutic approach–surgical or nonsurgical. Postoperative isokinetic conditioning is by far the more complicated and more debated topic and therefore deserves particular attention. Where conservative treatment is concerned, the incorporation of isokinetics follows the general principles of progressive resistive exercise (PRE) or its variants (see, for instance, Knight 1979), except, of course, where it is contraindicated.

Some models regarding the most suitable stage for introducing an ICP into postoperative rehabilitation have been proposed. Notably, none of the models was based on a methodical exploration of this problem and therefore should be viewed with caution; to quote Zarins et al (1985):

Not all patients are rehabilitated uniformly, and a great deal of variability exists following arthroscopic surgery. . . Therefore an arbitrary time frame for rehabilitation. . . . is not recommended. Rather, each patient should progress from one stage of rehabilitation to the next, based on objective knee findings.

Hence, time per se should not serve as a criterion for introducing an ICP.

Quadriceps endurance as criterion

Sherman et al (1983) compared two methods of rehabilitation of patients following an open procedure for removal of the medial meniscus. The criterion for introduction of isokinetic conditioning was a level of quadriceps endurance which was equivalent to 8 sets × 10 repetitions of knee extension with 20 lb, using an NK table. The authors neither explained nor discussed the choice of this particular criterion which had been equally applicable to both experimental groups: one with knee immobilization and one without. Based on the above criterion, the ICP started 2 and 4 weeks after the operation, in the former and latter group respectively.

Phase of healing

A four-phase general rehabilitation program following surgery of the knee (Table 4.4) has been

Table 4.4   Phases of postoperative knee rehabilitation: the program of Zarins et al (1985)

Phase	Description	Characteristics	Exercises
I	Immediate postoperative period	Incision, bleeding, pain, quadriceps, inhibition	Quadriceps setting, straight-leg-raising, hamstring resistance, ambulation ± external support
II	Early healing	Less pain, effusion, muscles weak, 90° of motion	Active ROM, continue isometrics, ambulate, cycle
III	Late healing	No pain, effusion ± weakness, 120° of motion	Walk, cycle, swim, functional exercise, high speed isokinetics
IV	Late rehabilitation and conditioning	Full ROM, no effusion, muscle weakness, not returned to sports	Isotonic, functional activities, running, jumping, gradual return to sports, all speeds isokinetics

proposed by Zarins et al (1985). This program was also designed specifically for the rehabilitation of patients following open or arthroscopic meniscectomy, although the authors maintained that it was appropriate for other knee arthrotomy procedures.

According to this program, isokinetic conditioning may start as soon as early healing (phase II) is over. It should be noted that 'late healing' was characterized by less pain and effusion and hence less likelihood of quadriceps inhibition (De Andrade 1965). Thus the criterion for introducing isokinetic conditioning is clinical and subjective.

Clinical exercise progression of Davies (1992)

A general approach to clinical exercise progression has been proposed by Davies (1992). The principles of patient safety and overloading are the basis of this method. The program is conducted sequentially:

Stage I   multiple-angle, submaximal isometrics
Stage II   multiple-angle, maximal isometrics
Stage III short arc, submaximal isokinetics
Stage IV   short arc isotonics
Stage V   short arc, maximal isokinetics
Stage VI   full ROM, submaximal isokinetics
Stage VII full ROM, isotonics (if not contraindicated)
Stage VIII full ROM, maximal isokinetics.

According to this model isokinetic conditioning may be introduced fairly early and the criterion for its initial introduction is a safe performance of maximal, multiple-angle isometric contractions. The introduction of submaximal isokinetic before isotonic contractions is somewhat surprising, unless the former can be maintained at load values lower than the latter. Even more notable is the obscurity of the term 'submaximal'; its quantitative significance is never spelled out, although the author maintains elsewhere that:

the minimum sub-maximal threshold to produce a training response with isokinetics is unknown at the present time. Therefore there is need for research in this area.

Another weakness of this model and of the others mentioned is the apparent omission of the eccentric model; it is not obvious whether 'isokinetics' refers to both contraction modes. The present author is not aware of any conditioning model that deals directly with this problem.

Suggested criteria for ICP introduction

To summarize, there are three general approaches to the timing of ICPs:

1. Use of predominantly clinical signs and estimation of the status of healing (Zarins et al 1985).
2. Use of a muscle performance criterion (Sherman et al 1983).
3. The sequential approach of Davies (1992).

Undoubtedly, where postoperative conditioning is concerned, the stage of tissue healing (which will reflect surgical procedure/s) is the single most important criterion for deciding whether to refrain from, or initiate, an ICP. Obviously the exertion of high loads on an as yet unhealed tissue could set the healing process back or even undermine the surgical objective. On the other hand, a progressive build-up of stress is essential for healing. Hence the optimal stage for introducing an ICP can probably be determined using a combination of the three approaches.

Assuming normal tissue recovery, patient compliance and the availability of reasonable physical therapy, introduction of submaximal isokinetic conditioning should be based on isokinetic testing. Testing of the involved versus the contralateral sound structure/s may be carried out when there is a reasonable level of healing (end of phase II as defined by Zarins et al) and after full active ROM is achieved. With these considerations in mind, the following procedures are suggested. Although based on postmeniscectomy conditioning, they may provide a convenient basis for future clinical exploration of this issue.

1. Testing should preferably be performed in a nongravity plane.

2. Uninvolved side concentric and eccentric testing should be carried out to full capacity.

3. Involved side concentric-only testing should be performed at a submaximal level and an upper moment limit be set at 30% of the contralateral peak moment; this may be judged too low but it leaves a comfortable safety margin of 70%. This criterion incorporates the design of Sherman et al (1983) which was based on a 20 lb resistance load in an endurance test. Assuming a lever of 30 cm this load is equivalent to about 30 N m. Normative values for knee extensor isokinetic strength (Freedson et al 1993) provide a basis for comparison. For example the extension moment at 180 °/s, corresponding to the 50th percentile of the male age group 31–40 was about 110 N m (120 N m and

100 N m for the 21–30, 41–50 age groups respectively). Therefore the relative exertion here is $(30/110) \times 100 = 27\%$. This figure (27%) should also be valid for women.

4. At this level of exertion the level of pain, rated according to any common and applicable pain rating system, should be recorded; discomfort or other negative signs should also be recorded.

5. A pain level expressed by a statement such as 'it is really painful' (for instance 5 on the Borg (1982) modified 0–10 pain scale) may signify that the tissues are not yet ready to negotiate such a load and hence isokinetic conditioning should be deferred to a later date; the same logic applies to other signs.

6. Upon the positive completion of the test, a short conditioning protocol consisting of a single set of 10 repetitions may be attempted in order to assess the patient's ability to sustain these exertions satisfactorily, and an ICP may then follow.

7. Eccentric isokinetic conditioning may be introduced once the concentric peak moment has reached 50% of that of the sound side. This figure is based on an eccentric/concentric strength ratio of 1.33. This is a rough average of muscle performance at medium velocities (Albert 1991).

As mentioned, this procedure is but one way to rationally introduce isokinetic conditioning. Similar programs have to be worked out individually for specific therapeutic interventions.

CONDITIONING PROTOCOLS

This section deals with a number of problems concerning optimal isokinetic conditioning within the framework of a single set. These problems concern, for instance, the choice of high versus low velocity conditioning, or the use of a velocity spectrum design as advocated by Davies (1992). The scientific rationale for choosing an optimal protocol is virtually nonexistent, a situation generally characteristic of isokinetic conditioning at large. The order of presentation of the following is not an indication of the relative importance of the problems.

Minimal initial contraction intensity for ICPs

This question may be phrased: what is the minimal magnitude of moment required to induce changes in strength? There are two approaches to this problem. One, proposed by Young et al (1985), maintains that the intensity of the neural drive, rather than the magnitude of the load, may represent the stimulus for increasing strength. The other states that the major determinant of the adaptive strength response is indeed the tension generated by the muscle. It seems, from the relevant literature, that the latter hypothesis prevails. For instance, it has been shown that at training loads below approximately 66% of the maximum, no increase in the maximal voluntary contraction (MVC) was obtained even if up to 150 contractions/day were used (McDonagh & Davies 1984). Though none of the available studies is directly relevant to isokinetics, they do provide a frame of reference.

Thus submaximal conditioning must on the one hand be limited by an upper moment value, and on the other, it must not fall below a certain minimum if change is to be induced. The present author suggests that an isokinetic endurance test, at a medium velocity, of the contralateral limb is carried out. The findings should be indicative of the desired potential of the involved muscles and/or associated structures. A reasonable initial 'performance ceiling' (nonsurgical) would then be at a level of 50% of the above maximal force. Increases in this parameter should follow the usual course of PRE (see also below). This takes into consideration the fact that the patient is already well into the rehabilitation process.

High versus low velocity conditioning

This topic has been addressed in a clinical context by Thomee et al (1987) in a study of isokinetic conditioning following reconstruction (procedure unspecified) of the ACL. The ICP was initiated, on average, after a 6-month postoperative period, during which knee casts and conventional physical therapy had been used. Two patient groups participated in the study, one trained at 60 °/s and the other at 180 °/s. Both knee extensors and flexors were trained. The conditioning regimens were: 8 w × 3 d × (3–10) sets (10 repetitions max) and 8 w × 3 d × (3–10) sets (15 repetitions max) for the slower and faster velocity group respectively. Compared with the contralateral limb, the increases in strength were from 56 to 74% and 78 to 102% for the quadriceps and hamstring respectively. However, upon testing along a velocity spectrum of 30 to 300 °/s, no significant differences were noted between the two groups, although there was a slight tendency towards velocity specificity.

Considering the ACL surgical procedure as sufficiently representative of a number of knee interventions, in terms of soft tissue damage and intensity of rehabilitation, it can be concluded that if a concentric ICP is to be based on a single velocity, then a medium velocity is preferable to a low velocity. This has three benefits:

1. A shorter exposure time to the mechanical loads imposed due to the muscle/s contraction force.
2. A smaller contraction force as illustrated by the moment–angular velocity relationship.
3. No loss of generality, because of an excellent downwards physiological overflow, which may extend isometric strength.

It should however be pointed out that if the patient finds it difficult to accelerate the distal segment forcefully enough to reach the preset velocity, adjusting the latter is necessary. Hence it may be beneficial to start at 120 °/s and observe the angular sector of the ROM required to develop isokinetic conditions. If this takes up more than one-third of the ROM, it means that the patient is virtually performing a submaximal isotonic contraction. This in turn will require the use of an even lower velocity, 60–90 °/s.

As indicated below, modern protocols involve more than one velocity yet the use of the medium/higher end of the velocity spectrum, in the context of isokinetic conditioning (rather than testing), is still the more logical one.

Rest intervals and sets

The optimal numbers of repetitions and sets, and the length of rest intervals, are of prime importance to the design of an ICP, but there are few studies relating to these topics.

Number of repetitions

The optimal number of repetitions required for improvement of knee flexor and extensor total contraction work, contractional power, and endurance ratios was investigated by Davies et al (1985a, b). The study regimen was: 6 w × 3 d × 3 sets with 5, 10, 15 or 20 repetitions at 180 °/s. With respect to total contractional work and endurance ratios, it was found that the best results were obtained using 15 or 20 repetitions for the quadriceps (although 10 repetitions also yielded significant improvements), and 10 for the hamstring. The contractional power of both muscles increased maximally following a 10-repetition protocol.

The studies suggest that with these regimens, 10 repetitions, is overall, the optimal number. Although this is a very convenient parameter, a fixed number of repetitions is not essential.

Sherman et al (1982) have proposed that the termination of an individual set should be decided by reference to a fatigue ratio, i.e. it should be ended when the peak moment of a contraction is only 50% of the initial moment. Although functionally it is a sounder parameter, technical difficulties prevent the wider use of this criterion.

Inter-set and inter-velocity spectrum intervals

Ariki et al (1985) have studied the optimal intervals for inter-set and inter-spectrum time. The inter-spectrum time refers to the time period between two identical full spectrums consisting of the velocities: 180, 210, 240, 270 and 300 °/s. The optimal inter-set and inter-spectrum time intervals were 90 s and 3 min respectively.

In his book, Davies (1992) claims correctly that a 90 s interval may be too long since a typical clinic may not have more than one isokinetic system. Therefore, unless the patient is uncomfortable or exhausted this period can be reduced to 30–60 s. On the other hand, a 3 min inter-spectrum period is appropriate.

Optimal number of sets

Determination of the optimal number of sets may be the most difficult question since this largely depends on the design of the protocol. However, a reasonable solution to this problem is to use the percentage reduction in peak moment as has already been suggested with regard to the number of intra-set repetitions. Such a solution was indeed reported in a case study (Timm & Patch 1985) with respect to a full velocity spectrum program.

A reasonable way for establishing the number of sets is to have the subject perform a trial set of 10 repetitions and compare the mean of the peak or average moment (PM or AVM) of the last three (L) with the corresponding figure for the first three (F) repetitions. In the absence of pain the suggested rule is: if $L/F > 50\%$ proceed to the next set otherwise terminate conditioning.

Once the number of sets is determined, progression to the next phase should not be problematical.

Total contraction output

A study by Lesmes et al (1978) raised an important question regarding the total contraction output needed for an effective ICP. It was indicated that a significant improvement, 5–25% in knee extensor and flexor force, could be derived from a protocol consisting of 4 minutes of conditioning per week(!). Therefore the relatively large volume prescribed for isokinetic conditioning in other methods is much in question.

Discharge from conditioning programs

Discharge from an ICP is based on achieving near or perfect bilateral parity. The 'near' approach is represented, for instance, by Tegner et al (1983), and indeed by most of the advocates of accelerated rehabilitation following ACL reconstruction (for a detailed discussion see Chapter 6). The 'perfect' approach, which has been advocated by Sherman et al (1982), may not be a realistic one, particularly with respect to ligament reconstruction surgery.

SELECTED PROTOCOLS

In theory, if not in practice, there is an infinite number of possible ICPs. Since the scientific and clinical bases of even the most commonly used ICPs have never been subjected to a rigorous comparative analysis, it is difficult to single out any particular ICP as a better, let alone the best option. As mentioned more than once, the variety of clinical situations, coupled with the individual differences among patients makes the selection of an appropriate ICP quite problematic. If in addition

the issue of eccentric conditioning is considered, this problem becomes intractable.

Principles of ICP design

The principles governing ICP design have been laid out in this Chapter. They are based on consideration of:

1. the nature of the pathology or dysfunction
2. the status of tissue healing and repair and the level of pain
3. the extent of the joint/s ROM
4. the load intensity sustained by the joint/s before initiation of the ICP
5. the correct application of the various phenomena associated with the specificity of muscle performance, particularly with regard to velocity and contraction mode
6. the correct integration of the abovementioned protocol-related issues.

The protocols shown in Table 4.5, which have been successfully applied in clinical situations, are described in order to demonstrate the use of the above. They refer to different pathologies, some nonorthopaedic. The suitability of each may be judged according to the above points.

DELAYED ONSET MUSCLE SORENESS DUE TO ISOKINETIC CONDITIONING

This problem has been dealt with at length in a number of studies (Albert 1991). It was suggested that exercises of a predominantly eccentric character were more liable to cause delayed onset muscle soreness (DOMS) than concentric exercises. This assumption has recently been investigated by Fitzgerald et al (1991) using isokinetic dynamometry. The research design was based on two experiments one in which subjects exercised at the same power level, and another in which they exercised at maximal effort level.

Findings indicated that there was no change in muscle soreness between pre- and postexercise periods with regard to the first experiment. Greater increases in muscle soreness were indicated by subjects in the second experiment. The result suggested intensity rather than contraction type was linked with soreness.

The significance of this study in this context

Table 4.5 Protocols illustrating principles of isokinetic conditioning program (ICP) design

	Sherman et al (1982)*	Bennett & Stauber (1986)	Jensen & Di Fabio (1989)	Knutsson & Martensson (1991)
Objective	Rehabilitation after knee surgery (meniscectomy)	Rehabilitation of anterior knee pain	Rehabilitation of patellar tendinitis	Rehabilitation of spastic paresis
Muscles	Knee extensors and flexors	Knee extensors	Knee extensors	Knee extensors
Termination	Full strength parity	Pain relief	Time-based	Time-based
Protocol Weeks	Until termination criterion achieved	Until pain relief (usually 2–4)	8	6
Days/week	3–4	3	3	2
Sets	2	3	Week 1–6 / Weeks 2–8: 4 at each velocity	2 at submaximal followed by 5–15 at maximal intensity
Repetitions	Until peak moment is 50% of initial	10/set	5/set	10/set
Inter-set rest	3–5 min	Patient-adjusted		
Effort intensity in contraction	Maximal	Maximal (pain-limited)	Maximal	Submaximal, maximal (see Sets)
Contraction mode	Concentric	Eccentric	Eccentric	Concentric in one, eccentric in contralateral
Velocities	Anchor: 60–120 °/s (may be implemented immediately) 180, 240, 300 °/s within 1–2 weeks	30, 60, 90 °/s	Incremental: 30–70 °/s Week 1 30 °/s 2 30, 35 °/s 3 30, 35, 40 °/s 4 30, 40, 45 °/s 5 30, 40, 50 °/s 6 30, 45, 60 °/s 7 30, 50, 65 °/s 8 30, 50, 70 °/s	30, 60, 120 180 °/s

* Program initiated following phase I healing.

cannot be overestimated. Eccentric action in itself is probably not responsible for the phenomenon of DOMS. Rather it is the intensity of eccentric contractions that overloads the muscle and contrib-

utes to the sensation of pain. Thus the setting of an upper limit for maximal eccentric effort could provide a solution.

REFERENCES

Albert M 1991 Eccentric muscle training in sports and orthopaedics. Churchill Livingstone, New York

Ariki P, Davies G J 1985 Rest interval between isokinetic velocity spectrum rehabilitation sets. Physical Therapy 65: 733–734 (abstract)

Bennett G J, Stauber W T 1986 Evaluation and treatment of anterior knee pain using eccentric exercise. Medicine and Science in Sports and Exercise 18: 526–530

Bishop K, Durrant E, Allsen P, Merrill G 1991 The effect of eccentric strength training at various speeds on concentric strength of the quadriceps and hamstring muscles. Journal of Orthopaedic and Sports Physical Therapy 13: 226–230

Borg G 1982 A category scale with ratio properties for intermodal interindividual comparisons. In: Geissler G H, Petzold P (eds) Psychophysical judgement and the process of perception. VEB Deutscher Verlag der Wissenschaften, Berlin

Caiozzo V J, Perrine J J, Edgerton V R 1981 Training-induced alterations of in vivo force–velocity relationship of human muscle. Journal of Applied Physiology 51: 750–754

Costill D L, Coyle E F, Fink W F, Lesmes G R, Witzmann A F 1979 Adaptations in skeletal muscle following strength training. Journal of Applied Physiology 46: 96–99

Cote C, Simoneau J-A, Lagasse P, Boulay M, Thibault M-C, Marcotte M, Bouchard C 1988 Isokinetic strength training protocols: do they induce skeletal muscle fiber hypertrophy? Archives of Physical Medicine and Rehabilitation 69: 281–285

Coyle E F, Feiring D C, Rotkis TC 1981 Specificity of power improvements through slow and fast isokinetic training. Journal of Applied Physiology 51: 1437–1442

Davies G J (ed) 1992 A compendium of isokinetics in clinical usage. S & S Publishers, Onalaska, Wisconsin

Davies G J, Bendle S R, Wood K L, Rowinski M J, Price S, Halbach J 1985a The optimal number of repetitions to be used with isokinetic training to increase average power. Physical Therapy 65: 794 (abstract)

Davies G J, Bendle S R, Wood K L, Rowinski M J, Price S, Rose D E 1985b The optimal number of repetitions to be used with isokinetic training to increase total work and endurance ratios. Physical Therapy 65: 794 (abstract)

De Andrade J R 1965 Joint distension and reflex muscle inhibition in the knee. Journal of Bone and Joint Surgery 47A: 313–318

De Niccio D K, Davies G J, Rowinski M J 1991 Comparison of quadriceps isokinetic eccentric and isokinetic concentric data using a standard fatigue protocol. Isokinetics and Exercise Science 1: 81–86

Duncan P, Chandler J, Cananaugh D, Johnson K, Buehler A 1989 Mode and speed specificity of eccentric and concentric exercise training. Journal of Orthopaedic and Sports Physical Therapy 11: 70–75

Enoka R M 1988 Muscle strength and its development: new perspectives. Sports Medicine 6: 146–168

Esselman P C, De Lateur B J, Alquist A D, Questad K A, Giaconi R M, Lehmann J F 1991 Torque development in isokinetic training. Archives of Physical Medicine and Rehabilitation 72: 723–728

Ewing J L, Wolfe D R, Rogers M A, Amundson M L, Alan Stull G 1990 Effects of velocity of isokinetic training on strength, power, and quadriceps muscle fiber characteristics. European Journal of Applied Physiology 61: 159–162

Fitzgerald G K, Rothstein J M, Mayhew T P, Lamb R L 1991 Exercise-induced muscle soreness after concentric and eccentric exercise. Physical Therapy 71: 505–513

Freedson P S, Gilliam T B, Mahoney T, Maiszewski A F, Kastango K 1993 Industrial torque levers by age group and gender. Isokinetics and Exercise Science 3: 34–42

Grimby G, Gustafsson E, Peterson L, Renstrom P 1980 Quadriceps function and training after knee ligament surgery. Medicine and Science in Sports and Exercise 12: 70–75

Hakkinen K, Komi P V, Tesch P A 1981 Effect of combined concentric and eccentric strength training and detraining on force–time, muscle fibre and metabolic characteristics of leg extensor muscles. Scandinavian Journal of Sports Science 3: 50–58

Jenkins W L, Thackaberry M, Killian C 1984 Speed-specific isokinetic training. Journal of Orthopaedic and Sports Physical Therapy 6: 181–183

Jensen K, Di Fabio R 1989 Evaluation of eccentric exercise in treatment of patellar tendinitis, Physical therapy 69: 211–216

Knight K L 1979 Knee rehabilitation by daily adjusted progressive resistive exercise. American Journal of Physical Medicine 7: 336–340

Knutsson E, Martensson A 1991 The effect of concentric and eccentric training in spastic paresis. In: Eriksson E, Grimby G, Knutsson E, Thorstensson A (eds) Dynamic dynamometry in research and clinical work, Karolinska Institute, Stockholm, Sweden

Komi P V 1986 Training of muscle strength and power: interactions of neuromotoric, hypertrophic and mechanical factors. International Journal of Sports Medicine 7 (suppl): 10–15

Komi P V, Burskirk E R 1972 Effect of eccentric and concentric muscle conditioning on tension and electrical activity of human muscle. 15: 417–434

Lesmes G R, Costill D L, Coyle E F, Fink W J 1978 Muscle strength and power changes during maximal isokinetic training. Medicine and Science in Sports and Exercise 10: 266–269

Luthi J M, Howald H, Classen H, Rosler K, Vock P 1986 Structural changes in skeletal muscle tissue with heavy-resistance exercise. International Journal of Sports Medicine 7: 123–127

Lyndberg K, Danneskiold-Samsoe B, Ramsing B U, Nawrocki A, Harreby M 1991 Isokinetic knee extension training in rheumatoid arthritis. In: Eriksson E, Grimby G, Knutsson E, Thorstensson A (eds) Dynamic dynamometry in research and clinical work, Karolinska Institute, Stockholm, Sweden

Mannion A Q F, Jakeman P M, Willan P 1992 Effects of isokinetic training of the knee extensors on isometric strength and peak power output during cycling. European Journal of Applied Physiology 65: 370–375

McDonagh M J, Davies C T 1984 Adaptive response of

mammalian skeletal muscle to exercise with high loads. European Journal of Applied Physiology 52: 139–155

Milner-Brown H S, Stein R B, Lee R G 1974 The contractile and electrical properties of human motor units in neuropathies and motor neurone disease. Journal of Neurology and Neuropsychiatry 37: 670–676

Moritani T, De Vries H A 1979 Neural factors versus hypertrophy in the time course of muscle strength gain. American Journal of Physical Medicine 58: 115–130

Nicely K, Schultz C, Porter S, Allen F, Hanten W 1988 Effects of training using isokinetic–concentric, isokinetic–eccentric and isometric contractions on the peak torque of the knee extensors. Physical Therapy 68: 799

Perrin D, Lephart S, Weltman A 1989 Specificity of training on computer obtained isokinetic measures. Journal of Orthopaedic and Sports Physical Therapy 12: 495–498

Petersen S, Bagnall K, Wegner A, Reid D, Castor W, Quinney H 1989 The influence of velocity-specific resistance training on the in vivo torque–velocity relationship and the cross-sectional area of the quadriceps femoris. Journal of Orthopaedic and Sports Physical Therapy 12: 456–462

Petersen S, Wessel J, Bagnall K, Wilkins H, Quinney A, Wegner H 1990 Influence of concentric resistance training on concentric and eccentric strength. Archives of Physical Medicine and Rehabilitation 71: 101–105

Petersen S, Bell G, Bagnall K, Quinney A 1991 The effects of concentric resistance training on eccentric peak torque and muscle cross-sectional area. Journal of Orthopaedic and Sports Physical Therapy 13: 132–137

Sale D G 1988 Neural adaptation to resistance training. Medicine and Science in Sports and Exercise 20: S135–S145

Shelbourne K D, Nitz P 1990 Accelerated rehabilitation after anterior cruciate ligament reconstruction. American Journal of Sports Medicine 18: 292–299

Sherman W M, Pearson D R, Plyley M J, Costill D L, Habansky A J, Vogelgesang D A 1982 Isokinetic rehabilitation after surgery. American Journal of Sports Medicine 10: 155–161

Sherman W M, Pearson D R, Plyley M J, Habansky A J, Vogelgesang D A, Costill D L 1983 Isokinetic rehabilitation after meniscectomy: a comparison of two methods of training. The Physician and Sports Medicine 11: 121–133

Stauber W T (1989) Eccentric action of muscles: physiology, injury and adaptation. Exercise and Sports Science Review 19: 157–185

Stone M H 1988 Implications for connective tissue and bone alterations resulting from resistance exercise training. Medicine and Science in Sports and Exercise 20: S162–S168

Tegner Y, Lysholm J, Lysholm M, Gillquist J 1993 Strengthening exercises for old cruciate ligament tears. Acta Orthopaedica Scandinavica 57: 130–134

Tesch P A 1988 Skeletal muscle adaptations consequent to long-term heavy resistance exercise. Medicine and Science in Sports and Exercise 20: S132–S134

Thomee R, Renstrom P, Grimby G, Peterson L 1987 Slow or fast isokinetic training after knee ligament surgery. Journal of Orthopaedic and Sports Physical Therapy 8: 475–479

Timm K E 1987 Investigation of the physiological overflow effect from speed-specific isokinetic activity. Journal of Orthopaedic and Sports Physical Therapy 9: 106–110

Timm K E 1988 Postsurgical knee rehabilitation: a five year study of four methods and 5381 patients. American Journal of Sports Medicine 16: 463–468

Timm K E, Patch D G 1985 Case study: use of the Cybex II velocity spectrum in the rehabilitation of postsurgical knees. Journal of Orthopaedic and Sports Physical Therapy 6: 347–349

Tomberlin J P, Basford J R, Schwen E E, Orte P A, Scott S G, Laughman R K, Ilstrup D 1991 Comparative study of isokinetic eccentric and concentric quadriceps training. Journal of Orthopaedic and Sports Physical Therapy 14: 31–36

Wilk K E, Andrews J R 1992 Current concepts in the treatment of anterior cruciate ligament disruption. Journal of Orthopaedic and Sports Physical Therapy 15: 279–293

Young K, McDonagh M J, Davies C T M 1985 The effects of two forms of isometric training on the mechanical properties of the triceps surae in man. Pflugers Archives 405: 384–388

Zarins B, Boyle J, Harris B A 1985 Knee rehabilitation following arthroscopic meniscectomy. Clinical Orthopaedics and Related Research 198: 36–42

Isokinetics of the hip muscles

In the field of isokinetic research, the hip is probably the most neglected among the major joint systems, after the elbow. A search of the literature yields only a handful of papers relating to testing procedures and representative values, and offering little of clinical significance. Considering the important role of hip muscles in locomotion and posture this poverty is rather surprising. Moreover, the suggested contribution of the hip extension mechanism to the initial phase of lifting (see Chapter 8) could have been expected to stimulate considerable research into the relationship between hip and trunk extension functions.

This short chapter, therefore, mostly concerns procedures. As will be shown, these are far from definitive, and this may be a reason for the tardy development of a comprehensive database for hip muscle performance under isokinetic conditions.

PART 1
ISOKINETIC TESTING OF HIP JOINT MUSCLES

The hip joint affords lower limb movement about three independent axes, resulting in sagittal, frontal and axial motions. Isokinetic measurement of the performance of the muscles involved in executing these motions must take into account:

1. the tested range of motion (ROM)
2. positioning and stabilization
3. alignment of the biological and mechanical axes
4. positioning of the force pad
5. the test angular velocities.

The significance of these elements is discussed in the context of the three types of motion.

SAGITTAL PLANE MOTION

Range of motion

Movement in the sagittal plane is normally described in terms of flexion and extension. There are considerable discrepancies concerning norms for hip joint ROM in all planes. For instance whereas in one study the norm for extension was 10° (Boone & Azen 1979) in another it was 50° (Dorinson & Wagner 1948).

In one of the first instrumented analyses of hip muscle strength, Jensen et al (1971) indicated that, from multiple-point isometric measurements, the peak of the force vs. angular position curve was located at an angle of about 30° of flexion, for flexion and extension alike. The curve was approximately symmetrical for extension, with the recorded forces diminishing very rapidly towards the initial (dependent lower limb) and final position (at about 80°). In flexion there was a comparable reduction in force towards the initial position but a much milder decline up to 90° of flexion.

In the most comprehensive study of hip musculature available to date (Cahalan et al 1989) the authors suggested that 45° should be a standard angle for isometric testing in the upright position. Consequently for strength measurements the recommended tested ROM in the upright position (see below) is 60–75° from the neutral (dependent) lower limb position.

The upright position

Sagittal, and also frontal motion testing, should be performed with the subject in the upright position, for two reasons:

1. Most of the functional activities involving the hip, like walking, running and stair climbing, are performed while the body is in the upright position. It also means that the activation patterns of the muscles which take part in these movements will basically be maintained during the test.

2. The gravitational factor in any other position, particularly supine, is quite considerable, and it is likely that some subjects will find it difficult or even impossible to generate sufficient moment to lift the lower limb.

Stabilization

Stabilization in the upright position requires a special attachment, whose potential bulk may be the reasons why the nonphysiological supine or sidelying testing positions are recommended by a few manufacturers of isokinetic systems. Failure to properly stabilize the subject in the upright position is likely to result in poor reproducibility.

Cahalan et al (1989) designed a fixed special attachment for a Cybex II dynamometer, which allowed stabilization of the upper limbs and pelvis. Figures 5.1 and 5.2 show positioning for hip flexors and extensors testing respectively. The subject stands on a special platform designed by the author (not shown) which is compatible with the specific dynamometer in use. To prevent substitution the subject is strapped at various levels, including the contralateral shank and thigh as well as the upper pelvis.

Knee position, particularly when full extension is maintained throughout the test, is important for two reaons:

1. The resulting gravitational moment of the shank is higher than in testing where flexion is allowed.
2. Rectus femoris contraction, because of the combined hip flexion–knee extension, may

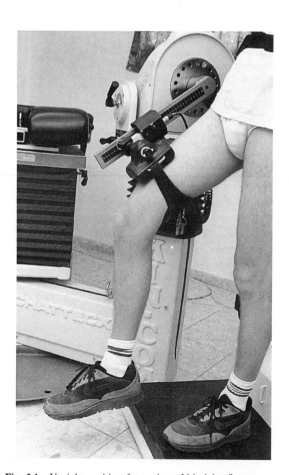

Fig. 5.1 Upright position for testing of hip joint flexors.

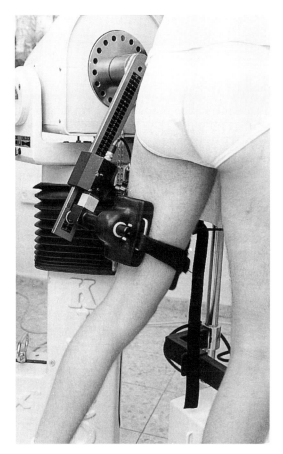

Fig. 5.2 Upright position for testing of hip joint extensors.

result in variations in the strength curve of either the flexors or extensors.

Therefore it is suggested that when hip sagittal motion is tested the knee should be allowed to flex passively, i.e. as a result of gravity.

Axes alignment and force pad position

Alignment of the biological and mechanical axes is achieved by placing the axis of the actuator against the greater trochanter which serves as the anatomical marker for the hip joint axis.

The resistance pad should be placed slightly above the superior pole of the patella.

Angular velocities

There is a lack of information regarding the most appropriate angular velocities for hip muscle testing, although the work of Cahalan et al (1989) is an

important reference. There is a temptation to use velocities derived from walking or running but these are, par excellence, activities where conditions are not isokinetic.

As patients may find that lifting the lower limb through a ROM of 60–75° involves considerable effort, concentric testing may be more comfortably performed at slow velocities. Indeed two studies which concentrated on hip flexion and extension strength chose to stay at this end of the spectrum. Burnett et al (1990) used 30 and 90 °/s as their test velocities (supine position) and found that the strength of extensors, flexors, abductors and adductors was similar at both velocities. Tis et al (1991) used 20 °/s as the test velocity (upright position) but did not compare it with other velocities.

On the other hand, Cahalan et al (1989) studied a spectrum of velocities consisting of 30, 90, 150 and 210 °/s. The latter authors indicated that the moment curves at the two higher velocities were characterized by overshoot inconsistencies, and hence recommended testing only at 30 and 90 °/s.

The use of 60 °/s as a single test velocity, or 30 and 90 °/s as more comprehensive performance indicators is therefore recommended.

FRONTAL PLANE MOTION

ROM in the frontal plane

Movement in this plane is described in terms of abduction and adduction. The accepted ROM for abduction is 45°, whereas for adduction there is a very wide variation among different sources; however 25° may be considered a representative ROM (Miller 1985). The tested ROM may be much smaller, depending on both the position of peak moment (Donatelli et al 1991) and the functional demands. In the case of side-lying testing there is also a mechanical block, which prevents an adduction angle of more than 5° in the contralateral direction.

Upright position in frontal plane testing

Although testing in the supine or side-lying positions has been reported, the upright position is preferred for frontal plane testing, as with the sagittal plane, and for the same reasons. Figure 5.3 shows upright positioning during abduction/adduction testing.

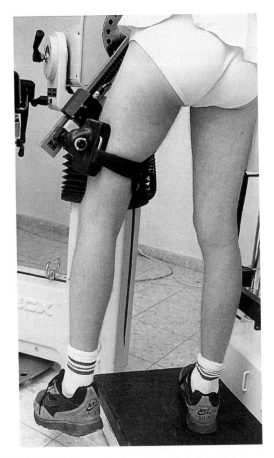

Fig. 5.3   Upright position for testing of hip joint abductors.

Test ROM   The test ROM of abduction in this position is 0–30°.

Positioning and stabilization   Stabilization is centered on the contralateral hip region since there is a conspicuous tendency particularly during abduction to laterally flex the trunk towards the tested side. This tendency, which results from movement of the iliac crest towards the femur because of gluteus medius activity, causes a protrusion of the greater trochanter of the contralateral side, which detrimentally affects the length–tension relationship of this muscle. The opposite applies to adduction testing where the pelvis tends to move towards the tested side. The knee joint should be kept passively at full extension as only negligible motion is afforded in the frontal plane.

Alignment of axes   This is performed by placing the actuator axis opposite the hip joint at a coronal level about 1 cm medial to the anterior superior iliac spine

The resistance pad   This should be placed on the lateral side of the thigh at the same level as that for sagittal testing.

Side-lying position

Though the supine position has been employed in one study (Olson et al 1972) its applicability seems limited. However, testing in the side-lying position, as reported by Burnett et al (1990) and Donatelli et al (1991), is more popular.

Positioning and stabilization   The single most important advantage of this position is the stabilization provided by the plinth, although strapping of the waist, pelvis and the untested lower limb is necessary (Fig. 5.4).

Resistance pad position and alignment of axes   These are similar to those of upright testing. Prevention of discomfort, or even slight improvement in moment generation, may be accomplished using a dual, thigh–shank pad as described in Donatelli et al (1991).

Angular velocites in the frontal plane

Those employed in frontal plane testing have ranged from 30 to 210 °/s (Cahalan et al 1989) but in two other papers velocities of 30, 60 and 90 °/s (Burnett et al 1990, Donatelli et al 1991) were regarded as adequate. In view of the very limited functional ROM it is suggested that one velocity, i.e. 30 °/s, may suffice for demonstrating frontal strength values.

AXIAL MOTION TESTING

Range of motion

Internal and external rotation of the hip joint are considered by most sources to span equal ROMs of 45° (Miller 1985). However, isokinetic testing of the muscles responsible for these movements can reliably reflect their major performance parameters using a much shorter arc. Although this arc has not been explicitly defined, it does seem that a ROM of 30°, from 5° of internal rotation to 25° of external rotation, is sufficiently comprehensive.

Positioning and stabilization

The most reliable source concerning positioning in axial motion testing of the hip is a study by Lindsay

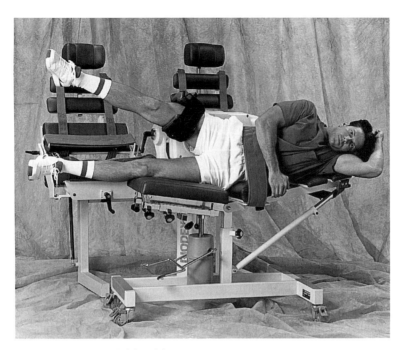

Fig. 5.4 Side-lying position for testing the hip joint abductors.

et al (1992). This reported the comparison of three distinct positions: seated with the knee flexed at 90°; supine with knee flexed to 90°, and supine with knee extended. In all three positions stabilization was provided by straps around the distal thigh, across the pelvic crests and across the chest.

Findings indicated that the seated position was associated with the highest internal and external rotation strength scores, followed by the abovementioned second and third positions respectively. Figure 5.5 depicts the seated position and stabilization as recommended in this paper.

Alignment of axes and resistance pad positioning

Alignment of axes was carried out with reference to the long axis of the femur in the study of Lindsay et al. The resistance pad was placed immediately above the lateral malleolus.

Angular velocities

The test velocity which was used by Lindsay et al was 60 °/s, whereas Cahalan et al (1989) have reported their axial strength findings using a spectrum of velocities.

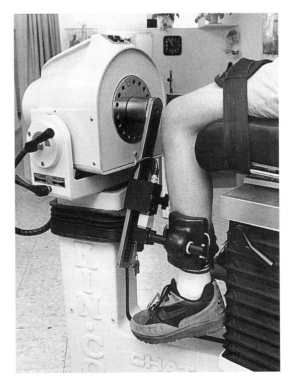

Fig. 5.5 Seated position for testing of hip joint rotators.

The recommended testing velocity is either 30 or 60 °/s depending on the degree of compliance of the patient.

TESTING OF ECCENTRIC MODE

It should be noted that though most of the sources quoted in this section refer to concentric testing, the eccentric activity of hip muscles is conspicuous, notably in the walking cycle. Hence if an active dynamometer is available testing in eccentric mode is essential.

PART 2
REPRODUCIBILITY OF HIP PERFORMANCE

The dearth of information regarding hip muscles is reflected in reproducibility studies. Furthermore, no single study has incorporated all movements of the hip joint; such a study is obviously very much needed.

Studies of normal subjects

Two studies have dealt with reproducibility of normal subjects. Burnett et al (1990) tested the strength of the flexors, extensors, abductors and adductors in a group of children 6–10 years old. There were two testing sessions, one week apart, using the velocities of 30 and 90 °/s. Testing was conducted in supine and side-lying positions for sagittal and frontal movements respectively. Intraclass correlation coefficients (ICCs) were employed to determine reproducibility, which was found to be acceptable (ICC = 0.84) only for the extensors at 90 °/s. The corresponding ICCs for the other muscle groups were consistently lower, particularly in the case of abductors and adductors, where the range was 0.49–0.59. Some procedural factors, such as a definite lack of similarity between the conditions for testing and retesting, were mentioned as potential sources for the low reproducibility.

The major implication of this study is that, at present, there is no evidence for the reproducibility of test findings relating to the flexors, extensors, abductors and adductors of the hip joint in children. Consequently, follow-up measurements of muscle

performance status in specific pathologies, such as Duchenne muscular dystrophy, cannot be relied upon.

In a study of the axial rotator muscles (Lindsay et al 1992) it was indicated that intra-session reproducibility was very good, exceeding 0.90 at each of the three positions employed, and for both internal and external rotation. However, as pointed out in Chapter 4, intra-session reproducibility does not provide a sufficiently strong basis for predicting inter-session variation. Thus these findings do not establish reproducibility of rotator performance in the wider sense. On the other hand, the acceptable intra-session reproducibility of this particular group of muscles, allows interpretation relating to the effort factor, i.e. to what extent the subject cooperates in the examination.

Study of arthritic individuals and controls

In a study of knee flexors and extensors and hip flexors in control and arthritic individuals (Giles et al 1990) it was found that the inter-session reproducibility of the hip measurements, as expressed by the coefficient of variation, was greater than that of the knee. In this instance, hip flexors were tested in the supine position without the incorporation of a gravity correction. The authors have suggested that change may be inferred if there is a variation beyond the very wide margin of 20%. The present author suggests that this study does not help to determine the reproducibility of hip muscle performance in isokinetic dynamometry.

Conclusion

From the studies mentioned above, it will be seen that unless new evidence proves otherwise, it would be wrong to make any clinical inferences based on isokinetic testing of the hip muscles. The only exception is when a single examination reveals bilateral differences of at least 30%.

PART 3
REPRESENTATIVE VALUES FOR HIP STRENGTH

The database relating to hip muscles is particularly poor. For instance, the largest uniform sample consisted of 42 male subjects (Donatelli et al 1991), and other studies have based their findings on between 15 and 30 subjects. On the other hand, a growing awareness regarding the adoption of strict protocols of testing has been demonstrated in recent years. This is reflected in very acceptable reproducibility scores for groups of subjects (Lindsay et al 1992), which means that findings based even on small samples may sometimes serve as excellent guidelines. Attention should however be given to the type of dynamometer used to collect the test information.

The following tables outline strength values, means and standard deviations, of the six principal movemnets of the hip joint.

Flexion and extension

Table 5.1 refers to flexion and extension and is solely based on findings obtained by Cahalan et al (1989).

Unfortunately further flexion and extension findings by Tis et al (1991) were expressed in force (N) rather than moment (N m) units and hence cannot be compared with those of Cahalan et al. However, two findings of Tis et al are worth mentioning:

1. The mean force in extension was only slightly higher than that in flexion. The discrepancy between this finding and the significant variations found by Cahalan et al probably resulted from different stabilization used by Tis et al.

2. The eccentric/concentric ratios, which are unit-independent, were 1.13 and 1.19 for hip extension and flexion respectively.

Table 5.1 Hip flexor and extensor concentric strength*, based on Cahalan et al (1989)

Motion and angular velocity	Women		Men	
	20–40 years	40–81 years	20–40 years	40–81 years
Flexion				
30 °/s	91(24)	67(21)	152(50)	113(21)
90 °/s	70(26)	46(17)	126(50)	84(21)
Extension				
30 °/s	110(37)	101(27)	177(42)	157(22)
90 °/s	97(41)	70(26)	163(49)	132(32)

* mean (SD), in N m.

Abduction and adduction

Table 5.2 incorporates findings obtained by Cahalan et al (1989) and Donatelli et al (1991), regarding abduction and adduction. The significant variations noted between these two sources arise from the use of different positions and stabilization, and different measurement systems, Cybex and Merac respectively.

Table 5.2 Hip adductor and abductor concentric strength*, based on Cahalan et al (1989) and Donatelli et al (1991)

Motion and angular velocity	Women			Men		
	20–40 years	21–32 years[†]	40–81 years	20–40 years	21–32 years[†]	40–81 years
Adduction						
30 °/s	82(26)		63(17)	121(26)		99(18)
60 °/s		146(28)			207(63)	
90 °/s	62(32)		44(19)	103(32)		83(28)
Abduction						
30 °/s	66(19)		48(14)	103(26)		75(18)
60 °/s		58(9)			86(20)	
90 °/s	54(20)		38(13)	79(20)		63(19)

* Mean (SD), in N m
[†] Based on Donatelli et al (1991)

Internal and external rotation

Table 5.3 shows findings by Cahalan et al (1989) and Lindsay et al (1992) for internal and external rotators. In this case also, there are significant variations which may be explained by different stabilization methods as well as the differing

Table 5.3 Hip internal and external rotator concentric strength* based on Cahalan et al (1989) and Lindsay et al (1992)

Motion and angular velocity	Women			Men		
	18–30 years[†]	20–40 years	40–81 years	18–30 years[†]	20–40 years	40–81 years
Internal rotation						
30 °/s		47(13)	34(9)		72(17)	61(21)
60 °/s	87(16)			139(21)		
90 °/s		36(14)	22(7)		53(19)	41(16)
External rotation						
30 °/s		43(13)	32(11)		65(24)	50(15)
60 °/s**	53(10)			84(16)		
90 °/s		31(12)	21(8)		49(24)	38(12)

* Mean (SD), in N m.
[†] Based on Lindsay et al (1992).

measurement systems, Cybex II and Cybex 340 respectively.

Strength ratios

The reciprocal strength ratios for frontal and axial movements are shown in Table 5.4.

Table 5.4 Reciprocal strength ratios: frontal and axial motions

	Women	Men
Adduction/abduction		
Donatelli et al (1991)	2.46	2.09
Lindsay et al (1992)	1.64	1.65
Internal/external rotation		
Cahalan et al (1989)		
30 °/s	1.08	1.11
90 °/s	1.16	1.09

PART 4
INTERPRETATION OF HIP ISOKINETICS

BILATERAL COMPARISONS

The integrity of function of the muscles moving the involved hip joint may be judged primarily against the performance of their contralateral counterparts. This assumes that performance, which hitherto was confined to strength measurements (i.e. no parameters other than strength, such as contractional work or power, was calculated), is generally equal on both sides. Surprisingly, there is only incidental reference to this issue, apart from in the study by Lindsay et al (1992), where axial rotations were compared. In the seated position with the knee flexed at 90°, the bilateral difference in both internal and external rotation was less than 1%. In the other two positions (supine with knee flexed to 90°, and supine with knee extended) the bilateral difference was less than 3%. One may reasonably assume that with proper positioning and stabilization, these figures apply for other hip muscle groups, though it should be clear that this is not completely certain.

Clinical findings

In an early study (Nicholas et al 1976), thigh muscle weakness was studied in relation to various unilateral pathological states of the lower extremity, including disorders of the knee (patellofemoral, intraarticular, ligamentous and arthritic); ankle and foot (chronic sprains and anatomical abnormalities), and the back. The strength of hip flexors, abductors and adductors, and knee flexors and extensors was assessed bilaterally.

It was found that significant weakness in abduction and adduction was associated with ankle and foot disorders. Significant weakness of the hip flexors was associated with patellofemoral disorders. The latter finding could be attributed to a possible inhibition of the rectus femoris which operates simultaneously in the movements of hip flexion and knee extension.

Total leg strength

In additon to investigation of single muscle groups, the total leg strength, which is the composite score of the individual strength of knee extensors and flexors and hip flexors, adductors and abductors, was compared between the affected and unaffected sides. It was indicated that in all those lower limb pathology groups which consisted of a sufficiently large sample, there was a highly significant total leg strength deficiency in the affected side. Table 5.5 outline the results of this analysis.

Table 5.5 Total leg strength scores (N m) in various pathologies (Nicholas et al 1976)

Pathology	n	Mean total leg strength (N m) Affected side	Unaffected side	Deficit
Ankle and foot disorders	14	431	576	26*
Back	19	462	515	10*
Ligamentous instability	23	518	602	14*
Intraarticular defects	14	496	557	11*
Patellofemoral disorders	16	462	523	12*
Arthritis	5	405	492	18

$\star$ $p < 0.01$

Further findings

In an extension of the study of Nicholas et al (Gleim et al 1978) it was indicated that there was a definite deficit in muscle strength, which amounted to more than 5%, when the affected and unaffected sides were compared in the above disorders. However these deficiencies were not limited to the affected side. Often a weakness associated with a single muscle group also appeared in the contralateral side. However in most subjects, the total leg strength was deficient in the affected side. It was also observed that large standard deviations were characteristic of single muscle groups, whereas for the total leg strength they were much smaller. The authors suggested that, in view of these findings, 5 and 10% could be considered a significant deficit in total leg strength and single muscle groups respectively. Given the lack of evidence concerning the reproducibility of hip muscle testing, this conclusion must be reevaluated.

TESTING OF OTHER MUSCLE GROUPS

If hip muscle testing is indicated, there is a good reason to proceed with knee and, perhaps, even ankle testing. The global or total leg strength may reveal whether the deficiency is confined to the hip or whether it affects other areas as well. Conversely, particularly where the ankle complex is concerned, frontal plane hip testing may be justified.

THE STRENGTH ORDER OF HIP MUSCLES

Consideration of the strength order of hip muscles is likely to assist in interpreting findings. As highlighted by Cahalan et al (1989) the order, from the strongest to the weakest, is: extensors, flexors, adductors, abductors, internal rotators and external rotators. This order was strictly preserved throughout the spectrum of test velocities used in this study.

Therefore, a relative 'within-side' deficiency may be brought to light upon testing the entire musculature of the hip joint. Such testing is not difficult to apply in the upright position and using the stabilizing frames mentioned earlier. Hence, testing at the initial phase (preoperative, or at the beginning of treatment, or for general assessment) and the final phase should include the three principle planes of the hip.

REFERENCES

Boone D C, Azen S P 1979 Normal range of motion in male subjects. Journal of Bone and Joint Surgery 61A: 756–759

Burnett C N, Filusch Betts E, King W M 1990 Reliability of isokinetic measurements of hip muscle torque in young boys. Physical Therapy 70: 244–249

Cahalan T D, Johnson M E, Liu S, Chao E Y S 1989 Quantitative measurements of hip strength in different age groups. Clinical Orthopaedics and Related Research 246: 136–145

Donatelli R, Catlin P A, Backer G S, Drane D L, Slater S M 1991 Isokinetic hip abductor to adductor torque ratio in normals. Isokinetics and Exercise Science 1: 103–111

Dorinson S M, Wagner M L 1948 An exact technique for clinically measuring and recording joint motion. Archives of Physical Medicine 29: 468–470

Giles B, Henke P, Edmonds J, McNeil D 1990 Reproducibility of isokinetic strength measurements in normal and arthritic individuals. Scandinavian Journal of Rehabilitation Medicine 22: 93–99

Gleim G W, Nicholas J A, Webb J N 1978 Isokinetic evaluation following leg injuries. Physician and Sports Medicine 6: 74–82

Jensen R H, Smidt G L, Johnston R C 1971 A technique for obtaining measurements of force generated by the hip muscles. Archives of Physical Medicine and Rehabilitation 52: 207–215

Lindsay D M, Maitland M E, Lowe R C, Kane T J 1992 Comparison of isokinetic internal and external rotation torque using different testing positions. Journal of Orthopaedic and Sports Physical Therapy 16: 43–50

Miller P J 1985 Assessment of joint motion. In J M Rothstein (ed) Measurement in physical therapy, Churchill Livingstone, Edinburgh

Nicholas J A, Strizak A M Veras G 1976 A study of thigh muscle weakness in different pathological states of the lower extremity. American Journal of Sports Medicine 4: 241–248

Olson V L, Smidt G L, Johnston R C 1972 The maximum torque generated by the eccentric isometric and concentric contractions of the hip abductor muscles. Physical Therapy 52: 149–158

Tis L L, Perrin D H, Snead D B, Weltman A 1991 Isokinetic strength of the trunk and hip in female runners. Isokinetics and Exercise Science 1: 21–24

CHAPTER 6 Isokinetics of the knee muscles

It may safely be claimed that, at one time, more than 75% of all papers which dealt with any aspect of isokinetics – theory, methodology or clinical applications – were based on a single joint system: the knee. In fact, during the early period of research in isokinetics and until the late 1970s, the relevant medical and physiological literature was strictly knee-related. This trend is still evident, although the knee no longer enjoys the same degree of exclusivity. Rather, research on knee isokinetics has come of age, in the sense that an increasing number of papers deal with the clinical aspects of this technology. This, among other things, is a reflection of the significant progress made in recent years in knee surgery and rehabilitation, conservative or postoperative. In addition, the basic design of isokinetic dynamometers (except for special purpose trunk units) has not changed since the original Cybex instrument became available in the late 1960s. This design is still better suited for knee testing and rehabilitation than it is for other joints.

Clearly, much of the voluminous literature on the knee, is not directly relevant to this chapter. For instance, a large number of papers describe parameters of knee muscle performance in relation to general methodological problems such as reproducibility. Others relate to the athletic rather than the clinical setting. The main objective of this chapter is the description and critical analysis of topics of clinical relevance to knee isokinetics. However procedural issues and normative values are first discussed.

The issue of reproducibility has been covered in detail in Chapter 4.

PART 1
ISOKINETIC TESTING PROCEDURES FOR THE KNEE

As with the trunk and the shoulder, testing of the knee involves particular consideration of:

1. the alignment of the biological and mechanical axes
2. positioning and stabilization
3. position of the resistance pad, and
4. test angular velocities.

ALIGNMENT OF THE BIOLOGICAL AND MECHANICAL AXES

The knee has two major articulations, the tibiofemoral and the patellofemoral. However, since patellar motion per se is irrelevant in the context of isokinetic testing, tibiofemoral alignment only is discussed. For testing in the usual, sitting, position, assuming minimal femoral motion because of distal stabilization of the thigh, a convenient alignment axis extends through the lateral femoral epicondyle. However the center of rotation for sagittal tibial motion is not fixed on this axis. In fact it has been shown that for sagittal tibial motion, in a normal tibiofemoral joint, the center of rotation itself moves in the shape of an arc (Smidt 1973). This means that the length d_e (see Fig. 1.2) between the resistance pad and the center of rotation in the joint changes during the movement (Nisell 1985). The strength (maximal moment) of the quadriceps or the hamstrings can be obtained from the data, using the relationship, maximal moment = force registered × lever-arm length. However, calculation of the actual force developed requires an additional set of length parameters derivable from radiological analysis of the joint. This issue is even more significant when interpreting knee muscle forces in patients afflicted with unstable knees.

Alignment in the leg press test

For multijoint lower limb testing, as exemplified by the leg press test, the greater trochanter is used as a convenient marker for alignment. Though the quadriceps is a major contributor in this activity, its exact share in developing the force recorded by the dynamometer cannot, at the moment, be obtained from any of the available isokinetic dynamometers.

POSITIONING AND STABILIZATION

Three positions may be used for testing the knee joint: the seated (Fig. 6.1), the supine and the prone. The first position is by far the most common.

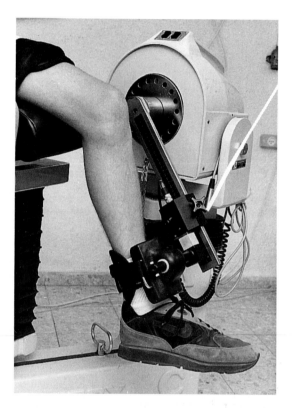

Fig. 6.1 Seated position for knee testing, particularly for quadriceps performance.

The seated position

The subject sits with her/his back slightly reclined, and the thighs well supported by the seat. In this position, the knee is tested along a ROM which extends from 75–90° of flexion, towards maximal allowable extension.

The angle of recline

It has been indicated that the angle of recline has a differential effect on the strength of the quadriceps and the hamstring (Bohannon et al 1986). While quadriceps strength was not significantly different between the upright and semireclined positions, hamstring scores were significantly higher in the upright position. Thus upright sitting (back at approximately 80°) is probably the optimal position for testing both the extensors and flexors, at least in terms of testing time.

Stabilization in the seated position

Though stabilization in the seated position is normally accomplished using femoral and pelvic strapping, the optimal set-up is probably more involved and has been the subject of a number of papers. Hart et al (1984) have shown that adding thoracic strapping improved quadriceps strength significantly.

Magnusson et al (1992) explored the effect of four stabilization methods on knee flexion and extension strength. Stabilization of the back and hands was compared with stabilization of the back, the hands and no stabilization. Findings revealed a significant effect of method: back and hands stabilization and no stabilization were associated with the highest and lowest scores respectively.

On the other hand, Hanten & Ramberg (1988) failed to find such differences while applying 'maximal' and 'minimal' stabilization. 'Maximal' stabilization consisted of thoracic, pelvic and femoral straps. In 'minimal' stabilization subjects were instructed only to grip the sides of the testing table. These authors concluded that with gripping, the subject's weight and backrest support were sufficient to ensure scores similar to those obtained in maximal stabilzation.

The gripping of the table is therefore an important factor, and this had already been highlighted with respect to isometric testing (Currier 1977). Its effect is mainly explained by the counterforce that the handles exert against the forearm. Ultimately, this force works to stabilize the thorax. However, since gripping cannot be applied to all subjects with the same efficiency (Bohannon et al 1986) most isokinetic dynamometers do not offer this option. Therefore stabilization in sitting is normally confined to the pelvic and thigh segments.

The supine position

In the supine position stabilization should be provided at the pelvic level using straps. The contralateral (untested) knee should be maintained in the flexed position in order to reduce somewhat the stresses on the lumbar spine.

The prone position

In the prone position the subject is also stabilized with straps at the pelvic level. There is the added benefit that the table's surface helps prevent excessive thigh movement.

The prone position is particularly suitable for hamstring testing. A comparison between the supine and prone position (Barr & Duncan 1988) demonstrated that if gravity correction was performed, the moments generated by the hamstring in the prone position were significantly higher than in the supine position. In the study of Worrell et al (1990), hamstring strength was significantly higher in the prone, as compared to the sitting position. These authors suggested that the beneficial effect of the prone position could be attributed to a neurophysiological mechanism: the tonic labyrinthine reflex. This reflex is believed to increase flexor tone in both the iliopsoas and the hamstring, thus significantly amplifying the moment about the hip and knee.

In another study Worrell et al (1989) tested the hamstring and quadriceps in the seated and supine positions. Although the seated position yielded higher moments for both muscle groups, the authors suggested that the supine position should be used for testing. This was because, in the many athletic activities which involve running, the position of the hip is closer to that tested in the supine position rather than the seated. However, as one of the main objectives of isokinetic testing is to expose the maximal potential of a given muscle, the above proposal might not be followed.

The present author recommends that the hamstring is preferably tested in the prone position, or alternatively, in the less demanding seated position.

POSITION OF THE RESISTANCE PAD

In the testing of normal subjects, the resistance pad is normally placed at a level immediately superior to the medial malleolus. In a study of the optimal placement of the pad, more than 70% of the subjects, women and men, preferred this position most while the rest reported that a position at two-thirds of the usable leg length was more comfortable (Kramer et al 1989).

When using the selected location the examiner should ensure that the subject is free to maximally dorsiflex the ankle, and that the strap around the lower part of the shank is not overtight.

A number of studies have shown that variations in the site of the resistance pad may result in significant differences in the moment generated by knee muscles. Siewert et al (1975) indicated that the strength of both the extensors and the flexors became successively smaller as the resistance pad was placed nearer to the knee joint. This trend was apparent at all test velocities. In a later study, in which parallel findings were obtained, the authors (Taylor & Casey 1986) suggested that the reason for this phenomenon was compression of the soft tissues which in turn caused divergence of the knee axis away from the actuator's axis.

The latter argument was also supported by Kramer et al (1989) whose findings were similar. Moreover, it was argued that shortening of the dynamometer application arm increased the angle between the arm and the shank. These mechanical factors interacted with a number of neurophysiologic inhibitory mechanisms, such as reduced motor unit activation, discomfort or pain to account for the general reduction in quadriceps strength.

Consistency in the position of the resistance pad is therefore crucial both for bilateral and follow-up comparisons.

Anterior cruciate ligament deficiency and siting of the resistance pad

In patients with an ACL disorder, the resistance pad is positioned differently. In this case there is a need to reduce the anterior (translocating) force of the rotatory component of the quadriceps. To control this force, Johnson (1982) designed a dual pad (the 'anti-shear device'), which consisted of distal and proximal pads. Another version was described by Brown et al (1992). The proximal pad in Johnson's design supplies a compressive force component which balances off the abovementioned rotatory component.

The use of this accessory has been validated (Timm 1985), and its incorporation in testing and

rehabilitation of patients after ACL repair/reconstruction, or those suffering from anterior laxity is strongly recommended.

TEST ANGULAR VELOCITIES

The hamstring and, even more, the quadriceps have been tested or conditioned using an extensive range of angular velocities. For instance, in a study of normative values of extension and flexion strength, Borges (1989) chose the extremely low value of 12 °/s for one of the criterion velocities. On the other hand Ghena et al (1991) and Hall & Roofner (1991) tested subjects at velocities as high as 450 and 500 °/s respectively.

Use of high angular velocities

It is debatable whether the use of high (greater than 180 °/s) velocities, particularly for knee testing, yields findings that significantly enhance interpretation.

First, it is unclear whether a reasonable sector of the ROM is covered at a constant velocity. This may be determined only through the use of an objective external velocity measuring device. Such measurement is seldom undertaken, but one study which dealt with this problem (Kues et al 1992) showed that even at a velocity as low as 90 °/s there was one case in which nonisokinetic conditions prevailed throughout the first and last 15° of the tested 90° of knee ROM. With a dramatic increase in the test velocities, the acceleration and deceleration phases would occupy such a large proportion of the ROM as to make the effort basically 'isotonic'.

Second, in their study, Ghena et al (1991) demonstrated only a very slight (3 N m) and nonsignificant difference between the concentric strength of the hamstring at 300 and 450 °/s. For the quadriceps, there was a significant decrease (33 N m) in peak moment between these velocities, but it was small compared to the difference between 120 and 300 °/s (74 N m).

Third, the findings by Hall & Roofner (1991) reveal a moment–angular velocity curve which may easily be defined in mathematical terms and hence prediction of strength values at high velocities would be possible.

It seems therefore that in testing, very high

velocities would provide no useful information, unless there was a good reason to believe that the main deficiency was associated with high speed muscle performance. Moreover, other than for professional athletes, high velocities do not seem to simulate any purposeful activity.

For muscle conditioning, a velocity of 450 °/s may constitute a genuine stimulus, and this has indeed been recommended by Mangine & Noyes (1992). However, at the time of writing, no quantitative information concerning the use or validity of very high velocities was available.

Recommended range of test angular velocities

A reasonable and comfortable range for test velocities would be between 60 and 180 °/s. It also seems to meet the essential requirement of test validity and the need for information about muscle performance at the functional range. An added benefit is the very wide usage of this range in numerous studies.

The use of the very low velocities mentioned earlier is contraindicated in ligamentous or patellofemoral disorders, unless the purpose of the test is the provocation of a specific reaction like a 'break' in the moment curve (see Patellofemoral dysfunctions section below).

PART 2
REPRESENTATIVE VALUES FOR THE KNEE

In view of the vast research on knee muscle testing, one could justifiably assume that much work had been done to determine performance norms. This however, is not the case. The establishment of norms requires a large database, consisting of subjects who share a number of 'descriptors'. These descriptors may be classed as subject-linked (gender, age, activity level, fiber types, health status, anthropometric factors), protocol-linked (contraction mode, angular velocities, testing procedures) and measurement-linked (measurement device, and the measured variables i.e. peak moment, average moment, power etc.). Given this variety of factors, it becomes almost impossible to provide a coherent and dependable normative framework.

NORMS ASSOCIATED WITH SPORTING ACTIVITIES

If the requirement of a large and age-stratified sample size is waived, numerous studies can provide some guidelines. These refer to specific sporting activities such as ice hockey (Smith et al 1981), football (Gilliam et al 1979), middle and distance running (Morris et al 1983), cross country skiing (Davies et al 1980), ballet (Kirkendall et al 1984) and soccer (Constantin & Williams 1984).

Ghena et al (1991)

Since isokinetics is a very commonly used tool in the testing and rehabilitation of athletes, a 'normative' database for this group is highly desirable. A relevant database is found in a study by Ghena et al (1991) who based their findings on subjects representing various athletic branches. A total of 100 male athletes, aged 18–25, were tested using their dominant limb, for quadriceps and hamstring concentric strength at 60, 120, 300 and 450 °/s, and eccentric strength at 60 and 120 °/s. The findings are outlined in Table 6.1.

Table 6.1 Peak moments of knee extensors and flexors in male athletes, based on Ghena et al (1991)

Muscle group	Mode	Angular velocity, °/s	Mean peak moments* (SD), N m
Extensors	Concentric	60	260(59)
	Concentric	120	219(40)
	Concentric	300	146(27)
	Concentric	450	113(20)
	Eccentric	60	257(36)
	Eccentric	120	260(38)
Flexors	Concentric	60	142(28)
	Concentric	120	126(24)
	Concentric	300	88(20)
	Concentric	450	92(27)
	Eccentric	60	166(40)
	Eccentric	120	168(39)

* Rounded to nearest integer.

GENERAL POPULATION NORMS

Murray et al 1980

With respect to the general population, one of the first reports of normative isokinetic values for the knee was by Murray et al (1980), dealing with flexor and extensor strength. A total of 72 normal men, aged between 20 and 86 years, without any neuromuscular or skeletal dysfunction, took part in the study. A single test velocity, 36 °/s, was used and the strength findings, which were angle-based, related to three age groups. The use of a slow velocity, the relatively insensitive resolution and the absence of an acceptable performance parameter, such as the peak moment, limited the usefulness of this source.

Freedson et al (1993)

The most comprehensive study, at least in terms of the population size was by Freedson et al (1993) who tested 4541 subjects, 1196 women and 3345 men. Subjects were drawn from 20 companies which carried out medium to heavy physical work. All participants passed a standard physical examination and were considered free of injury at the time of evaluation. Tests used three angular velocities, and the peak moments of the extensors and flexors were recorded, apparently without gravity correction.

Findings for men and women are presented as percentiles and according to age, in Tables 6.2 and 6.3. There was a faster strength loss with age in women, as compared to men.

Borges (1989)

In another comprehensive study of 280 subjects, the

isokinetic strength of women's knee flexors and extensors was compared with that of men using a test protocol with three angular velocities (Borges 1989).

The data, which are outlined in Tables 6.4 and 6.5, revealed a significant decrease in strength between the ages of 20 and 30 years in men and between 40 and 50 years in women. There was another decrease in strength, for both genders between the ages of 60 and 70 years. There were no significant differences between the right and left limbs. Most importantly, both isokinetic and isometric strength were not significantly different between moderately active and inactive subjects, for both women and men. This finding widens the applicability of these norms.

COMPARISON OF SWEDISH AND AMERICAN DATA

Though analysis of the findings from the comparable age groups in the Borges (1989) and Ghena et al (1991) studies already mentioned must be made with extreme caution, it is interesting to note that there is a signifcant measure of similarity. The youngest men's group in the Swedish study (Borges 1989), with an average age of 20 years, may be compared with the American group, whose mean age was 20.13 years. Weight and height, both of which are important factors in strength (Gross et al

Table 6.2 Normative values (in N m) of flexion (F) and extension (E) in men, for angular velocities of 60, 180 and 300 °/s, based on Freedson et al (1993)

Angular velocity	Percentile	<21 years F	<21 years E	21–30 years F	21–30 years E	31–40 years F	31–40 years E	41–50 years F	41–50 years E	>50 years F	>50 years E
60 °/s	90	163.7	255.2	171.5	267.8	163.5	256.3	159.3	240.0	143.7	222.0
	70	139.0	225.2	149.8	233.2	143.7	218.7	139.0	214.1	129.1	198.0
	50	126.1	203.4	133.6	209.5	130.2	196.6	125.2	189.8	111.9	171.9
	30	113.9	185.1	120.7	188.5	116.1	177.6	118.0	172.5	101.8	152.8
	10	101.8	156.3	103.7	162.7	98.9	152.3	97.1	148.5	88.1	126.9
180 °/s	90	114.9	150.5	118.0	153.2	111.2	142.1	109.7	133.6	94.4	115.7
	70	98.3	129.5	102.4	132.9	96.3	122.0	91.5	111.9	81.8	101.6
	50	89.5	116.6	92.2	118.7	87.5	108.5	83.0	99.7	71.9	90.9
	30	73.9	105.1	82.0	106.4	78.6	95.6	72.5	89.0	67.1	74.2
	10	67.5	90.9	69.2	90.9	63.1	79.3	61.7	73.9	53.3	59.0
300 °/s	90	97.2	107.4	96.7	108.8	90.2	101.0	85.4	92.9	76.3	86.5
	70	81.4	92.9	81.4	91.5	76.6	84.1	73.2	76.6	65.1	70.4
	50	71.9	82.0	71.9	80.7	67.8	72.5	64.4	65.8	59.0	60.7
	30	63.1	72.5	63.7	70.5	59.0	63.1	55.6	56.3	50.3	46.2
	10	51.3	61.0	52.2	58.7	47.4	50.9	43.4	45.4	40.0	34.6

Table 6.3 Normative values (in N m) of flexion (F) and extension (E) in women, for angular velocities of 60, 180 and 300 °/s, based on Freedson et al (1993). F, Flexion; E, extension

Angular velocity	Percentile	<21 years F	<21 years E	21–30 years F	21–30 years E	31–40 years F	31–40 years E	41–50 years F	41–50 years E	>50 years F	>50 years E
60 °/s	90	101.2	160.0	108.5	176.3	109.8	167.9	105.8	152.3	93.2	120.4
	70	90.2	144.4	94.2	149.8	94.1	148.2	91.8	129.5	77.0	109.7
	50	82.7	132.9	86.8	135.6	84.1	131.5	84.1	120.7	69.2	106.4
	30	74.6	120.0	79.3	123.4	76.6	118.7	73.9	109.6	55.5	91.8
	10	62.4	103.1	67.8	105.1	64.8	100.8	61.7	98.0	46.5	67.1
180 °/s	90	71.2	90.2	71.2	92.2	69.6	87.5	62.1	75.5	51.1	60.7
	70	60.3	78.0	64.4	80.4	60.3	73.9	55.6	63.7	47.7	51.8
	50	54.9	70.5	57.6	71.9	53.3	65.1	50.2	56.3	39.3	40.0
	30	48.1	65.1	51.5	63.1	47.9	57.0	45.4	50.2	30.4	35.0
	10	40.0	52.9	42.0	52.7	38.6	47.2	36.2	42.8	14.1	23.3
300 °/s	90	57.0	63.1	59.0	63.2	54.9	58.7	50.0	50.0	42.8	42.3
	70	48.8	52.9	50.2	53.6	46.6	47.5	44.3	40.7	39.5	32.5
	50	43.4	46.8	44.7	46.8	40.7	40.7	38.0	38.0	29.2	23.7
	30	37.3	41.4	38.6	40.7	35.9	34.6	33.2	29.8	25.1	19.0
	10	28.5	34.6	31.9	32.5	28.5	27.8	25.8	25.1	11.9	6.8

Table 6.4 Normative peak moments of knee extensors* (in N m), at three angular velocities, based on Borges (1989)

	Age (years)	12 °/s Right	12 °/s Left	90 °/s Right	90 °/s Left	150 °/s Right	150 °/s Left
Women	20	183(34)	172(31)	143(25)	137(24)	110(18)	106(19)
	30	169(34)	163(30)	138(22)	134(20)	108(19)	107(15)
	40	172(28)	161(26)	134(20)	131(20)	105(15)	102(14)
	50	153(30)	143(26)	122(18)	114(17)	94(16)	92(14)
	60	145(20)	126(24)	113(13)	99(15)	84(10)	79(12)
	70	128(28)	120(25)	98(17)	93(15)	74(12)	70(11)
Men	20	289(44)	269(47)	231(32)	217(27)	180(24)	179(22)
	30	258(45)	243(47)	207(38)	196(35)	158(34)	160(28)
	40	248(29)	238(42)	203(27)	197(31)	158(24)	155(26)
	50	226(51)	220(45)	186(36)	177(32)	145(27)	143(30)
	60	223(48)	212(40)	179(34)	169(32)	142(28)	136(22)
	70	188(36)	183(37)	143(24)	145(30)	113(22)	113(21)

* Findings expressed as mean (SD).

1989) were also very similar: 75 and 76 kg and 180 and 182 cm for the Swedish and American groups respectively.

Since the velocities used were different, the average of the findings relating to 90 and 150 °/s in the Swedish study (Tables 6.4 and 6.5) may be compared with the isokinetic findings at 120 °/s in the American study (Table 6.1). Therefore, average quadriceps strength was 205 N m in the general population (Swedish) and 219 N m in athletes (American). The average hamstring strength was 109 N m and 126 N m respectively. The difference is hence about 6% in quadriceps and 14% in hamstring strength.

If this very simple analysis is any lesson, it indicates that strength may not be a primary differentiating factor between athletes and non-athletes and therefore the applicability of Borges's findings may be even wider.

PREDICTION OF INDIVIDUAL PERFORMANCE FROM NORMATIVE VALUES

In view of the growing interest in using high velocity knee testing and rehabilitation, the work of Hall & Roofner (1991) offers original information and a practical approach to determining individual performance from equations based on normative

Table 6.5 Normative peak moments of knee flexors* (in N m), at three angular velocities, based on Borges (1989)

	Age (years)	12 °/s Right	12 °/s Left	90 °/s Right	90 °/s Left	150 °/s Right	150 °/s Left
Women	20	100(20)	95(20)	68(21)	66(17)	49(19)	46(16)
	30	90(18)	88(18)	61(15)	58(13)	46(14)	42(12)
	40	93(20)	91(18)	62(14)	61(13)	46(14)	46(13)
	50	76(24)	75(20)	52(13)	51(13)	36(13)	38(11)
	60	77(14)	74(17)	53(12)	47(13)	38(11)	35(12)
	70	65(12)	59(13)	39(13)	38(13)	28(8)	25(9)
Men	20	155(28)	144(27)	122(21)	113(21)	96(19)	91(19)
	30	150(28)	143(35)	113(23)	108(29)	91(26)	87(25)
	40	149(22)	144(24)	112(18)	106(21)	87(16)	83(15)
	50	142(32)	129(30)	98(24)	91(25)	82(23)	76(25)
	60	130(38)	133(34)	95(29)	86(30)	78(24)	75(25)
	70	109(30)	109(32)	78(26)	77(23)	61(23)	60(26)

* Findings expressed as mean (SD).

values. The authors used a sample of 60 normal subjects, 30 women and 30 men, of 20–62 years of age, and velocities of 60, 180, 300, 400 and 500 °/s. The measured parameters included quadriceps strength (peak moment), average work and power.

It was suggested that the descriptive statistics obtained and the following equations, enable the prediction of these performance parameters from age, weight and sex data. At 180 °/s the latter factors may account for 80, 74 and 51% of the differences in quadriceps strength, average work and average power respectively.

Strength = 54.607 – (age × 1.187) + (sex × 32.905) + (weight × 0.378)

Average work = 113.534 – (age × 1.617) + (sex × 58.471) + (weight × 0.371)

Average power = – 1.107 – (age × 2.102) + (sex × 11.264) + (weight × 1.296)

where sex has the value 1 for men and 0 for women.

ECCENTRIC PERFORMANCE

Eccentric muscle performance was not widely reported until the late 1980s though its significance for knee activity is now firmly established.

A study by Highgenboten et al (1988) reported on the concentric and eccentric average strength of knee flexors and extensors in a group of 127 normal subjects, women and men, ranging in age between 15 and 34 years. Both knees were tested, and

strength scores were pooled. The activity status of the subjects was not specified. A single test velocity, 50 °/s, was used and the units of strength were normalized for bodyweight (N m/kg). Flexor strength was tested in the supine position. Table 6.6 outlines the findings.

The choice of hamstring test position, test velocity and units of measurement precludes comparison between the norms derived from this study and those mentioned earlier.

Table 6.6 Normalized strength at 50 °/s of knee extensors and flexors* as a ratio of peak or average moment/bodyweight (N m/kg), based on Highgenboten et al (1988)

Peak moment	Concentric Extensors	Concentric Flexors	Eccentric Extensors	Eccentric Flexors
Women				
15–24 years	2.19(0.51)	0.87(0.16)	2.37(0.90)	1.06(0.26)
25–34 years	1.98(0.49)	0.85(0.18)	2.36(0.77)	1.11(0.28)
Pooled	2.12(0.51)	0.85(0.17)	2.36(0.85)	1.06(0.26)
Men				
15–24 years	2.98(0.57)	1.21(0.24)	3.09(0.88)	1.44(0.33)
25–34 years	2.49(0.66)	1.08(0.28)	2.67(0.82)	1.37(0.32)
Pooled	2.76(0.66)	1.16(0.26)	2.88(0.86)	1.40(0.33)
Average moment				
Women				
15–24 years	1.26(0.30)	0.59(0.12)	1.31(0.53)	0.70(0.22)
25–34 years	1.22(0.37)	0.58(0.12)	1.38(0.51)	0.72(0.21)
Pooled	1.25(0.32)	0.58(0.12)	1.34(0.52)	0.70(0.22)
Men				
15–24 years	1.78(0.42)	0.85(0.29)	1.87(0.62)	1.01(0.32)
25–34 years	1.48(0.45)	0.73(0.18)	1.71(0.57)	0.95(0.26)
Pooled	1.66(0.45)	0.80(0.26)	1.81(0.60)	1.00(0.29)

* findings expressed as mean (SD).

SUMMARY

Assuming that the required normative parameter is the concentric strength (peak moment) of the quadriceps and hamstring (tested in the seated position), the present author would recommend using the findings by Freedson et al (1993) or by Borges (1989) as general normative sources. For eccentric tests, the findings by Highgenboten et al (1988) may serve as an adequate source, providing one converts the units accordingly.

Users of these norms should however be aware that findings based on isokinetic dynamometers of different makes are not compatible (see Chapter 3 for detailed analysis). Consequently reasonable error margins should be used.

PART 3
SELECTED DISORDERS OF THE KNEE

The great majority of studies of isokinetic aspects of knee muscle dysfunction, concern either ligamentous or patellofemoral disorders. Among the former, the anterior cruciate ligament has received almost exclusive attention, whereas interest in disorders of the posterior, medial and lateral collateral ligaments has been negligible. This reflects not only the major role of the anterior cruciate ligament in maintaining a normally functioning knee, and the incidence of partial or complete rupture, but also the dramatic progress made during recent years in anterior cruciate ligament reconstruction and rehabilitation.

'Patellofemoral dysfunctions', is a collective term for a number of pathologies.

Muscle involvement in other fairly common disorders of the knee, such as torn menisci, have been studied also, and relevant findings will be presented.

ANTERIOR CRUCIATE LIGAMENT DISORDERS

As mentioned above, work on the anterior cruciate ligament (ACL) comprises the lion's share of research into ligamentous disorders. A constructive approach to the testing of ACL patients and to the interpretation of findings emerges from consideration of the following questions:

1. At a given time, postinjury or postoperatively, how does the strength of the involved side compare with that of the sound side (bilateral comparison) and is there a general decline relative to the expected norm?
2. Will isokinetic performance parameters other than strength assist in interpretation of the findings?
3. What is the significance of the hamstring/quadriceps ratio (HQR)?
4. Is there an objective, isokinetically measurable goal at which rehabilitation or steady state performance should be aimed?

The answers to these questions depend to an extent on the history of the patient. Some will suffer from 'chronic' ACL deficiency, i.e. the torn ligament has not been surgically rectified, while others have undergone surgical repair of the ACL. Following loss of the ACL, in chronic patients, a steady state neuromuscular performance, at a lower level than previously, is normally achieved. The time-span post-injury, for reaching this plateau is not known, but is regarded as years rather than months.

BILATERAL COMPARISONS
Chronic ACL deficiency

Concentric and eccentric testing, at 30 °/s, of chronic ACL patients who had declined surgery, was performed by Dvir et al (1989) approximately one-and-a-half years postinjury. Comparing data for the involved and uninvolved sides, concentric strength deficits were on average, 21 and 14% for the quadriceps and hamstring respectively, whereas the corresponding eccentric deficits were 18 and 15%.

Tegner et al (1986) tested patients with 'old' tears of the ACL (the period postinjury was not specified). The group consisted of predominantly chronic patients and a few who suffered from instability in spite of an operation. Concentric isokinetic tests at 30 and 180 °/s revealed that, compared to the sound side, the quadriceps strength deficiency was, on average, 21 and 16% at these velocites. The corresponding hamstring deficiencies were 8 and 4% respectively.

Bonamo et al (1990) studied various factors associated with conservative treatment of 59 active but noncompetitive recreational athletes with ACL deficiency. Using isokinetic testing (60 and 240 °/s), performed more than 4 years following injury, these authors reported quadriceps deficits of 11–14%, and deficits of 3–4% for the hamstring. It was however suggested that conservative treatment meant significant activity modification.

Kannus & Jarvinen (1991) tested subjects with partial tear of the ligament, 8 years postinjury. The tests revealed that except for a significant decrease in quadriceps strength at the low velocity of 60 °/s there were no significant differences between the involved and sound knee.

Conclusions

These and other studies indicate therefore that in the chronic ACL patient:

1. In spite of conservative intervention, significant quadriceps strength deficits, of approximately 20%, exist during at least the first year following tear of the ligament.
2. These deficits subside quite sharply in the longer term but a change in activities is sometimes inevitable.
3. The effect of the tear on hamstring strength is significantly less conspicuous than for the quadriceps. Providing proper attention has been given to flexor function, full recovery of hamstring strength in the involved side may be expected.

Chronic partial tears and hamstring strength

Interestingly, in a group of patients with chronic partial tears of the ACL, with or without medial collateral ligament rupture, the hamstring strength was generally more compromised than that of the quadriceps (Kannus et al 1992). This trend was even more pronounced with an increase in the velocity.

Besides the possibility of a more selective atrophy of type II fibers, another explanation of this finding may be that a partially functioning ACL does not stimulate an increase in hamstring strength to the same extent that the absence of the ACL does.

Reconstructed ACL and bilaterial comparisons

A different situation obtains where patients have undergone surgical repair of their torn ACL. For example, patients are expected to regain muscle function within a relatively short period of time. On the other hand, the particular operative technique and the rehabilitation regimen especially are crucial factors affecting the rate of improvement. Although it is not the intention here to review the procedures and complexities associated with surgery of this ligament, Table 6.7 shows variables affecting rehabilitation after ACL reconstruction, as identified by Wilk & Andrews (1992).

Among these variables, the type of surgical procedure has been mentioned in connection with isokinetic performance of thigh muscles. For instance, Seto et al (1988) indicated that 5 years postoperatively, there was a significant correlation between the increase in quadriceps strength on the operated side and a return to functional activity, in

Table 6.7 Variables influencing rehabilitation of patients after ACL reconstruction, based on Wilk & Andrews (1992)

1. Type of surgical procedure 　Arthrotomy 　Arthroscopic assisted 　Endoscopic	5. Graft tensioning
	6. Tourniquet time
2. Tissue type used 　Patellar tendon 　Semitendinous 　Iliotibial band	7. Concomitant surgeries 　Collateral ligament 　Meniscal lesions 　Posterior cruciate 　ligament (PCL) 　injuries 　Condral lesions 　Surgical notchplasty 　Capsular deficiencies
3. Graft fixation 　Screw 　Button 　Staple 　Suture	
4. Graft placement 　Isometric 　Nonisometric	8. Patient variables 　Size 　Alignment 　Activity level 　Compliance

patients with intraarticular, but not extraarticular, ACL reconstruction. However, this author is not aware of any comparative, systematic, long-range study that discusses surgical procedure and isokinetic performance in a satisfactory manner. Rather, most studies consider either the postoperative time-span or the rehabilitation program, e.g. accelerated or nonaccelerated, in relation to the isokinetic data.

Nonaccelerated rehabilitation: up to 2 years postoperatively

Some studies have investigated the variations over a period of time in thigh muscle function following ACL reconstruction.

Murray et al (1984) compared patients who were treated conservatively with those who underwent reconstruction following 6 months of nonaccelerated rehabilitation. Isokinetic tests were carried out bilaterally at 30 and 180 °/s. Quadriceps strength deficits in both groups were significant: 17% for reconstruction and 7% for conservative treatment, but the difference was not statistically significant between the groups. Deficits in the hamstring were similar in the two groups, and generally less conspicuous than the quadriceps deficit.

Elmqvist et al (1989) increased the span of assessment, testing bilateral extensor function at 90 °/s in patients before, and at 14, 20, 34 and 52 weeks after, ACL reconstruction (for technique see Marshall 1979). Following cast immobilization, patients underwent intensive nonaccelerated reha-

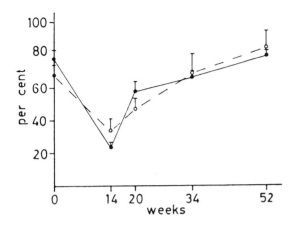

Fig. 6.2 Relative strength (isokinetic strength as percentage of noninjured leg strength) at 90 °/s of the quadriceps of the injured leg in 17 patients with ACL reconstruction. Patients trained either isokinetically (solid circles) or using isometrics and PRE (open circles). (From Elmqvist et al 1989).

bilitation. Preoperatively, there were significant strength (21%) and total work (27%) deficiencies. Figure 6.2 illustrates the variation in strength during the first year. Despite isometric or isokinetic conditioning administered during the first year after the operation, quadriceps strength of the involved knee was still approximately 20% lower than that of the contralateral knee.

Elmquist et al (1988) also investigated quadriceps strength 2 years after ACL reconstruction. The findings were similar, i.e. there was a 20% deficit compared to the uninjured limb. These results are very similar to those of Murray et al (1984) though the operative procedures, rehabilitation protocols and testing velocities were not identical.

Lopresti et al (1988) Using the 'bone–patellar tendon–bone graft' procedure, Lopresti et al (1988) reported deficits of, on average, 12 and 20% in quadriceps strength in men and women respectively, at both 60 and 120 °/s. There were no detectable deficits in hamstring strength.

Rosenberg et al (1992), who also used the central third of the patellar tendon, showed that 12–24 months postoperatively, there was still a quadriceps deficiency of 18% (measured concentrically at 60 °/s) whereas hamstring deficiency stood at 10%.

Halperin & Dvir (1993) Finally, a 13% concentric deficit and a 4% eccentric deficit were found in the quadriceps and hamstring respectively 2 years after a semitendinosus and gracilis ACL

reconstruction. It is worth noting that although a significant component of the hamstring was used for the reconstruction, the eccentric force of this muscle, which controls the anterior motion of the tibia, was regained in its entirety.

Conclusions Therefore during a period of up to 2 years post ACL reconstruction, and following a nonaccelerated rehabilitation program, a quadriceps deficit of 15–20% compared with the uninvolved side should be expected. There is however a negligible deficit of hamstring strength.

Nonaccelerated rehabilitation: long-term results

Only a limited number of studies describe long-term postoperative results of ACL reconstruction (greater than 2 years) related to thigh muscle strength. Yasuda et al (1992), who used the bone-patellar tendon–bone graft technique, suggested that quadriceps strength of the operated side, reached 85% of that of the sound side at final follow-up (3–7 years) in men and 70% in women, while hamstring strength was fully recovered.

Seto et al (1988) used a 5-year post ACL reconstruction period. In the extraarticular reconstruction group, quadriceps deficiency at 120 °/s was still a significant 14%, whereas hamstring strength was practically identical in both limbs. It should however be emphasized that a considerable extensor deficit, 33%, existed in the intraarticular group.

At a period of about 8 years post ACL reconstruction Arvidsson et al (1981) found significant quadriceps strength deficits in two groups of patients whose functional capacity was rated as 'fair' or 'poor', but quadriceps strength was not significantly different from that of the sound side in the 'good' and 'excellent' groups.

Conclusions The performance level of thigh muscles long after an ACL reconstruction is still characterized by a significant reduction in extensor strength. A reduced activity level and/or a permanent impairment to the extensor mechanism, due to harvesting of the graft, are probably the main factors behind this deficit.

Accelerated rehabilitation

The concept of accelerated rehabilitation was first introduced by Shelbourne & Nitz (1990). It is used following surgery based on an intraarticular bone–patellar tendon–bone graft. Two factors stimulated this change in rehabilitation after ACL reconstruction (De Carlo et al 1992). First, noncompliant patients made faster progress than patients who rigidly obeyed a traditional, nonaccelerated protocol. Second, a certain percentage of patients experienced problems associated with quadriceps dysfunction when using a nonaccelerated protocol.

Briefly, accelerated rehabilitation emphasizes early terminal extension, early weight bearing, and the exclusive use of closed kinetic chain efforts for reconditioning of the quadriceps.

Comparison of accelerated and non-accelerated rehabilitation Using one of the most impressive databases ever reported in isokinetics-related research, De Carlo and his colleagues (1992) indicated that in terms of strength gains, and improved ROM, accelerated rehabilitation was significantly superior to nonaccelerated. Some of the findings are outlined in Table 6.8, and a consistent pattern of higher quadriceps and hamstring strengths is evident.

The difference in time taken for rehabilitation is most important. For instance, quadriceps strength at 3 months in the accelerated group was similar to that at 6 months in the nonaccelerated group. The more intensive rehabilitation therefore benefits the patient, allowing her/him to return sooner to normal activity.

Moreover, compared with nonaccelerated protocols which, after 1 year still result in an extensor deficit of about 20%, the accelerated regime brings the patient much closer to parity, with only a 13% deficit. Though the study of De Carlo et al refers only to the first postoperative year, extrapolation based on other studies shows that, with other factors being equal, the trend towards a continuous im-provement may not disappear.

Conclusion For the special case of accelerated rehabilitation, during the first year post ACL reconstruction a quadriceps deficit of 10–15% compared with the uninvolved side should be expected.

Margin of error

Variations for a given individual's scores may reach 5–10% within the same testing session. This margin of error should be used with the rehabilitation criteria (accelerated or nonaccelerated) when judging whether a rehabilitation objective has been achieved.

OTHER ISOKINETIC PERFORMANCE PARAMETERS

The use of parameters derived from strength, other than those related to endurance, has not helped to interpret test findings, since these parameters are so closely related to strength. The point has been demonstrated in studies dealing with the significance of total work during a series of contractions (Kannus 1988a,b, Elmqvist et al 1989), and of angular impulse or average power (Kannus 1990) in ligamentous disorders of the knee.

Therefore, the strength of the quadriceps and/or hamstring is sufficient for describing the basic mechanical capacity of these muscles, and other variables derived from the strength curve are redundant.

It should be mentioned that other parameters such as the rise time of the moment of the hamstring may be relevant. However, these are correctly derivable from isometric rather than isokinetic strength functions.

Table 6.8 The effect of accelerated vs. nonaccelerated rehabilitation on the postoperative strength variations in knee extensors and flexors (in percentage of strength of uninvolved side, at 180 °/s) based on De Carlo et al (1992)

Postoperative time (months)	Extensors		Flexors	
	Nonaccelerated	Accelerated	Nonaccelerated	Accelerated
3	63.9(2.3)	69.6(0.5)*	79.4(2.3)	92.7(1.1)†
6	71.5(1.2)	76.8(0.5)†	91.0(1.2)	97.8(0.5)†
12	80.0(1.5)	87.4(0.9)†	95.1(1.5)	98.7(0.9)

* $p<0.05$; † $p<0.01$

THE HAMSTRING/QUADRICEPS RATIO

This parameter has attracted a great deal of interest and was used as an indicator of normal balance between the extensor and flexor function in the knee. It became evident that the ratio was velocity-dependent: for low velocities the normal HQR was about 0.60, and for high velocities it was greater than one (Osternig 1983). However, the omission of a gravity correction in a number of studies means that their findings and conclusions must be viewed with reservation.

There has been some research on the role of the hamstring muscle group in controlling the unstable ACL-deficient knee, notably by Walla et al (1985) and Solomonow et al (1987). These authors have shown that instability is associated with increased reflex activity in the hamstring when the knee is exposed to extensor load.

The dynamic control ratio. Coactivation of the quadriceps and hamstring takes place through opposite contraction modes, the quadriceps contracting concentrically, and the hamstring eccentrically. Therefore in order to assess the balancing nature of the hamstring in the ACL-deficient knee the hamstring–quadriceps ratio should correctly be H_e/Q_c, i.e. the eccentric strength of the hamstring divided by the concentric strength of the quadriceps or the 'dynamic control ratio' (Dvir et al 1989).

However, almost all of the studies of the ACL-deficient knee and the HQR have been based on the concentric strengths of both muscles.

Kannus (1988a,b) studied the HQR in subjects with ACL-deficient knee 8 years after injury and found a high intersubject variability in this parameter of 23–205%. On the other hand, the HQR was significantly higher for the involved compared with the sound limb at the higher testing speed (180 °/s).

Lopresti et al (1988) reported HQRs of 0.66 vs. 0.75 in the involved and sound knees respectively and related the difference to a reduced quadriceps strength, as no detectable differences were indicated in the bilateral hamstring tests.

Dvir et al (1989) compared the values of the dynamic control ratio, H_e/Q_c, with the HQR, H_c/Q_c and H_e/Q_e at the test velocity of 30 °/s. The findings indicated that whereas the same contraction mode ratios, HQR and $H_e/Q e$, differed by no more than 3% between the involved and sound knees, there was a significant difference in the dynamic control ratio. A reduction of 11% in the concentric strength of the deficient side quadriceps accounted for this finding.

Interpretation of the HQR

It is therefore apparent that the hamstring–quadriceps ratio itself is a rather crude parameter whose relationship to ACL deficiency derives directly from the marked weakness of the quadriceps which is typical in this disorder. It is rather surprising that in the 'long chronic' patient, HQR still differs significantly between limbs (Kannus 1988a) since quadriceps weakness tends to diminish. However, the use of HQR for clinical inference may not be essential.

AN ISOKINETIC CRITERION FOR REHABILITATION IN ACL DISORDERS

There is a growing consensus among experts that the bilaterial ratio of quadriceps strength, the quadriceps/quadriceps ratio or QQR, may serve as a milestone for rehabilitation or long-term performance in ACL dysfunction. On the other hand, the timing of the tests and/or the postoperative phase in which they are performed is still a matter of controversy.

Usefulness of bilateral comparison

With regards to the isokinetic parameter, it has been shown by Kannus (1988a,b) that what matters in the long run is the extent to which performance of the muscles of the involved knee approximates that of the uninvolved knee. For instance, regarding the relevance of the HQR, it was claimed that neither did this parameter correlate with the long-term outcome, and nor could an optimal magnitude of HQR be recommended generally as a target for rehabilitation (Kannus 1988a,b). Rather 'a suitable HQ ratio may be the HQ ratio of the patient's uninvolved knee'. Therefore, comparison with the uninvolved side provides a comfortable and a reasonable goal for the steady-state phase, either in the chronic or postoperative patient.

The performance of the extensor mechanism in patients with chronic ACL tear was assessed, among other parameters, relative to the bilateral strength ratio of the quadriceps at a test velocity of

30 °/s (RQ30) by Tegner et al (1986). The authors suggested that the aim of rehabilitation should be to reach an RQ30 of 90% in view of the significant improvements in strength, performance, knee score and activity level associated with this value. The omission of any flexor component is notable.

Progression and discharge in rehabilitation

Another, perhaps more pressing problem is the decision whether to progress to a more advanced stage or to discharge a patient from rehabilitation following surgical correction of ACL tear. There are three commonly accepted mechanical parameters which guide clinicians in making such a decision: range of motion, knee joint stability and muscle performance. To these should be added the level of function which ultimately may be the most important.

Thigh muscle performance under isokinetic conditions can be measured very accurately and with acceptable repoducibility. Given that the choice of criteria is important for the success of the operation, it is tempting to rely upon isokinetically-based standards when deciding to vary the rehabilitation regimen.

Morever, bearing in mind the prevailing trends in medical malpractice litigation, the end-product of the testing, a clear, quantitative and graphical document, which describes the performance of the patient throughout the rehabilitation process, may constitute a significant tool.

Use of the QQR in rehabilitation

Baseline measurements

Irrespective of the rehabilitation protocol, accelerated or nonaccelerated, a preoperative test furnishes an important baseline (Elmqvist et al 1989). In the absence of any contraindication such a test should be performed.

The QQR in a nonaccelerated program

One of the most frequently quoted nonaccelerated rehabilitation protocols was designed by Paolos et al (1983). This protocol was also used by De Carlo et al (1992) in a comparative study of accelerated and nonaccelerated regimens. In this design isokinetic tests are initiated 6 months postoperatively, protecting the knee with the Johnson antishear device (1982) and blocking extension at 20°. The tests are carried out at medium to high velocities (180–240 °/s). Tests should be performed, at monthly intervals, after the first one.

Return to normal activity levels is allowed when the QQR reaches 80%; full ROM is gained; no pain or swelling are present, and successful completion of functional progression had been achieved.

Use of the QQR in accelerated programs

The accelerated rehabilitation regimen used by De Carlo et al differed considerably from the nonaccelerated, in the timing of the initial isokinetic test and the criteria applied. The first test was performed 5–6 weeks postoperatively under the same conditions as in the nonaccelerated system. If the QQR was greater than 70%, more demanding activities such as lateral shuffles, cariocas and rope jumping were incorporated. At 10 weeks another isokinetic evaluation was made, adding a slow test velocity of 60 °/s. At 16–24 weeks a QQR of 80% and successful completion of functional progression indicated return to sporting activities, including contact sports.

Wilk & Andrews (1992) have described another accelerated rehabilitation protocol, which allows athletes to return to sporting activities within 5–6 months following a patellar tendon–graft reconstruction. The protocol, in many respects similar to the one described by Shelbourne & Nitz (1990), is nevertheless less aggressive, notably with regard to the initiation of isokinetic testing as well as the velocities employed. The first testing session takes place 12 weeks postoperatively and velocities of 180 and 300 °/s are used. A test at 60 °/s is omitted as this velocity results in a greater amount of tibial translation compared to 180 and 300 °/s (Nisell et al 1989).

Wilk & Andrews do not regard a QQR of 70% as a criterion for progression to the next, 'light activity' phase even though it is implied that on average, such a score is indeed expected. The exact criterion for a 'satisfactory isokinetic test' is also not specified though at 6 and 12 months postoperatiively QQRs of around 75 and 90% are envisaged.

The QQRs and the bilateral hamstring ratios, obtained using the accelerated rehabilitation regimens of Wilk & Andrews and De Carlo et al, are compared in Table 6.9. It should be noted that

Table 6.9 The effect of accelerated ACL rehabilitation methods on strength variations in knee extensors and flexors (as a percentage of the strength of the uninvolved side)*

Postoperative time (months)	Wilk & Andrews (1992)		DeCarlo et al (1992)	
	Extensors	Flexors	Extensors	Flexors
3	69	94	70	93
6	73	97	77	97
12	91	110	87	99

* Tests performed at 180 °/s

other than a slight difference in hamstring strength 1 year postoperatively, the two designs result in almost identical strength increases.

Conclusions

The current isokinetic criterion for either progression or termination of conditioning in ACL deficiency, chronic or surgically corrected, is the bilateral ratio of quadriceps strength, the QQR. Tests should preferably be conducted at the medium velocity of 180 °/s, although addition of another test at 60 °/s may sometimes reveal specific deficiencies.

Accelerated rehabilitation Tests may be introduced as early as 5–6 weeks postoperatively, in which case:

• a QQR of 70% and above indicates progression to light functional activities.

Accelerated or nonaccelerated rehabilitation Assuming the scores representing other parameters (ROM, function etc.) are satisfactory:

• a QQR of 80% indicates the resumption of normal activity.

For ACL insufficiency, following reconstruction or conservative treatment:

• a QQR of 90% may be required to ensure a satisfactory level of functioning.

DISORDERS OF THE COLLATERAL LIGAMENTS

Isokinetic research regarding the medial and lateral collateral ligaments (MCL and LCL) has been very limited in spite of the fact that damage to the MCL

and medial capsular ligament may be the most common injury in sporting activities (Bergfeld 1979). However, the injury may not result in a complete rupture of the MCL (or LCL). In the latter cases, which are referred to as grade I and II, conservative treatment is exclusively prescribed, and it is sometimes used even for complete (grade III) rupture (Hastings 1980, Ballmer & Jakob 1988, Shelbourne & Porter 1992).

In systematic studies dealing with the collateral ligaments and thigh muscle performance, there is a conspicuous dearth of information regarding the short-term effects. Hence the extent of potential deficits and their significance cannot be specified.

On the other hand, the long-term effect of grade II (partial tear) insufficiency of the MCL, 8 years postinjury was studied by Kannus (1991). Tests were performed at 60 and 180 °/s. Strength deficits were minimal: on average 4 and 2% for the quadriceps and hamstring respectively. Systematically higher strength deficits were noted in the higher velocity indicating possibly greater atrophy in Type II fibers.

In another study, the long-term effects of grade II and III (complete tear) of the LCL were studied (Kannus 1988b). The reduction in the quadriceps strength of the involved side, 8 years postinjury was still significant, being between 10 and 13% (using the mean scores which appear in the paper). In other words the QQR was about 87–90%. Bilateral hamstring strength scores were almost identical.

Consequently, chronic collateral ligament injuries result in some strength deficit in the quadriceps but minimal deficit in the hamstring.

No research has been found which describes short-term variations in thigh muscle performance following isolated injuries to the collateral ligaments.

PATELLOFEMORAL DYSFUNCTIONS

Patellofemoral dysfunction (PFD) is one of the most common problems of the knee encountered by rehabilitation clinicians. It has been defined as 'pain, inflammation, imbalance and/or instability of any component of the extensor mechanism of the knee from congenital, traumatic or mechanical stresses' (Shelton & Thigpen 1991). It therefore encompasses a broad range of syndromes notably patellofemoral malalignment and pain, chondromalacia patella, patellar instability, plica syndrome, quadriceps and patellar tendinitis.

PFD has a particular significance in the physiotherapeutic setting since, unless there is an explicit indication otherwise, conservative management is generally accepted. Indeed, in an analysis of the results of extensor mechanism reconstruction, Cerullo et al (1988) suggested:

In dealing with a stable knee cap or so-called 'anterior knee pain', it is better to use conservative treatment, since the pathologic basis of the clinical syndrome is still obscure. In the absence of a diagnosis, the rationale for performing any operation is also suspect when the patient has all or some of the predisposing physical findings (high and lateral patella, vastus medialis obliquus dysplasia, increased Q angle) but has a stable patella.

Classification by cartilage damage

Pain is a very common consequence of many PFDs, though not necessarily of a magnitude commensurate with the degree of damage. In his classic paper on patellar pain, Insall (1981) described eight, well recognized causes of patellar pain. His classification was based on the extent to which the articular cartilage was damaged.

General damage appears in grade I-III chondromalacia where the cause of pain is believed to be mostly increased pressure due to maltracking, though in some patients the pain arises directly from the pathology (basal degeneration). Osteoarthritis (grade IV chrondromalacia), direct trauma and osteochondral fracture and osteochondritis are the other causes typical of the general damage group.

Variable cartilage damage is associated with malalignment syndromes which may produce pain through overloading and incorrect fit.

Pain may also be provoked in knees with usually normal cartilage, due to overuse syndrome, sympathetic dystrophy, or peripatellar causes like plica and tendinitis.

Patellofemoral pain syndrome

Those PFDs associated with anterior knee pain where there is no disruption to the cartilage are often referred to collectively as patellofemoral pain syndrome (PFPS). The malalignment of the patellofemoral joint which probably accounts for PFPS

results from a number of sources: abnormal anatomical architecture; extensor mechanism malalignment; retinacular restraints, and muscular imbalance and strength (Sczepanski et al 1991).

The muscular factors are of considerable importance as they are the basis of the conservative approach to the initial management of PFD. The mechanism by which conditioning the quadriceps alleviates the pain is not entirely clear, but its efficacy is unquestionable in a great number of cases (Insall 1981). An imbalance between the moments generated by the vastus medialis obliquus (VMO) and vastus lateralis (VL) has been suggested as a causative factor of patella maltracking (Mariani & Caruso 1979, Taunton et al 1987). Insufficiency of the VMO could lead to excessive lateral pull by the VL and exposure of the lateral facet of the patella, increased friction, erosion of the cartilage and pain. Additionally, lateral displacement of the patella could adversely affect the patellar retinacular structures, eventually leading to the need for surgical realignment procedures.

The nature of quadriceps atrophy

The nature and extent of quadriceps atrophy in PFDs, particularly in PFPS, has therefore theoretical as well as clinical implications. Current technology cannot show the individual contributions of the parts of the quadriceps. Consequently, the problem of imbalance between the VMO and VL has been studied semiquantitatively using electromyography. Though one study (Moller et al 1986) indicated that the quadriceps as a whole was weak in patients with PFPS, a yet older study (Mariani & Caruso 1979) and, particularly, a recent study by Souza & Gross (1991) showed that the VMO/VL ratio, as measured by integrated EMG, was significantly greater in normal subjects than in those with PFPS.

PFD AND QUADRICEPS PERFORMANCE

Dependence on test velocities

Studies of quadriceps performance, under isokinetic conditions, in patients with PFD show a definite dependence on the test velocity. This relationship is evident not only in the strength scores but also in the shape of the strength curve particularly at slow testing velocities (see below).

In a validation study of clinical (including isokinetic) parameters versus arthroscopy for diagnosis of chondromalacia (Elton et al 1985), the authors failed to reveal significant concentric strength differences between the affected and nonaffected knee. The tests were carried out at 180 °/s 'to avoid the risk of causing patellofemoral damage. This might account for [the] inability to find torque curve abnormalities in [the] subjects'.

In another study no significant differences in either the concentric or eccentric strength of the quadriceps, were indicated upon comparing women with PFPS and a control group (MacIntyre & Wessel 1988). Again, the reason for this finding might have been the high velocity, 200 °/s, at which the test was carried out.

The use of medium/high velocities means that:

1. The joint is exposed for a shorter time to the external resistance, leading to a lower load on the patellofemoral joint and hence reduced potential inhibition
2. The reflex arc may be too slow to react and inhibit the quadriceps.

On the other hand, concentric tests performed at the lower end of the velocity spectrum told a different story. Hoke et al (1983) using a test velocity of 30 °/s, indicated quadriceps strength curve variations in patients with chondromalacia. In a prospective study of quadriceps strength, the pre- and postoperative scores were compared in patients who underwent advancement osteotomy of the tibial tuberosity due to patellofemoral chondromalacia and osteoarthrosis (Nordgren et al 1983). Tests were performed at velocities of 6, 12, and 60 °/s. Table 6.10 outlines some of the findings:

1. Compared with matched normal subjects, both women and men demonstrated a highly significant reduction in strength. Considering the full spectrum of velocities, this reduction amounted to 34 and 22% in women and men respectively.
2. Quadriceps strength, in the involved knee improved significantly following the operation (no significant differences were noted for the sound knee).
3. Using the averages quoted in the study, the estimated average preoperative QQRs were 66 and 59% for women and men respectively.

Contraction mode and QQR

In a later study, Dvir et al (1990) tested a mixed group of young women and men presenting with PFPS. Bilateral concentric and eccentric tests were performed at 30, 60 and 120 °/s. Table 6.11 outlines the results, normalized for body weight. Compared with healthy subjects, women and men with PFPS had a reduction in strength of 35 and 27% respectively. In addition:

1. The reduction in eccentric contractions was

Table 6.10 Pre- versus postoperative findings* for pain and knee extensor strength. Based on Nordgren et al 1983 copyright © Springer-Verlag.

Angular velocity		Peak moment (N m)			Pain value (0–9 Lund Scale)		
			Involved knee				
	n	Uninvolved	Preoperative	Postoperative	n	Preoperative	Postoperative
60 °/s							
Women	16	133 (31)	86 (36)	106 (36)	13	3.85 (2.00)	2.02 (2.03)[‡]
Men	11	228 (77)	131 (52)	186 (49)[†]	9	5.01 (1.63)	2.22 (2.20)[‡]
12 °/s							
Women	17	139 (32)	84 (34)	109 (38)[†]	13	3.71 (2.05)	1.92 (1.86)[‡]
Men	11	207 (94)	112 (38)	174 (38)[‡]	9	4.89 (1.41)	2.19 (2.05)[‡]
60 °/s							
Women	17	125 (23)	79 (32)	92 (31)	17	2.28 (1.72)	0.87 (1.29)[†]
Men	13	188 (73)	109 (31)	147 (41)[†]	9	3.40 (2.05)	1.78 (1.92)

* Shown as mean (SD).
[†] $p < 0.05$.
[‡] $p < 0.01$.

Table 6.11 Concentric and eccentric knee extensor strength (in N m/kgbw)*: controls vs. patients with patellofemoral pain syndrome (PFPS) patients. Based on Dvir et al (1990)

Group	Contraction mode	n	Angular velocity (°/s) 30	60	120
Women					
Control	Concentric	15	2.47(0.49)	2.41(0.47)	1.93(0.37)
PFPS	Concentric	21	1.69(0.40)	1.55(0.79)	1.22(0.90)
Men					
Control	Concentric	15	3.02(0.51)	2.77(0.52)	2.43(0.41)
PFPS	Concentric	34	2.00(0.49)	1.93(0.60)	1.97(0.44)
Women					
Control	Eccentric	15	3.39(0.70)	3.23(0.70)	3.20(0.63)
PFPS	Eccentric	21	2.04(0.73)	1.87(0.70)	1.67(0.72)
Men					
Control	Eccentric	15	3.80(0.92)	3.65(0.83)	3.66(0.67)
PFPS	Eccentric	34	2.29(0.64)	2.27(0.60)	2.34(0.62)

* Shown as mean (SD).

larger than in concentric contractions: 44 vs. 35% in women, and 41 vs. 27% in men.

2. The average QQR was very stable at about 65 and 67% in women and men (concentric) and 60 and 62% (eccentric). (The close correspondence in the strength scores between this study and that of Nordgren et al is notable.)

Conclusions

Two principles thus emerge from the above analysis:

1. Slow test velocities, 30–60 °/s, may be used for PFD testing
2. Chronic PFPS may result in a significant reduction in the QQR, of greater than 30%.

Regarding the first point, though the policy of avoiding excessive pressure on the patellofemoral joint is entirely justified, the present author believes that a sounder interpretation of findings, based on low speed testing, can more than offset the potential risk from a set of 3–4 consecutive maximal contractions performed once every 2–3 weeks.

CORRELATION BETWEEN PAIN AND ISOKINETIC MEASUREMENTS IN PFPS

Clinical examination of patients suffering from patellofemoral pain frequently reveals that one of the most common mechanisms of avoiding pain is 'a reluctance, whether voluntary or involuntary, to initiate and maintain a strong quadriceps contrac-

tion' (Wild et al 1982). Both static and dynamic contractile activity may be avoided. Pain is probably the main obstacle to normal force generation when quadriceps strength in PFPS patients is measured. Moreover, improvement in the symptoms is often accompanied by an improved quadriceps performance, thus recording the pain level, as well as quadriceps strength, is of paramount importance in PFPS testing and rehabilitation.

Quadriceps strength and pain rating

The association of pain and patellofemoral stressing under isokinetic conditions was first reported by Nordgren et al (1983). Patients used the Lund 9-point scale to rate the pain perceived after each contraction, pre- and postoperatively. The significant reductions in anterior knee pain rating correlated with a significant increase in quadriceps concentric strength and the general functional level. In a later paper, Lysholm (1987) studied the combined effect of drug therapy and activity modification on quadriceps strength and knee pain in 25 subjects with patellar tendinitis.

A significant negative correlation was indicated between the pain, as measured by a visual analog scale, and peak moment. The negative correlation was more pronounced at 30 (– 0.59) than at 180 °/s (– 0.40). The closer association between pain and strength at the lower velocity testing could mean that the pain magnitude reflected either the higher moment generated at 30 °/s or the longer exposure during a slower test.

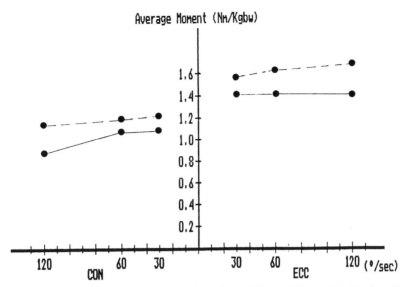

Fig. 6.3 Normalized average moment–angular velocity curves in patients with patellofemoral dysfunction. (From Dvir et al 1991a Isokinetics and Exercise Science 1: 26–30, with permission of Butterworth-Heinemann.) Solid lines—females; broken lines—males.

Contraction mode, load, and perceived pain

In a recent study of patients with PFPS, the association between concentric and eccentric quadriceps strength and perceived pain was analyzed (Dvir et al 1991a). Pain was assessed using the 10-point Borg modified pain scale. Figure 6.3 shows the average moment–angular velocity relationship. Figure 6.4 shows that the variations in the pain scores did not correspond to variations in

strength, at least with respect to eccentric efforts, as the levelling-off of the eccentric strength curve is not reflected in a similar shape for the pain curve.

Pain and load However, variation in the load, or impulse, which is the product of two distinct variables, the magnitude of the moment generated by the muscle and the period of time the joint is exposed to the contractile activity, is closely correlated with changes in the pain (Fig. 6.5). Therefore,

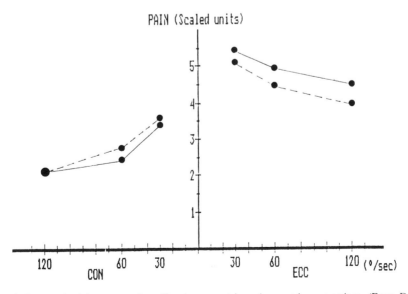

Fig. 6.4 Pain scores during maximal knee extension effort in concentric and eccentric contractions. (From Dvir et al 1991a Isokinetics and Exercise Science 1: 26–30, with permission of Butterworth-Heinemann.) Solid lines—females; broken lines—males.

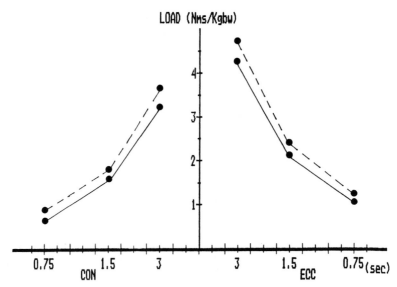

Fig. 6.5 Impulse (load) vs. angular velocity during maximal knee extension effort in concentric and eccentric contractions. (From Dvir et al 1991a Isokinetics and Exercise Science 1: 26–30, with permission of Butterworth-Heinemann.) Solid lines—females; broken lines—males.

the pain perceived by patients with PFPS was predominantly dictated by the load on the joint.

Eccentric contractions and pain mechanisms. Eccentric contractions resulted in significantly higher pain ratings ($p < 0.005$) than concentric contractions. Two possible causes are suggested. Higher moments are generated during eccentric contractions which result in greater patellofemoral forces and therefore greater pain. The other mechanism lies in patellar kinematics. During concentric activity, the area of contact between the patella and the femoral notch diminishes with greater extension (Goodfellow et al 1976). On the other hand, during eccentric activity, the knee flexes and the contact area becomes larger. Although this may result in an improved pressure distribution, the total area exposed to friction increases, leading potentially to the greater intensity of pain. It is of interest that in a recent study no observable relationship between perceived pain and quadriceps force output was indicated (Conway et al 1992). As shown above, such a relationship may indeed not exist unless load is used instead of moment and a spectrum of velocities rather than a single test velocity.

PFPS AND THE SHAPE OF THE QUADRICEPS MOMENT CURVE

Normally, an isokinetic moment curve which is derived from a perfectly sound joint–muscle unit should consist of a relatively smooth 'inverted-U' shape (Ch. 2). When there is either a sudden and considerable change in the muscle's lever or a 'shut-off' of its contractile activity this curve may assume an irregular shape. Here irregularity does not refer to common oscillatory phenomena (Hart et al 1985) but to single, sometimes double or triple, conspicuous 'dents' in the curve.

The 'break' in PFPS moment curves

Such an irregularity in the moment curve of the quadriceps is a striking expression of PFPS, obtained during low velocity isokinetic testing. Nordgren et al (1983) were among the first to document this phenomenon. Figure 6.6 (Nordgen et al 1983) shows three different quadriceps moment curves from the same patient on three occasions: preoperatively, under intraarticular anesthesia and during (supposedly) a later rehabilitation phase. This irregularity which was termed 'break' by Grace et al (1984) was later mentioned in other papers (Bennett & Stauber 1986, Lysholm 1987).

In the first quantitative analysis of this phenomenon in patients with PFPS (Dvir et al 1991b) a break was defined as a perturbation in the curve which exceeded a drop of 10% or more in the magnitude of the pre-break moment. (See Figure 6.7 for explanation.)

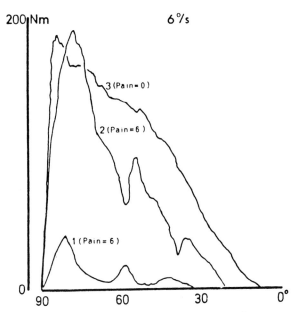

Fig. 6.6 Maximal isokinetic knee extension strength in a woman with chondromalacia of the patella. 1, before the operation; 2, before the operation and after intraarticular anesthesia; 3, at the follow-up. Rating of pain was made according to the Borg-Lindblad scale. (From Nordgren et al 1983 copyright © Springer-Verlag.)

In this study, whose design has been described earlier (Dvir et al 1991a), breaks occurred exclusively during eccentric contractions. Nearly 50% of the subjects had at least one break during the series of tests.

The break was associated with a partial relief of pain in the patellofemoral joint, at about 45° flexion, close to the value reported by Hart et al (1985), but not at 75°, which has been calculated to coincide with maximal patellofemoral joint reaction force (Kaufman et al 1991, Nisell & Ericson 1992). Whether, therefore, a different pain mechanism operates during eccentric contractions is not known at present. However, since the concentric loads, which at 30 °/s were greater than the eccentric loads at 60 °/s, were not associated with breaks, one could speculate that the underlying reason for the breaks was not the load imposed on the joint. Breaks occured predominantly during the 30 °/s test, which had the longest exposure time.

To further analyze the pain–break relationship, the average pain scores in tests which showed breaks were compared with tests which did not. Though the former were consistently higher in both genders throughout the entire spectrum of velocities, the differences were not significant. On the other hand, using an alternative analysis, it was evident that the pain provoked during a 'break contraction' was most frequently perceived as the most intense among the eccentric tests. As already mentioned in this study, the break phenomenon occured exclusively during eccentnric activity, a finding which was in accordance with Hart et al (1985) and Bennett & Stauber (1986) but at variance with the finding of Nordgren et al (1983). The reason for this discrepancy is probably the very low test velocities employed in the latter study which led to exceedingly long exposures.

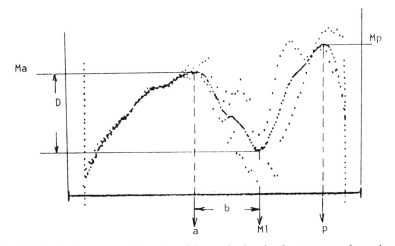

Fig. 6.7 An example of the break phenomenon. Ma—value of the maximal prebreak moment; a—the angle at which Ma occurs; ML—value of the minimal within–break moment; b—the angular displacement from a to the angle at which ML occurs; D—the difference between Ma and ML; Mp—the value of the maximal post-break moment; p—the angle at which Mp occurs.

ISOKINETIC TESTING IN PFPS
A PRELIMINARY MODEL

A combination of the three factors, significantly reduced quadriceps strength, pain, and the break phenomenon has been utilized to set up a preliminary model for analysis and interpretation of PFPS based on isokinetic testing (Dvir & Halperin 1992). Each of these factors was assigned a positive or negative value according to certain criteria, so that every subject was classified according to the following triad: strength $(+/-)$, pain $(+/-)$ and break $(+/-)$. For instance, the description '$+ + -$' meant that the subject demonstrated significant strength reduction and pain but no break. A relatively high percentage of patients, 27%, were classified as negative on all factors but this might have reflected the stringency of the criteria (Sherman et al 1987). On the other hand, 24% of the subjects were categorized as '$+ + +$' and when those classed as '$+ - +$' and '$+ + -$' were added, the percentage of patients rose to about 40%. This value is on a par with the clinical tests employed, reflecting an empirical impression among clinicians that most of the accepted techniques in diagnosing PFD are no more powerful than this. This conclusion is however very tentative and much more research is required on the interdependence of morphological, pathological and functional variables, of which muscle strength, pain and irregularity in the moment curve form an important subset.

Need for pain assessment

But even without validation of the above, or other, models, clinicians are advised that testing patients with PFPS should be supplemented with some form of pain assessment. Considerably more may be learned, clinically and functionally, than from assessment of strength or pain alone. The location of breaks and attention given to their continued presence or disappearance, during a rehabilitation process, also significantly assists in judging outcome. Figure 6.7 provides a good demonstration of this practice.

MENISCAL DISORDERS

Meniscal disorders have been studied using isokinetics, particular concerning the effect of the sur-

gical technique. During recent years, arthroscopy has become exceedingly popular for treating some of the typical meniscal disorders. In order to prove its efficacy in terms of muscle function, isokinetic analyses of thigh muscles have been performed. One of the first reports (Patel et al 1982) indicated a QQR of 88% and a much smaller hamstring deficit of 5%, one month following meniscectomy. Hamberg et al (1983) studied the effect of open and closed (arthroscopic) meniscectomy and found that:

1. Compared to the preoperative levels at the same side, there was a 40% decrease in quadriceps strength, 1 week following the operation, in patients who underwent partial or total closed meniscectomy. Normal function was recovered 8 weeks later.
2. Open meniscectomy resulted in 70% loss of quadriceps strength at 1 week and recovery was not complete after 8 weeks.
3. Flexor function was recovered one month following the intervention.

Somewhat less drastic effects but showing the same trends were reported by Prietto et al (1983). Mariani et al (1987) reported a QQR of better than 90% only 2 weeks after arthroscopic meniscectomy for medial bucket-handle tears. Flexor strength remained at preoperative levels throughout rehabilitation. The differences between the studies of Patel et al and Mariani et al, and between those of Hamberg et al and Prietto et al, may be explained by the nature of the cases involved and differing rehabilitation procedures. However, according to the available sources:

1. Arthroscopic meniscectomy is significantly less detrimental to quadriceps function compared with the open approach.
2. With the closed technique, the immediate and sharp decrease in QQR should be recovered within a period of 4–8 weeks.
3. Flexor function should not be compromised.

PART 4
ISOKINETICS FOR KNEE MUSCLE CONDITIONING

Most of the published literature concerning the isokinetics of the knee concerns muscle testing.

Less has been written concerning the application of isokinetics to muscle conditioning in clinical situations. The principles governing this aspect of isokinetics namely submaximal versus maximal muscle tension, pretensioning and grading of velocities were described in detail in Chapter 4. This section will therefore concentrate on the use of a specific modality, eccentric conditioning, which has been studied with particular respect to PFPS. The treatment, as opposed to the testing, of ACL deficiency increasingly uses functional activities. Correspondingly, there is a growing emphasis on the use of closed kinetic chain exercises involving multiple joint efforts, which has only recently been recognized by manufacturers of isokinetic systems. An attachment, for this purpose (leg press) is illustrated in Figure 6.8.

ECCENTRIC MODE TRAINING

Rationale

A novel approach to the treatment of anterior knee pain was described by Bennett & Stauber (1986). The basic tenet of their approach was that:

Errors in control of muscle function during the performance of negative work (expressed as depressed muscle forces during muscle lengthening activities) might cause varying degrees of soft tissue trauma, especially in those situations where no well-defined orthopaedic disorder could be identified.

According to this theory, a (neurophysiological) deficiency existed and its removal could alleviate the pain.

Patient selection and protocol

The clinical basis for selection of patients, other than the presence of anterior knee pain was vague. The isokinetic criterion was moment-based strength, measured at 30 °/s. The eccentric moment of the muscle, Q_{ecc}, was compared with its concentric counterpart, Q_{con}, and only those with a score of 85% or less for the ratio: Q_{ecc}/Q_{con} (at any point throughout the tested ROM) were admitted to the study group. The rehabilitation program was based on eccentric training which consisted of 3 sets of 10 repetitions at each of the velocities, 30, 60 and 90 °/s, with three sessions per week until pain was relieved.

Results

Figure 6.9 shows the relative moment–position curve for the uninvolved knee; Figure 6.10 the findings for the symptomatic knee, pretreatment, and Figure 6.11 the postreatment symptomatic knee findings. A success rate of 93% was claimed by the authors with a full reversal of the eccentric deficiency.

Though the authors were not able to offer a rigorous explanation for their findings, it was suggested that the rapid reversal of the symptoms pointed to an 'error' in the use of the eccentric component of the vastus medialis. Though the exact nature of this error was not elucidated, it was rectified by appropriate training.

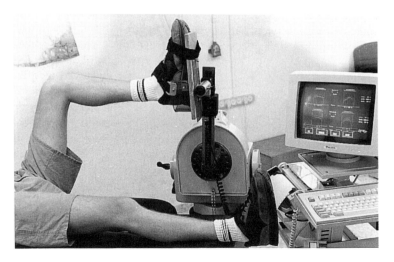

Fig. 6.8 The leg press attachment and testing position.

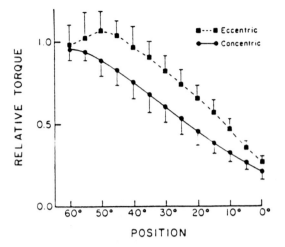

Fig. 6.9 Relative knee extension moment as a function of knee position in the unsymptomatic knee. (From Bennett & Stauber 1986 Evaluation and treatment of anterior knee pain using eccentric exercise. Medicine and Science in Sports and Exercise 18: 526–530.)

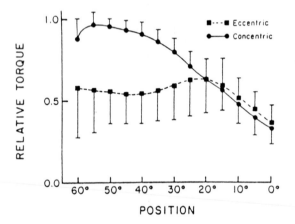

Fig. 6.10 Relative knee extension moment as a function of knee position in the symptomatic knee before treatment. (From Bennett & Stauber 1986 Evaluation and treatment of anterior knee pain using eccentric exercise. Medicine and Science in Sports and Exercise 18: 526–530.)

Limitations of the patient selection criterion

The use of the 85% Q_{ecc}/Q_{con} criterion has since been criticized (Trudelle-Jackson et al 1989), on the grounds that 35–54% of normal subjects demonstrate such deficiency. On the other hand, Conway et al (1992) have claimed that in their experimental group which consisted of 30 patients with PFPS, the Q_{ecc}/Q_{con} was never less than 0.95. In view of this, it might be concluded that Bennett & Stauber's protocol is particularly suitable for patients with a conspicuous eccentric deficency.

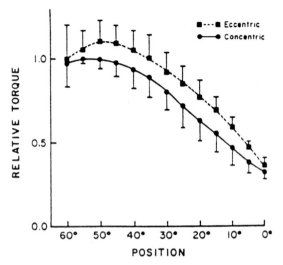

Fig. 6.11 Relative knee extension moment as a function of knee position in the symptomatic knee after treatment. (From Bennett & Stauber 1986 Evaluation and treatment of anterior knee pain using eccentric exercise. Medicine and Science in Sports and Exercise 18: 526–530.)

Support for eccentric conditioning approach

Although the patient selection process and rehabilitation protocol, of the Bennett & Stauber study are still controversial, it is one of the most innovative and intriguing among the many studies which have attempted to incorporate isokinetics as a therapeutic means. Obviously there must be support from research and accumulated experience before this approach can gain acceptance.

A study by Jensen & Di Fabio (1989) has already given some backing. These authors compared patients with patellar tendinitis with control subjects. Each group was divided into a subgroup that performed home muscle stretching exercises only, and one which received additional eccentric isokinetic exercises. The intensity of the isokinetic exercise was enhanced by gradually increasing the velocity of contraction from 30 to 70 °/s (a protocol which is not necessarily supported by current knowledge regarding the moment–angular velocity relationship). The isokinetic performance parameter was the QQR of the work done during 5 consecutive concentric–eccentric contractions at 50 °/s. The intensity and occurrence of pain were assessed.

The results indicated that subjects with patellar tendinitis increased their QQR following eccentric input, but that this increase was not significant compared with the matched group which received only stretching input. The authors have attributed this finding to pain inhibition since there was a high negative correlation between pain frequency (-0.80) and occurrence (-0.78) and QQR (work).

Severity of injury and the gender composition of the sample were also implicated. The achievement of optimal strength increases was therefore hampered by pain.

REFERENCES

Arvidsson I, Ericsson E, Haggmark T 1981 Isokinetic thigh muscle strength after ligament reconstruction in the knee joint: results from 5–10 year follow-up after reconstruction of the anterior cruciate ligament of the knee joint. International Journal of Sports Medicine 2: 7–11

Ballmer P M, Jakob R P 1988 The non-operative treatment of isolated complete tears of the medial collateral ligament of the knee. A prospective study. Archives of Orthopaedic and Traumatic Surgery 107: 273–276

Barr A E, Duncan P W 1988 Influence of position on knee flexor peak torque. Journal of Orthopaedic and Sports Physical Therapy 9: 279–283

Baugher W H, Warren R F, Marshall J L, Joseph A 1984 Quadriceps atrophy in the anterior cruciate insufficient knee. American Journal of Sports Medicine 12: 192–195

Bennett J G, Stauber W T 1986 Evaluation and treatment of anterior knee pain using eccentric exercise. Medicine and Science in Sports and Exercise 18: 526–530

Bergfeld J 1979 First, second and third degree sprains. American Journal of Sports Medicine 7: 207–209

Bohannon R W, Gajdosik R L, LeVeau B F 1986 Isokinetic knee flexion and extension torque in the upright sitting and semicircled sitting positions. Physical Therapy 66: 1083–1086

Bonamo J, Colleen F, Firestone T 1990 The conservative treatment of the anterior cruciate deficient knee. American Journal of Sports Medicine 18: 618–623

Borges O 1989 Isometric and isokinetic knee extension and flexion torque in men and women aged 20–70. Scandinavian Journal of Rehabilitation Medicine 21: 45–53

Brown L E, Whitehurst M, Bryant J R 1992 A comparison of the LIDO sliding cuff and the tibial control system in isokinetic strength parameters. Isokinetics and Exercise Science 3: 101–109

Cerullo G, Puddu G, Conteduca F, Ferretti A, Mariani P 1988 Evaluation of the results of extensor mechanism reconstruction. American Journal of Sports Medicine 16: 93–96

Colliander E B, Tesch P A 1989 Bilateral eccentric and concentric torque of quadriceps and hamstrings muscles in females and males. European Journal of Applied Physiology 59: 227–232

Constantin R, Williams A K 1984 Isokinetic quadriceps and hamstring torque level of adolescent female soccer players. Journal of Orthopaedic and Sports Physical Therapy 5: 196–200

Conway A, Malone T R, Conway P 1992 Patellar alignment/tracking: effect on force output and perceived pain. Isokinetics and Exercise Science 2: 9–17

Crocker B, Stauber W T 1989 Objective analysis of quadriceps force during bracing of the patellae: a preliminary study. Australian Journal of Medicine and Science in Sport 10: 25–28

Currier D P 1977 Positioning for knee strengthening exercises. Physical Therapy 57: 148–151

Davies G J, Halbach J W, Carpenter M A 1980 A descriptive muscular strength and power analysis of the US cross-country ski team. Medicine and Science in Sports and Exercise 12: 141

De Carlo M S, Shelbourne K D, McCarroll J R, Rettig A C 1992 Traditional versus accelerated rehabilitation following ACL reconstruction: a one-year follow-up. Journal of Orthopaedic and Sports Physical Therapy 15: 309–316

Dvir Z, Halperin N 1992 Patellofemoral pain syndrome: a preliminary model for analysis and interpretation of isokinetic and pain parameters. Clinical Biomechanics 7: 240–245

Dvir Z, Eger G, Halperin N, Shklar A 1989 Thigh muscle activity and anterior cruciate ligament insufficiency. Clinical Biomechanics 4: 87–91

Dvir Z, Shklar A, Halperin N, Robinson D 1990 Concentric and eccentric torque variations of the quadriceps femoris in patellofemoral pain syndrome. Clinical Biomechanics 5: 68–72

Dvir Z, Halperin N, Shklar A, Robinson D 1991a Quadriceps function and patellofemoral pain syndrome. Part I: pain provocation during concentric and eccentric isokinetic contractions. Isokinetics and Exercise Science 1: 26–30

Dvir Z, Halperin N, Shklar A, Robinson D 1991b Quadriceps function and patellofemoral pain syndrome. Part II: the break phenomenon during eccentric contractions. Isokinetics and Exercise Science 1: 31–35

Elmqvist L-G, Lorentzon R, Langstrom M, Fugl-Meyer A R 1988 Reconstruction of the anterior cruciate ligament: long term effects of different knee angles at primary immobilization and different modes of early training. American Journal of Sports Medicine 16: 455–462

Elmqvist L-G, Lorentzon R, Johansson C, Langstrom M, Fagerlund M, Fugl-Meyer A 1989 Knee extensor muscle function before and after reconstruction of anterior cruciate ligament tear. Scandinavian Journal of Rehabilitation Medicine 21: 131–139

Elton K, McDonough K, Savinar E, Jensen G 1985 A preliminary investigation: History, physical and isokinetic exam results versus arthroscopic diagnosis of chondromalacia patella. Journal of Orthopaedic and Sports Physical Therapy 7: 115–121

Figoni S F, Christ C B, Massey B H 1988 Effects of speed, hip and knee angle, and gravity on hamstring to quadriceps torque ratio. Journal of Orthopaedic and Sports Physical Therapy 9: 297–291

Fillyaw M, Bevins T, Fernandez L 1986 Importance of correcting isokinetic peak torque for the effect of gravity when calculating knee flexor to extensor muscle ratios. Physical Therapy 66: 23–29

Freedson P S, Gilliam T B, Mahoney T, Maliszweski A F, Kastango K 1993 Industrial torque levels by age group and gender. Isokinetics and Exercise Science 3: 34–42

Fu F H, Woo S, Irrgang J 1992 Current concepts for rehabilitation following anterior cruciate ligament reconstruction. Journal of Orthopaedic and Sports Physical Therapy 15: 270–278

Ghena D R, Kuth A L, Thomas M, Mayhew J 1991 Torque characteristics of the quadriceps and hamstring muscles during concentric and eccentric loading. Journal of Orthopaedic and Sports Physical Therapy 14: 149–154

Gilliam T B, Sandy S P, Freedson P S 1979 Isokinetic torque levels for high school football players. Archives of Physical Medicine and Rehabilitation 60: 110–114

Goodfellow J, Hungerford D S, Zindel M 1976 Patellofemoral joint mechanics and pathology. Part I: Functional anatomy of the patellofemoral joint. Journal of Bone and Joint Surgery 58B: 287–290

Grace T G, Sweetser E R, Nelson M A, Ydens L R, Skipper B J 1984 Isokinetic muscle imbalance and knee joint injury. Journal of Bone and Joint Surgery 66A: 734–740

Grana W A, Kriegshauser L A 1985 Scientific basis of extensor mechanism disorders. Clinics in Sports Medicine 4: 247–257

Gross M T, McGrain P, Demilio P, Plyler L 1989 Relationship between multiple predictor variables and normal knee torque production. Physical Therapy 69: 54–62

Hageman P A, Gillaspie D M, Hill L D 1988 Effects of speed and limb dominance on eccentric and concentric isokinetic testing of the knee. Journal of Orthopaedic and Sports Physical Therapy 10: 59–65

Hall P S, Roofner M A 1991 Velocity spectrum study of knee flexion and extension in normal adults: 60 to 500 deg/sec. Isokinetics and Exercise Science 1: 131–137

Halperin N, Dvir Z 1993 Arthroscopic hamstring loop reconstruction combined with ITB strip tenodesis. In: The Ninth International Jerusalem Symposium on Sports Injuries

Hamberg P, Gillquist J, Lysholm J, Oberg B 1983 The effect of diagnostic and operative arthroscopy and open meniscectomy on muscle strength in the thigh. American Journal of Sports Medicine 11: 289–292

Hanten W P, Ramber C L 1988 Effect of stabilization on maximal isokinetic torque of the quadriceps femoris muscle during concentric and eccentric contractions. Physical Therapy 68: 219–222

Hart D L, Stobbe T J, Till C W 1984 Effect of trunk stabilization on quadriceps femoris muscle torque. Physical Therapy 64: 375–380

Hart D L, Miller L C, Stauber W T 1985 Effect of cooling on voluntary eccentric force oscillations during maximal contractions. Experimental Neurology 90: 73–80

Hastings D E 1980 The non-operative management of collateral ligament injuries of the knee joint. Clinical Orthopaedics and Related Research 147: 22–28

Highgenboten C L, Jackson A W, Meske N B 1988 Concentric and eccentric torque comparisons for knee extension and flexion in young adult males and females using the Kinetic Communicator. American Journal of Sports Medicine 16: 234–237

Hoke B, Howell D, Stack M 1983 The relationship between isokinetic testing and dynamic patellofemoral compression. Journal of Orthopaedic and Sports Physical Therapy 4: 150–153

Insall J 1981 Patellar pain. Journal of Bone and Joint Surgery 64A:147–152

Jensen K, Di Fabio R 1989 Evaluation of eccentric exercise in treatment of patellar tendinitis. Physical Therapy 69: 211–216

Johansson C, Lorentzon R, Fugl-Meyer A R 1989 Isokinetic muscular performance of the quadriceps in elite ice hockey players. American Journal of Sports Medicine 17: 30–34

Johnson D 1982 Controlling anterior shear during isokinetic knee extension exercise. Journal of Orthopaedic and Sports Physical Therapy 4: 10–15

Kannus P 1988a Ratio of hamstring to quadriceps femoris muscles' strength in the anterior cruciate ligament insufficient knee: relationship to long term recovery. Physical Therapy 68: 961–965

Kannus P 1988b Knee flexor and extensor strength ratios with deficiency of the lateral collateral ligament. Archives of Physical Medicine and Rehabilitation 69: 928–931

Kannus P 1990 Relationship between peak torque, peak angular impulse and average power in the thigh muscles of subjects with knee damage. Research Quarterly 60: 141–145

Kannus P, Jarvinen M 1991 Thigh muscle function after partial tear of the medial ligament compartment of the knee. Medicine and Science in Sports and Exercise 23: 4–9

Kannus P, Jarvinen M, Johnson R, Renstrom P, Pope M, Beynnon B, Nichols C, Kaplan M 1992 Function of the quadriceps and hamstring muscles in knees with chronic partial deficiency of the anterior cruciate ligament. American Journal of Sports Medicine 20: 162–168

Kaufman K R, An K, Litchy W J, Morrey B F, Chao E Y 1991 Dynamic knee joint forces during isokinetic exercise. American Journal of Sports Medicine 19: 305–316

Kirkendall D T, Berfeld I, Calbrese J A 1984 Isokinetic characteristics of ballet dancers and the response to a season of ballet training. Journal of Orthopaedic and Sports Physical Therapy 5: 207–211

Klopfer D A, Greij S D 1988 Examining quadriceps/hamstrings performance at high velocity isokinetics in untrained subjects. Journal of Orthopaedic and Sports Physical Therapy 10: 18–22

Kramer J F, Hill K, Jones I C, Sandrin M, Vyse M 1989 Effect of dynamometer application arm length on concentric and eccentric torques during isokinetic knee extension. Physiotherapy Canada 41: 100–106

Kues J M, Rothstein J M, Lam R L 1992 Obtaining reliable measurements of knee extensor torque produced during maximal voluntary contractions: an experimental investigation. Physical Therapy 72: 492–504

Leeuw G H F, Stam H J, Nieuwenhuyzen J F 1989 Correction for gravity in isokinetic dynamometry of knee extensors in below knee amputees. Scandinavian Journal of Rehabilitation Medicine 21: 141–145

Lopresti C, Kirkendall D T, Street G M, Dudley A W 1988 Quadriceps insufficiency following repair of the anterior cruciate ligament. Journal of Orthopaedic and Sports Physical Therapy 9: 245–249

Lysholm J 1987 The relation between pain and torque in an isokinetic strength test of knee extension. Arthroscopy 3: 182–184

Lysholm J, Nordin M, Ekstrand J, Gillquist J 1984 The effect of a patellar brace on performance in a knee extension strength test in patients with patellar pain. American Journal of Sports Medicine 12: 110–112

MacIntyre D, Wessel J 1988 Knee muscles torque in patellofemoral pain syndrome. Physiotherapy Canada 40: 20–24

Magnusson P, Geismar R, McHugh M, Gleim G, Nicholas J 1992 The effect of trunk stabilization on knee extension/flexion torque production. Journal of Orthopaedic and Sports Physical Therapy 15: 51–52

Malone T R, Garrett W E 1992 Commentary and historical perspective of anterior cruciate ligament rehabilitation. Journal of Orthopaedic and Sports Physical Therapy 15: 265–269

Mangine R E, Noyes F R 1992 Rehabilitation of the allograft reconstruction. Journal of Orthopaedic and Sports Physical Therapy 15: 294–302

Mariani P P, Caruso I 1979 An electromyographic investigation of subluxation of the patella. Journal of Bone and Joint Surgery 61B: 169–171

Mariani P P, Ferretti A, Gigli C, Puddu G 1987 Isokinetic

evaluation of the knee after arthroscopic meniscectomy: comparison between anterolateral and central approaches. Arthroscopy: 123–126

Marshall J L, Warren R F, Wickiewicz T L, Reider B 1979 The anterior cruciate ligament: a technique of repair and reconstruction. Clinical Orthopaedics 143: 97–104

Moller R N, Krebs R, Tidemand-Dal C, Aaris K 1986 Isometric contractions in the patellofemoral pain syndrome: an electromyographic study. Archives of Orthopaedic and Traumatic Surgery 105: 24–27

Morris A, Lussier L, Bell G 1983 Hamstring/quadriceps strength ratios in collegiate middle-distance and distance runners. The Physician and Sports Medicine 11: 71–77

Murray P M, Gardner G M, Mollinger L A, Sepic S B 1980 Strength of isometric and isokinetic contractions. Physical Therapy 60: 412–419

Murray S M, Warren R F, Otis J C, Kroll M, Wickiewicz T L 1984 Torque–velocity relationships of the knee extensor and flexor muscles in individuals sustaining injuries of the anterior cruciate ligament. American Journal of Sports Medicine 12: 436–440

Nisell R 1985 Mechanics of the knee: A study of joint load and muscle activity with clinical implications. Acta Orthopaedica Scandinavica, Supplement 216

Nisell R, Nemeth G, Ohlsen H 1986 Joint forces in extension of the knee. Acta Orthopaedica Scandinavica 57: 41–46

Nisell R, Ericson M O, Nemeth G, Ekholm J 1989 Tibio-femoral joint forces during isokinetic knee extension. American Journal of Sports Medicine 17: 49–54

Nisell R, Ericson M 1992 Patellar forces during isokinetic knee extension. Clinical Biomechanics 7: 104–108

Nordgren B, Nordesjo L-O, Rauschning W 1983 Isokinetic knee extension strength and pain before and after advancement osteotomy of the tibial tuberosity. Archives of Orthopaedic and Traumatic Surgery 102: 95–101

Nunn K D, Mayhew J L 1988 Comparison of three methods of assessing strength imbalances at the knee. Journal of Orthopaedic and Sports Physical Therapy 10: 134–137

Osternig L R, Hamill J, Sawhill J, Bates B T 1983 Influence of torque and limb speed on power production in isokinetic exercise. American Journal of Physical Medicine 62: 163–171

Paolos L E, Noyes F R, Grood E S 1983 Knee rehabilitation after anterior cruciate ligament reconstruction and repair. American Journal of Sports Medicine 9: 140–149

Patel D, Fahmy N, Sakayan A 1982 Isokinetic and functional evaluation of the knee following arthroscopic surgery. Clinical Orthopaedics and Related Research 167: 84–91

Pavonee E, Moffat M 1985 Isometric torque of the quadriceps femoris after concentric eccentric and isometric training. Archives of Physical Medicine and Rehabilitation 66: 168–170

Prietto C A, Caiozzo V J, Prietto P P, McMaster W C Closed versus open partial meniscectomy: postoperative changes in the force–velocity relationship of muscle. American Journal of Sports Medicine 11: 189–194

Rizzardo M, Bay G, Wessel J 1988 Eccentric and concentric torque and power of the knee extensors of females. Canadian Journal of Sports Sciences 13: 166–169

Rosenberg T D, Franklin J L, Baldwin G N, Nelson K A 1992 Extensor machanism function after patellar tendon graft harvest for anterior cruciate ligament reconstruction. American Journal of Sports Medicine 20: 519–526

Sczepanski T L, Gross M T, Duncan W P, Chandler J M 1991 Effect of contraction type angular velocity and arc of motion on VMO:VL EMG ratio. Journal of Orthopaedic and Sports Physical Therapy 14: 256–262

Seto J L, Orofino A S, Morrissey M C, Medeiros J M, Mason W J 1988 Assessment of quadriceps/hamstring strength, knee ligament stability, functional and sports activity levels five years after anterior cruciate ligament reconstruction. American Journal of Sports Medicine 16: 170–180

Shelbourne K D, Nitz P 1990 Accelerated rehabilitation after anterior cruciate ligament reconstruction. American Journal of Sports Medicine 18: 292–299

Shelbourne K D, Porter D A 1992 Anterior cruciate ligament – medial collateral ligament injury: nonoperative management of medial collateral ligament tears with anterior cruciate ligament reconstruction. American Journal of Sports Medicine 20: 283–286

Shelbourne K D, Klootwyk T E, DeCarlo M S 1992 Update on accelerated rehabilitation after anterior cruciate ligament reconstruction. Journal of Orthopaedic and Sports Physical Therapy 15: 303–308

Shelton G L, Thigpen K 1991 Rehabilitation of patellofemoral dysfunction: a review of literature. Journal of Orthopaedic and Sports Physical Therapy 14: 243–249

Sherman O H, Fox J M, Sperling H, Del Pizzo W, Friedman M J, Snyder S J, Ferkel R D 1987 Patellar instability: treatment by arthroscopic electrosurgical lateral release. Arthroscopy 3: 152–160

Siewert M W, Ariki P W, Davies G J, Rowinski M J 1975 Isokinetic torque changes based upon lever arm pad placement. Physical Therapy 65: 715

Smidt G L 1973 Biomechanical analysis of knee flexion and extension. Journal of Biomechanics 6: 79–92

Smith D J, Quinney H A, Wenger H A 1981 Isokinetic torque output of professional and amateur ice hockey players. Journal of Orthopaedic and Sports Physical Therapy 3: 42–47

Solomonow M, Baratta R, Zhou B H, Shoji H, Bose W, Beck C, D'Ambrosia R 1987 The synergistic action of the anterior cruciate ligament and thigh muscles in maintaining joint stability. American Journal of Sports Medicine 15: 207–213

Souza D R, Gross M T 1991 Comparison of VMO:VL integrated electromyographic ratios between healthy subjects and patients with patellofemoral pain. Physical Therapy 71: 310–320

Taunton J E, Clement D B, Smart C W, McNichol K L 1987 Nonsurgical management of overuse knee injuries in runners. Canadian Journal of Sports Science 12: 11–18

Taylor R L, Casey J J 1986 Quadriceps torque production on the Cybex II dynamometer as related to changes in lever arm length. Journal of Orthopaedic and Sports Physical Therapy 8: 148–152

Tegner Y, Lysholm J, Lysholm M, Gillquist J 1986 Strengthening exercises for old cruciate ligament tears. Acta Orthopaedica Scandinavica 57: 130–134

Thorstensson A, Grimby G, Karlsson J 1976 Force–velocity relations and fiber composition in human knee extensor muscles. Journal of Applied Physiology 40: 12–16

Timm K 1985 Validation of the Johnson anti-shear accessory as an accurate and effective clinical instrument. Journal of Orthpaedic and Sports Physical Therapy 7: 298–303

Timm K 1988 Postsurgical knee rehabilitation: a five year study of four methods and 5381 patients. American Journal of Sports Medicine 16: 463–468

Trudelle-Jackson E, Meske N, Highenboten C, Jackson A 1989 Eccentric/concentric torque deficits in the quadriceps muscle. Journal of Orthopaedic and Sports Physical Therapy 11: 142–145

Vegso J J, Genuario S E, Torg J S (1985) Maintenance of hamstring strength following knee surgery. Medicine and Science in Sports and Exercise 17: 376–379

Walla D J, Albright J P, McAuley E, Martin R K, Eldridge V, El-Khoury G 1985 Hamstring control and the unstable anterior cruciate ligament-deficient knee. American Journal of Sports Medicine 13: 34–39

Westing S H, Seger J Y, Karlson E 1988 Eccentric and concentric torque velocity characteristics of the quadriceps femoris in man. European Journal of Applied Physiology 58: 100–104

Wild J, Franklin T, Woods G 1982 Patellar pain and quadriceps rehabilitation: an EMG study. American Journal of Sports Medicine 10: 12–15

Wilk K E, Andrews J R 1992 Current concepts in the treatment of anterior cruciate ligament disruption. Journal of Orthopaedic and Sports Physical Therapy 15: 279–293

Worrell T W, Perrin D H, Denrgar C R 1989 The influence of hip position on quadriceps and hamstring peak torque and reciprocal muscle group ratio values. Journal of Orthopaedic and Sports Physical Therapy 11: 104–107

Worrell T W, Denegar C R, Armstrong S L, Perrin D H 1990 Effect of body position on hamstring muscle group average torque. Journal of Orthopaedic and Sports Physical Therapy 11: 449–452

Worrell T W, Perrin D H, Gansneder B M, Gieck J H 1991 Comparison of isokinetic strength and flexibility measures between hamstring injured and noninjured athletes. Journal of Orthopaedic and Sports Physical Therapy 13: 118–125

Wyatt M P, Edwards A M 1981 Comparison of quadriceps and hamstring torque values during isokinetic exercise. Journal of Orthopaedic and Sports Physical Therapy 3: 48–56

Yasuda K, Ohkoshi Y, Tanabe Y, Kaneda K 1992 Quantitative evaluation of knee instability and muscle thigh strength after anterior cruciate ligament reconstruction using patellar quadriceps tendon. American Journal of Sports Medicine 20: 471–475

CHAPTER 7

Isokinetics of the ankle muscles

Among the major articulations of the lower limb, the talocrural–subtalar joint complex has received moderate attention, more than that accorded the hip, but receiving less interest than the knee, which became the paradigm for isokinetics-related research and clinical practice. With its relatively short, polyarticulated distal 'segment', its variety of movements, and the number of muscles spanning it, the ankle poses difficulties not shared by the hip and knee. These problems are reflected in procedural issues like positioning and alignment of axes, and by substantive issues such as closed versus open kinetic chain testing.

Little work has been done on the clinical applicability of ankle isokinetics. This is indeed surprising, given the high incidence of trauma, particularly ankle sprains which account for 85% of all ankle injuries (Garrick 1977). (A total of 70% of young basketball players have a history of sprain with an 80% recurrence rate (Smith & Reischl 1986).) Some explanation may be found in the already mentioned problems of positioning and stabilization of patients suffering from ankle trauma. In addition, reconstructive surgery, which played a decisive role in the development of knee, isokinetics lags behind with respect to the ankle. It is also true that the muscular machinery of the knee is much simpler than that of the ankle; the difficulty in evaluating the separate contributions of the various muscles operating in the ankle is a substantial practical obstacle.

The topics covered in this chapter are: the procedures for testing the ankle complex; the reproducibility of test findings; representative values, and interpretation and clinical significance.

PART 1
ISOKINETIC TESTING OF ANKLE MUSCLES

Measurement of ankle performance involves testing of dorsiflexion and plantarflexion, commonly known as ankle (talocrural) movements, and inversion and eversion, the subtalar movements. The following elements are considered in this section:

1. the tested range of motion (ROM)
2. positioning and stabilization
3. alignment of biological and mechanical axes, and
4. test velocities.

TESTING OF DORSIFLEXION AND PLANTARFLEXION

Test ROM

The ROM for dorsiflexion and plantarflexion is measured relative to the neutral position (0°) of the foot. The values commonly quoted for measurement range from 10 to 30° for dorsiflexion, and from 40 to 65° for plantarflexion. The normative ROM for dorsiflexion is 20°, while for plantarflexion it is 45°–50° (Miller 1985). An isokinetic test ROM for dorsiflexion–plantar flexion movements has very seldom been mentioned. In one study (Herlant et al 1992), the full ROM was quoted as being between 55 and 75°, depending on the test velocity and the clinical status of the limb. Clearly the tested ROM in this study coincided with the normal ROM.

Angle of peak moment

Some studies have investigated the angular position of the ankle associated with peak moment, for healthy subjects or patients, and either dorsi- or plantarflexion. As already indicated, this information is essential for decisions regarding the extent of tested ROM.

In a study by Fischer (1982) the isometric strength was measured every 6° from the position of maximal dorsiflexion (here defined as 0°). It was found that the greatest isometric strength of the plantarflexors was achieved at maximal dorsiflexion, where the triceps surae was most lengthened. On the other hand, the dorsiflexors reached maximum strength at 36°, corresponding to approximately 16° of plantarflexion (measured from the neutral position).

Sjostrom et al (1978) indicated that in the unaffected leg of patients who were treated for Achilles tendon rupture, the angle of peak moment shifted towards 30° upon increasing the test velo-

city from 30 to 180°/s. Gerdle et al (1988) applied a similar experimental protocol in a study which involved healthy subjects. The corresponding range was between 24 and 31°, practically identical to the results of Sjostrom et al.

Recommended ROM for testing

Functionally the typical ankle ROM during walking, corresponds to 10° dorsiflexion and 20° plantarflexion (McPoil & Knecht 1985), and for running (Soutas-Little et al 1987) it is 20° dorsiflexion and 25° plantarflexion. It is clear that the tested ROM need not correspond to the total ROM. A ROM of 45°, starting from maximal dorsiflexion, is sufficient for strength and endurance testing of both dorsiflexors and plantarflexors. Failure to ensure maximal dorsiflexion will result in a submaximal score for the plantarflexors.

Positioning and stabilization

Positioning and stabilization are cardinal issues whose importance in the reproducibility and validity of ankle isokentic testing cannot be overstated. Almost the entire repertoire of the plantarflexors consists of coupled eccentric–concentric contractions. These take place during weight–bearing in activities such as the propulsive phases of walking and running, and stair climbing and descending. Additionally, at certain times during these activities, ankle plantarflexors are a component of a closed kinetic chain (CKC) comprising the knee and hip of the ipsilateral limb as well as all articulations of the contralateral limb.

Kinematic analysis of the lower limb in ambulation reveals that during the propulsive phase the knee is in a near extended position. This may not be equally applicable in stair climbing and descending, where the pitch of the individual step determines the extent of knee flexion, which can reach 60° (Diffrient et al 1974). However it should be borne in mind that even placing the ball of the foot on the stair allows significant dorsiflexion and this helps to offset the loss of gastrocnemius length. Consequently, testing in the position of slight/moderate knee flexion may be logical.

Positioning for plantarflexion

In principle, the plantarflexors could be tested in the upright position, although this would be very awkward and even impractical with most isokinetic systems. For this purpose, the resistance pad would be placed on the shoulders, and the subject would tiptoe (uni- or bilaterally) while the axial skeleton was kept fully erect and stabilized. Assuming minimal spinal arching and/or shoulder sagging, the force developed by the plantarflexors would be easily determinable. However, quite apart from other obstacles, there would be obvious difficulties where the patient could not exert sufficient force in order to tiptoe , or the net force was so small that a reliable measurement could not be obtained.

This means that testing must be performed in the supine or prone positions, since in the long-seated position hamstring tension would detrimentally affect the gastrocnemius. However, testing in the horizontal position has the conspicuous drawback that it bears no resemblance to the functional position of the plantarflexors: The element of weight-bearing and the CKC configuration are missing.

Positioning for dorsiflexion

Positioning for dorsiflexion is more straightforward since the dorsiflexors are not involved in weight-bearing. Moreover, their function, which is to prepare the foot for the initial contact of the stance phase of locomotion is strictly part of an open kinetic chain activity. Thus positioning for dorsiflexor testing is the same as that described for plantarflexors.

Research on positioning

The majority of studies of plantar- and dorsiflexor performance have used horizontal positioning (Fig. 7.1), predominantly supine, with varying hip and knee extension (Fulg-Meyer et al 1980, 1981, Nistor 1981, Karnofel et al 1989, Seymour & Bacharach 1990, Herlant et al 1992). The prone (Gerdle et al 1986, Oberg et al 1987) and seated (Wennerberg 1991, Bobbert & Van Ingen Schenau 1990) positions have also been used. In one study which specifically analyzed dorsiflexor strength, sitting with knees at 90° was the position of choice (Backman & Oberg 1989).

The effect of positioning and test velocity on the strength of plantarflexors was studied by Fugl-Meyer et al (1979) and more recently by Seymour &

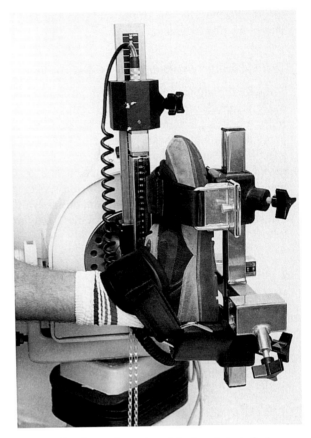

Fig. 7.1 Attachment for testing of dorsi- and plantarflexion muscles. Supine test position.

Bacharach (1990). In the former study it was found that at higher velocities strength was higher by 10–15% when the knee was in extension compared to 90° of flexion.

In the study of Seymour & Bacharach, three test positions were analyzed: (a) supine with knee extended; (b) supine with knee at 90°, and (c) prone with knee extended. Findings indicated that plantarflexion strength scores were highest when subjects were supine with knee in full extension. Strength was less in positions (b) and (c). This observation was valid at all three test velocities. The authors suggested that the low strength scores in supine/ knee flexed position resulted from shortening of the gastrocnemius.

However in another study, contrary to these findings, different knee positions did not result in any appreciable variations in plantarflexion strength (Svantesson et al 1991). These authors were not able to offer any explanation of their results but did speculate about the role of the soleus as the prime mover for plantarflexion.

Optimal position for testing plantar- and dorsiflexion

Though the supine/knee extended position obviously favors greater measured strength, it is currently not clear if and how supine (or semirecumbent) positioning with knee flexed at 45°, would affect the results, although some manufacturers recommend this position. In conclusion, the optimal position for plantar- and dorsiflexion testing is supine with the knee in full extension, or nearly full extension for subjects/patients who may find the former inconvenient.

Stabilization

The foot, shank and thigh must all be stabilized, and appropriate foot platforms, bolsters and straps are provided by manufacturers. If stabilization is not carried out properly higher strength scores may be obtained, possibly due to substitutions (Oberg et al 1987)

A recommended position for plantarflexion testing

One position which the present author has found to be both simple to apply and highly reproducible (unpublished data) relates to the performance of the plantarflexors (gastrocnemius in shortened position). The subject, in the seated position, exerts a maximal force against the resistance pad which rests on the knee (Fig. 7.2). The foot has an initial position of maximal, dorsiflexion adjustable by a screw located underneath the footplate. The range of motion is determined by asking the subject to maximally plantarflex the foot. Testing is very easily carried out in both concentric and eccentric modes.

Moreover, this set-up can be correctly described as a closed kinetic chain because of the fixed kinematic relationships of the various articulations, from the metatarsophalangeal up to the knee and the machine actuator axis.

Alignment of the biological and mechanical axes

The movements of plantar- and dorsiflexion do not pose any difficulties of alignment since the location

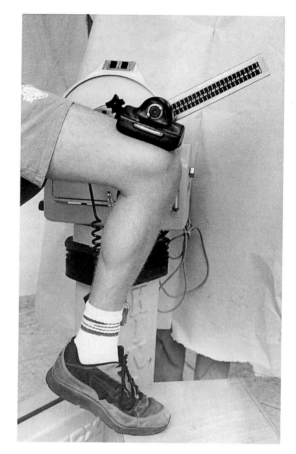

Fig. 7.2 Alternative position for testing of plantarflexion muscles.

of the biological axis is well defined. This axis is considered to pass through the malleoli (Inman 1976), forming an angle of approximately 80° with the longitudinal axis of the tibia.

Alignment should therefore be carried out with respect to an imaginary axis which connects the malleoli. A secondary alignment, to take into account the offset angle of 10° from the tibia, is, for all intents and purposes, unnecessary.

Test velocities

A fairly wide variety of velocities has been reported for plantar- and dorsiflexion testing. For instance Bobbert & Van Ingen Schenau (1990) measured plantarflexor strength at 30–300 °/s, while Backman & Oberg (1989) used the range 30–240 °/s to measure dorsiflexion strength. One reason for using high velocities is to make the testing situation comparable with the functional velocity. For instance, velocities of 150–200 °/s have been reported to occur during ankle plantarflexion in terminal stance (Sutherland et al 1980). However, the most commonly used velocities are within the range 30–180°/s.

Whether velocities higher than 30 °/s are required depends on the mechanical parameter (eg. peak moment or mean power) being used as the test criterion.

Peak moment as test criterion

In a study which compared plantarflexion strength at three different velocities, 0, 30 and 180 °/s it was found that the moment developed at 30 °/s exceeded the isometric moment. There was also a drastic reduction in the strength at 180 °/s (Seymour & Bacharach 1990). A parallel observation was made by Karnofel et al (1989), though with respect to a narrower range of velocities. Plantarflexor strength at 60°/s was almost twice that which was recorded at 120 °/s. Two possible reasons for these findings are that medium velocities (120–180 °/s) may be too high for plantarflexors, and the ROM may be too short.

Stretch–shortening cycle These arguments cannot fully explain the results obtained in a study by Svantesson et al (1991) which looked into the strength developed by the plantarflexors during a stretch–shortening cycle (SSC). The concentric plantarflexor strength was compared in two experimental situations: first as a result of a single concentric contraction and second, as a result of a concentric contraction which immediately followed (0.03 s) an eccentric contraction. It was found that the moments (near the neutral position of the ankle) in the second case were twice the moments developed by the single concentric contraction, for both angular velocities, 120 and 240 °/s. Moreover, plantarflexor moments in SSC-based concentric contractions were minimally affected by test velocity, whereas those developed during a single contraction showed a clear dependence on velocity. It should however be pointed out that, compared with other studies (e.g. Fugl-Meyer 1981) the magnitudes of the SSC moments were very small.

Dorsiflexor strength When the dorsiflexors are tested concentrically, the moment–angular velocity relationship shows a trend similar to that for the plantarflexors. Backman & Oberg (1989) examined this point in a group of children 6–15 years of age. The decline in concentric strength with an increase in test velocity was not as dramatic as in plantarflexor testing, but the general impression obtained from this study is of a similar effectiveness of testing using low velocities. It is unfortunate that eccentric testing of the dorsiflexors has not been properly reported, since this contraction mode is of particular importance in the loading response of the stance phase of locomotion.

Mean power as test criterion

However, mean power may be the test criterion, and its maximum is reached at medium/high velocities. In two studies (Fulg-Meyer et al 1982, Gerdle & Fugl-Meyer 1985), the mechanical output of the plantarflexors was examined in relation to the velocities employed and the electrical output (iEMG). It was found that although the strength and total work declined according to the usual moment–velocity relationship, the mean power peaked at 180 °/s. It thus appears that the velocity associated greatest mean power coincides with the velocity for functional demands, namely walking and running.

Conclusion

The above studies lead to the conclusion that: a strength-related protocol which does not incorporate SSC activity should consist of low test velocities. Alternatively, if the protocol is power-related or if testing is performed in SSC mode the velocities used could be in the medium range. (In the latter case the availability of an active dynamometer is taken for granted).

It is however clear that the use of very high velocities, i.e. exceeding 300 °/s, is of no especial relevance to the ankle complex.

TESTING OF INVERSION AND EVERSION

Test ROM

The movements of inversion and eversion take place in the subtalar joint. In more than one way they are more complex than dorsiflexion and plantarflexion. Inversion results from the combined foot movements of supination, adduction and plantarflexion which occur about the longitudinal, vertical and coronal axes respectively. Eversion is similarly a combination of pronation, abduction and dorsiflexion (Norkin & Levangie 1983). Large individual variations exist in the inclination of the inversion–eversion axis, but a commonly accepted description is that of Manter (1946), according to whom this axis is inclined 42° superioanteriorly and 16° medially, from the transverse and sagittal planes respectively. The ROM about this axis has been described as being between 30 and 50° in inversion, and between 15 and 20° in eversion (Miller 1985). Surprisingly, only one study (Simoneau 1990) has referred explicitly to the tested ROM, quoting an average figure of 82°. Furthermore, there has been no indication regarding the specific angle at which the peak moment was recorded. On the other hand, the use of targets placed at both ends of the active inversion–eversion ROM has been shown to assist subjects in generating a more consistent maximal effort (Leslie et al 1990). In the absence of specific information, it is recommended that the test ROM is the patient's active ROM.

Positioning and stabilization for inversion and eversion

Correct positioning for inversion–eversion testing is as crucial as it is for dorsi- and plantarflexion although some of the difficulties of the latter are absent. In both movement patterns knee position has a significant effect. It has been shown that because of the location of their insertions and line of action, the lateral and medial hamstrings can exert a significant tibial torque component (Osternig et al 1980). This, in turn, may amplify the moment generated by the invertor and evertor muscles. It has been indicated that tibial rotation can be better restrained in the 'close-packed' position of the knee, which takes place near or at full extension (Frankel & Nordin 1980). Consequently, measurement of the moment of the evertors and invertors in this position is likely to be more accurate than testing in a 'loose-packed' position.

Close- or loose-packed positioning

To examine this theory, Lentell et al (1988) studied

the moments generated by the invertors and evertors in two different knee angles. In both testing conditions the subject was in the supine position with the hips flexed at 80°. However, whereas for the loose-packed ankle joint position the knee of the tested side was in 70° of flexion, in the close-packed position it was in 10° of flexion. This meant that in the latter case the leg was actually suspended. This was associated with a significant drop in hamstring motor unit activity as shown by EMG. It was suggested that testing in the loose-packed position results in artificially higher invertor–evertor strength because of considerable substitution from the hamstring and other tibial rotators. Hence testing of the invertors and evertors should be conducted in the close-packed position except when it is contraindicated, as in sciatica or tight hamstring.

A survey of studies dealing with isokinetic testing of these muscle groups reveals that the close-packed position was also employed by Karnofel et al (1989), Leslie et al (1990) and Cawthorn et al (1991). Testing in the loose-packed position was used by Wong et al (1984), Simoneau (1990) and Gross &

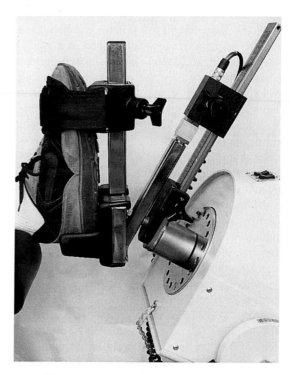

Fig. 7.3 Attachment for testing of inversion and eversion muscles. Supine test position.

Brugnolotti (1992). Since both, methods of positioning offer good to excellent reliability (Cawthorn et al 1991, Simoneau 1990) the decision on which method to employ is based on:

1. clinical contraindications as mentioned above
2. the higher validity of the closed-packed position
3. specific attachments provided by the manufacturer
4. the need to consult representative values and the methods employed in the respective sources.

Angle of plantarflexion

Another issue related to positioning concerns the angle of dorsi- or plantarflexion during the test. Inversion–eversion strength has been measured in three positions, 10° of plantarflexion, 0° (neutral) and 10° of dorsiflexion (Cawthorn et al 1991). In the supine/knee extended position, 10° of plantarflexion was not only associated with the greatest peak moments but the reproducibility of the test findings was highest, for both inversion and eversion. On the other hand, Leslie et al (1990) failed to find any significant variation in inversion–eversion strength between the positions of 0 and 20° of plantarflexion. The latter position probably produced an overlengthened configuration of the plantarflexors. Therefore, the question of ankle position in terms of the plantarflexion angle cannot be currently resolved, although it seems that slight plantarflexion would benefit strength production by these muscles.

Recommended positioning

To summarize, in the absence of limitations or contraindications a single evaluation of inversion–eversion performance should preferably be performed in the close-packed position. If follow-up is intended or other structures are involved the position, close or loose-packed should be determined according to the patient's safety and comfort. The ankle should be maintained at an angle of 10° of plantarflexion.

Stabilization

Stabilization of the subject, in both the supine or semirecumbent/seated position, involves positioning the foot in the attachment with the use of Velcro straps to ensure minimal movement of the foot. The lower leg and the pelvis should be stabilized, using similar means.

Alignment of the biological and mechanical axes

Because of the particular inclination of the inversion–eversion axis, it is debatable whether there is any possibility of proper alignment with current dynamometer designs. Hence, available attachments are based on approximations. One such attachment is shown in Figure 7.3.

To align the axes the dynamometer head is tilted away from the table/bench at an angle which corresponds to the offset of the biological axis. For instance, Lentell et al (1988), who used the Cybex' UBXT-Iv/Ev attachment–dynamometer combination, set this angle at 55°. The mechanical axis was made to extend through the superior edge of the lateral malleolus. The same basic configuration has been used by others, sometimes using other dynamometers (Simoneau 1990, Cawthorn 1991). No account was taken for the inclination of the other axis of the joint.

Test velocities for inversion–eversion

The range of test velocities for inversion–eversion testing has typically been 30–120 °/s. There is only one reported exception, the study by Cawthorn et al (1991), where the test velocity was 160 °/s. This was used in an attempt to stimulate subtalar motion during normal/walking. In some respects, the arguments for the use of lower velocities in dorsi- and plantarflexor testing, apply similarly for inversion–eversion testing. Moreover, for the purpose of normal walking/running, the mean power which is an important parameter in ankle motion may not be of parallel significance in subtalar motion.

However, if the main clinical problem is recovery of mechanical output after ankle complex sprain, medium velocity testing may be very relevant. If the concept of primary and secondary restraints as used in the knee, namely the ligamentous and muscular protection of the joint, is applied to the ankle, the speed with which the neuromuscular system reacts to a sudden external inverting force may affect the end-result of that force. One might therefore speculate that if the evertors come into play rapidly enough, and their eccentric performance is preserved, the chance for recurrence of injury is likely to be lower.

Admittedly isometric testing, using software routines provided with modern isokinetic systems, can yield valuable information regarding rapidity of mobilization. On the other hand such a test cannot demonstrate strength variations throughout the ROM, which may be vital. Consequently, the present author suggests that medium velocity inversion–eversion testing of patients with sprained ankle is advisable once all symptoms have subsided and normal activity has been resumed. The strength and the time within which the preset speed is reached are the parameters to observe.

PART 2
REPRODUCIBILITY OF ANKLE TESTING

DORSI- AND PLANTARFLEXION

Ostensibly, there is a lack of unanimity regarding this issue. Findings from four studies, with differing test–retest periods are discussed here.

Test–retest gap of at least 24 hours

Karnofel et al (1989) examined the reproducibility of strength findings in a group of 41 subjects. The protocol consisted of three different testing sessions, with at least 24 hours, between each one using 60 and 120 °/s as the test velocities (supine position). Intra-rater and inter-rater reproducibility, using the correlation coefficient Pearson's r, were in the ranges 0.86–0.94 and 0.87–0.94, respectively. No significant differences in strength values across the three test sessions were evident.

Test-retest period of 3 weeks

Reinking (1992) tested and retested strength and work, at the velocities of 30 and 90 °/s in a group of healthy subjects, a period of 3 weeks apart. The intra-class correlation coefficients (ICCs) ranged from 0.87, for peak concentric moment at 90 °/s, to 0.96 for peak eccentric moment at 30 °/s.

Retesting within 10 minutes

In another study, using the same dynamometer as Reinking 32 subjects took part in what might be described as an intra-session reproducibility assess-

ment (Wennerberg 1991). Retesting followed testing within 10 min. The test velocities were 30 and 120 °/s and the seated position was used.

Reproducibility as assessed by Pearson's r was below 0.8 for both dorsi- and plantarflexion and for both velocities. These are of course unacceptable values, especially given the very short retest period. The author suggested that the low correlations could derive from improper positioning, testing in bare feet, and possibly from fatigue because of the short pause between trials.

The points mentioned by Wennerberg raise doubts about the procedural rigor of his study, and stimultaneously help to validate the findings of the other two studies. It is indicated that a well defined protocol ensures acceptable reproducibility of dorsi- and plantarflexion strength scores.

Retesting after 2 years

Fugl-Meyer et al (1985) studied the reproducibility of strength and work in the context of plantarflexor endurance, using a Cybex II system. A group of 13 subjects were tested twice, years apart. Although no correlational analysis was presented, the shape of the endurance curves, peak moment and work vs. repetition number, was similar in both tests. Moreover, the differences between the two tests were consistently not significant, and less than 10 N m throughout the test, except for the last 20 of the 200 repetitions.

It was therefore concluded that 'in randomly selected middle-aged males with stabilized levels of physical activities, maximum supine isokinetic plantarflexor output varies only slightly'. Thus plantarflexion endurance, as well as strength, is a reproducible factor.

INVERSION AND EVERSION

In view of their complexity and their involvement in ankle sprain, the reproducibility of performance of the inventors and evertors is of obvious interest. However it was not until the late 1980s that studies were undertaken with contradictory results.

Karnofel et al (1989)

Alongside their analysis of dorsi- and plantarflexion, Karnofel et al (1989) examined the reproducibility of inversion–eversion, using the same protocol with velocities of 60 and 120 °/s with the exception that the subjects were seated. Intra-rater and inter-rater correlation coefficients (Pearson's r) ranged from 0.85 to 0.93 for inversion, and from 0.78 to 0.89 for eversion. Although the correlation coefficients varied only slightly with test velocity, where there was a difference, correlation was better at 120 °/s. Clearly the reproducibility level of invertor testing was on a par with that of dorsi- and plantarflexion, but eversion scores were more variable. The authors suggested that the difference derives from two sources: dorsi- and plantarflexion is a more commonly performed and a more functional activity, and inversion–eversion testing is more complicated. Nevertheless, the reproducibility of inversion testing is definitely acceptable, according to this study.

Simoneau (1990)

Quite opposite results were obtained by Simoneau (1990), who examined reproducibility based on three testing sessions, 1 week apart. Two velocities were used, 60 and 120 °/s and the test was conducted in the sitting position. The ICCs were consistently higher at the velocity of 60 °/s and greater in eversion. Reproducibility improved with additional test sessions. For eversion the ICCs were 0.82–0.93 for strength and 0.83–0.94 for total work. For inversion, the corresponding figures were 0.80–0.86 and 0.72–0.88. These findings indicate acceptability of eversion test findings. Two possible sources for the discrepancy between these studies are the use of different dynamometers, and different positioning and stabilization.

Cawthorn et al (1991)

These authors used a retesting period similar to Wennerberg's to examine inversion–eversion reproducibility. Only a few minutes were allowed until retesting was carried out. Apparently, reproducibility was not affected by the test velocity. The correlation coefficients were acceptable (0.87–0.94) but consistently higher for inversion.

Leslie et al (1990)

In another study, Leslie et al (1990) used a Cybex II system to examine the effect of ROM targets and ankle position of inversion–eversion reproducibility, using two sessions at least 24 hours apart. Tests

were performed at 30 and 120 °/s. With the use of these targets, 88% of the values of r were significant, compared to only 56% without ROM targets. In addition, a 50% increase in reproducibility, as judged by the number of significant r values, was observed in the test position of 20° plantarflexion. These correlation coefficients were greater than 0.8. No velocity effect on reproducibility was mentioned.

Conclusion

The studies of Cawthorn et al (1991) and Leslie et al (1990) do not help to resolve the contradictions, although it does seem that the reproducibility of inversion test findings is better than that of eversion testing. Moreover, testing in the close-packed position should yield more consistent results. Hence if the aim of the test is to reflect variations over time, the protocol of Karnofel et al (1989), at low angular velocities, is recommended.

PART 3
REPRESENTATIVE VALUES

There is a wide variation among different sources regarding the performance of ankle complex muscles. This is sometimes evident even between studies performed by the same group (see below). As with other joints, side dominance has not been proven to be a significant factor, at least with regard to strength (Fugl-Meyer et al 1980, Wong et al 1984, Leslie et al 1990, Simoneau 1990). Consequently the values refer, where applicable to the dominant side.

DORSI- AND PLANTARFLEXOR NORMS

Strength and angular velocity

Performance norms in terms of strength, as a function of the test angular velocity, are shown in Table 7.1. The entries are based on a series of studies by Fugl-Meyer and his colleagues. It should be noted that whereas considerable differences in plantarflexor strength were recorded between sedentary and trained subjects, the scores for dorsiflexors were very similar and hence quoted only for the former group.

Table 7.1 Dorsiflexor and plantarflexor concentric strength. Subjects were tested supine, with full knee extension

Velocity, °/s	Gender	Dorsiflexors*	Plantarflexors Sedentary*	Plantarflexors Trained[†]
30	F	26(8)	84(13)	140(19)
	M	33(6)	126(17)	183(24)
60	F	20(6)	64(12)	113(15)
	M	26(6)	96(19)	145(21)
120	F	15(5)	39(7)	75(13)
	M	18(5)	60(14)	95(26)
	F	12(6)	27(5)	52(9)
180	M	12(5)	41(10)	64(9)

* Fugl-Meyer et al (1980); [†] Fugl-Meyer et al (1981).

The findings by Karnofel et al 1989 were not incorporated since they did not distinguish between women and men, and the findings of all subjects, who covered a wide range of ages, were pooled together. The findings by Oberg et al (1987) were based, in the case of plantarflexion, on the uncommon prone position and consisted of a relatively small sample, and hence are not outlined here.

Variation of plantarflexion strength with age

Variations in plantarflexor strength as a function of age form an important component of any normative database. Thus although the size of each age category is small ($n = 15$), Table 7.2 which is based on the performance of sedentary Swedish subjects (Fugl-Meyer et al 1985) is of specific significance.

Prediction of peak moment and work

Using the above database, Fugl-Meyer et al (1985) derived the coefficients which appear in Table 7.3.

Table 7.2 Age variations of plantarflexor strength at three angular velocities*

Age group (years)	Gender	Planatarflexor strength, mean (SD), N m 30 °/s	60 °/s	180 °/s
40–44	F	108(13)	87(12)	41(8)
50–54	F	101(19)	78(14)	35(7)
60–64	F	78(15)	64(13)	30(5)
40–44	M	171(27)	133(22)	62(13)
50–54	M	154(21)	119(16)	57(11)
60–64	M	139(16)	106(14)	46(9)

* Based on Fugl-Meyer et al (1985).

Table 7.3 Coefficients for prediction formulae for plantarflexor performance. Based on Fugl-Meyer 1981 copyright © Springer-Verlag.

	Peak moment	Work (joules)
Gender coefficient (× 1 for men, × 0 for women)	39.2	23.4
Age group		
40–44	– 24.4	– 6.2
50–54	– 35.2	– 17.9
60–64	– 45.4	– 24.8
Crural circumference coefficient	3.1	1.8
r^2	0.79	0.63
SD	13.4	12.7

These enable the prediction of plantarflexion peak moment and work from gender (male = 1, female = 0), age and crural circumference. It is of interest to note that weight was not incorporated into the optimal formulae. In the following example the plantarflexor strength of a woman 41 years of age, with a crural circumference of 36 cm, is calculated:

Plantarflexor strength = gender coefficient +
age group coefficient +
(crural circumference ×
crural circumference
coefficient)
= (39.2 × 0) – 24.4 +
(36 × 3.1)
= 87.2 N m

INVERTOR AND EVERTOR NORMS

In this instance the sources of representative values are more versatile and up-to-date. As is evident from Table 7.4, there is a surprising compatibility among the three different sources even though the experimental conditions were dissimilar.

Table 7.5 stratifies the representative values in terms of age groups. The data are based on Gross & Brugnolotti (1992). It should be noted that these findings are somewhat higher than those quoted in Table 7.4. It is seen from Table 7.5 that:

1. Inverter–evertor strength in women is generally maintained at the same level throughout from 19 to 50 years, and only then declines
2. Inverter–evertor strength in men is maximal at the third decade and then declines, thereafter staying generally at the same level throughout the tested age spectrum.

Prediction formulae, derived from these findings,

Table 7.4 Invertor and evertor concentric strength (SD*, in N m)

Source	Velocity °/s	Women		Men	
		Invertors	Evertors	Invertors	Evertors
Wong et al (1984)	30	24(5)	20(3)	32(6)	28(6)
Leslie et al (1990)	30	25(3)	23(4)		
Wong et al (1984)	60	20(4)	16(2)	26(5)	24(6)
Simoneau (1990)	60	19(5)	17(4)		
Wong et al (1984)	120	16(3)	13(2)	22(4)	19(3)
Leslie et al (1990)	120	17(3)	13(3)		
Simoneau (1990)	120	14(4)	12(3)		

* To nearest integer.

Table 7.5 Age variations of invertor and evertor strength*, in N m to the nearest integer

	Age group (years)			
	19–30	30–40	40–50	50–62
Women				
Invertors				
60 °/s	23 (4)	25 (6)	23 (4)	20 (3)
120 °/s	20 (3)	21 (6)	18 (4)	17 (3)
Evertors				
60 °/s	20 (3)	18 (4)	20 (5)	16 (4)
120 °/s	16 (4)	14 (3)	13 (4)	13 (2)
Men				
Invertors				
60 °/s	36 (5)	31 (6)	29 (10)	30 (5)
120 °/s	32 (7)	26 (7)	25 (7)	23 (4)
Evertors				
60 °/s	29 (3)	25 (5)	25 (7)	24 (4)
120 °/s	23 (5)	19 (6)	18 (5)	18 (4)

* Based on Gross & Brugnolotti (1992).

for the strength of the invertors and evertors, at 60 °/s only are shown in Box 7.1.

STRENGTH RATIOS

The strength ratios, dorsiflexors plantarflexors and evertors/invertors, have been investigated and are tools for interpretation of isokinetic test data.

Ratio of dorsiflexor to plantarflexor strength

Fugl-Meyer (1981) studied the dorsiflexor/plantarflexor strength ratio in relation to activity level, using sedentary and trained subjects. The value of this ratio appears to be inversely proportional to the test velocity, for both activity groups and for women and men alike. The reason for this decline is a sharper reduction in plantarflexor strength compared with that of the dorsiflexors. This decline should not however be confused with the ability of the muscle to function at higher velocities, as indicated earlier. The variations in this ratio are outline in Table 7.6.

Ratio of evertor to invertor strength

The particular ratio of evertor/invertor strength was studied by Wong et al (1984), Nickson (1987) and Leslie et al (1990). The findings appear in Table 7.6. Whereas no velocity dependence is apparent from the study of Wong et al, there seems to be a certain decline in this ratio as indicated by that of Leslie et al.

Box 7.1 Prediction formulae for invertor and evertor strength at 60 °/s, based on Gross & Brugnolotti (1992)

Women
Invertors = 14.312 + (0.057 × weight) – (0.371 × % body fat) + (0.504 × shoe size)
Evertors = – 15.726 – (0.061 × age) + (0.977 × leg dominance) + (0.468 × height)

Men
Invertors = 9.188 – (0.114 × age) + (0.83 × weight)
Evertors = – 14.433 + (0.086 × weight) + (0.495 × leg girth) – (0.416 × % body fat) + (1.162 × shoe size)

Units: strength (peak moment), ft-lb; weight, kg; shoe size system, American; age, years; height; inches; leg girth, inches, measured at a point one third of the distance between the fibular head and the lateral malleolus distal to the former; leg dominance factor: dominant leg = 1, nondominant leg = 2.

Table 7.6 Ankle muscles strength ratios, as percentages

	30 °/s	60 °/s	120 °/s	180 °/s
Dorsiflexor/plantarflexor				
Fugl-Meyer (1981)				
Sedentary				
Women	30	32	38	45
Men	26	27	29	30
Trained				
Women	19	19	20	24
Men	19	19	21	28
Evertors/invertors				
Wong et al (1984)				
Women	81	80	82	
Men	87	90	86	
Nickson (1987)				
Women	79	80	80	
Men	79	76	74	
Leslie et al (1990)	80		63	

PART 4
INTERPRETATION AND CLINICAL SIGNIFICANCE

Interpretation of isokinetic test findings in the setting of ankle dysfunction has been based on the following principles:

1. bilateral comparisons
2. comparison of experimental (dysfunctional) vs. control groups.

Pre-and post-intervention comparisons, for either conservative or surgical management, are conspicuous by their absence.

The use of eccentric/concentric ratios for strength, work or power are also notably absent.

The lack of intervention comparisons probably derives from the fact that testing of patients with acute ankle sprain or rupture of the Achilles tendon is very difficult or impossible, because of pain and/or other contraindications. Also, elective surgery for correction of chronic instability or other dysfunctions is not as common in the ankle joint as it is with the knee. Hence there are few studies, especially of surgical outcomes, and those that exist have examined the postintervention phase.

To the best of the present author's knowledge, the use of eccentric/concentric ratios has been reported in one study only (Reinking 1992). It was indicated that, for the dorsiflexors, this ratio was between 1.45 and 1.50, at 30 and 90 °/s respectively. This value is somewhat high relative to those

quoted for other muscle groups, notably the quadriceps and hamstring, under the same conditions. The proportionally higher eccentric strength may reflect the role of eccentric dorsiflexor contraction in mediating the loading response during the stance phase of locomotion.

BILATERAL COMPARISONS

This method of interpretation has been most commonly applied to isokinetic test findings in patients suffering from rupture of the Achilles tendon.

Study of Sjostrom et al (1978)

In one of the first reports, Sjostrom et al (1978) tested/plantarflexor strength 2 years postoperatively, in 9 patients who were treated surgically for Achilles tendon rupture. The soleus was specifically investigated, and hence the patients were tested with the hip and knee at 90°.

The strength ratio, involved limb/uninvolved limb, ranged between 83 and 96% over the spectrum of velocities (30–180 °/s). These variations were not correlated with any morphometric data. One intriguing feature was a significant delay in reaching peak moment in the involved side, compared to the uninvolved side. This phenomenon can only be reliably demonstrated using isokinetic dynamometers.

The authors recommended that where Achilles tendon rupture is confirmed, and there is calf hypotrophy and plantarflexor weakness, objective strength measurement should be performed. One may assume that if, in such a case, the test reveals that the plantarflexor strength involved /uninvolved ratio is within the expected range, i.e. up to 17% reduction, there may not be sufficient grounds for intervention. Such an approach should by all means consider other factors such as the time after injury, age and the general level of activity. Moreover, the present author would also recommend investigation of the patient's plantarflexor power, to ascertain whether the expected rise in this parameter with higher velocities takes place. If it does not, conditioning of the plantarflexors is clearly indicated.

Shields et al (1978)

In another study Shields et al (1978) examined variations in dorsi- and plantarflexor strength and power, at 3 years, on average, following surgical repair of spontaneous Achilles tendon rupture. From tests performed at 30 °/s it was found that:

1. The injured/uninjured strength and power ratios of the plantarflexors were 83.5 and 82.5% respectively. The corresponding values for the dorsiflexors were 90 and 88.5%.
2. Earlier repairs were characterized by a lesser power loss compared to those cases were repair had been delayed.
3. Muscle strength ratios did not generally reach the above levels until 1 year after injury.

Hence these results favor earlier surgical intervention. They also support the findings of Sjostrom et al (1978) not only showing comparable values, but also indicating that the plantarflexors of the involved side are not likely to achieve parity with those of the unaffected side, under normal circumstances.

Conservative and surgical management of Achilles tendon rupture

In a later study, Nistor (1981) compared conservative and surgical treatment of Achilles rupture, using isokinetic testing of the plantarflexors as one of the clinical criteria. Tests took place 2.5 years, on average, after the treatment. The findings indicated:

1. Conservatively managed patients had higher (but not statistically significantly so) plantarflexor strength than surgical patients, both in the involved and uninvolved sides.
2. The estimated involved/uninvolved strength ratio ranged between 82 and 90% and between 84 and 90% in the surgical and conservative groups respectively. This finding correlates very closely with the figures already quoted.
3. The reduction in plantarflexor strength was not associated with any dysfunction of the injured side, and in fact seemed to have little clinical importance.

It was concluded that the conservative approach better served the needs of this particular population and was consequently the treatment of choice.

Conclusions

It therefore appears to be well established that a long-term effect of Achilles tendon rupture is a reduction in plantarflexor strength, and possibly power, of up to 20% compared to the unaffected limb. This reduction does not, however, interfere with normal activities.

COMPARISON WITH A CONTROL GROUP

When bilateral analysis is not relevant, i.e. when both limbs are involved, comparison with a control group may provide an alternative method of interpretation.

This was the approach of Gerdle et al (1986), to analyze the effect of peripheral arterial insufficiency with intermittent claudication (PAI–IC) on plantarflexor performance. Patients with this disorder may be referred for physical therapy in an attempt to alleviate the pain. In order to asses the severity of the symptoms, measuring of walking tolerance is conventionally carried out; a typical symptom is halting after a short distance due to pain. This can be done using a treadmill. However, in patients who also suffer from generalized arteriosclerosis with cardiac insufficiency, the treadmill test may be too stressful. Isokinetic strength and endurance testing can measure plantarflexor strength and endurance in a more selective way.

Strength testing of the plantarflexors was performed at 30, 60, 120 and 180 °/s. Endurance was assessed using repeated plantarflexions at 60 °/s, until leg pain, muscular fatigue or general exhaustion caused the patient to break off. Plantarflexor performance of patients with PAI–IC was compared with that of a normal, age-matched group.

It was indicated that patients were significantly weaker than controls in strength (70–75%) and contractional work (70%). They also endured the effort significantly less than control subjects. At 40 contractions, most of the patients could no longer proceed with the test while the remaining demonstrated a significant decline in strength (50%) and contractional work (55%). It was also revealed that that the isokinetic parameters were well correlated ($r = 0.89$) with the maximum walking capacity as measured in free walking.

Therefore isokinetic testing of the ankle may provide valuable information on a specific group of patients. This comparison with a control group not only helped subsantiate the validity of this method in PAI–IC, but would enable clinicians to assess the efficacy of various therapeutic regimens in treating these patients. Clearly a follow-up, or a pre- and post treatment analysis may thus be performed in a more accurate and revealing fashion.

ANKLE MUSCLE CONDITIONING AND BILATERAL COMPARISON

Improving ankle–foot muscle performance using isokinetic systems is probably very seldom attempted. This results from a number of factors including, among others, the difficulties associated with alignment, positioning and the determination of an appropriate protocol. It does not mean however that the use of isokonetics in ankle dysfunction should be discounted. From the excellent Swedish studies of Fugl-Meyer and colleagues it is obvious that the ingenious application of isokinetic systems may provide an effective tool for muscle conditioning.

Perhaps the only study relating isokinetic conditioning to ankle dysfunction is by Fugl-Meyer et al (1979). In this study two subjects who had undergone operations for Achilles tendon rupture, had conditioning for the plantarflexors, 1 and 4 years following surgery. The reasons for the rehabilitation were long-standing myopathic changes in the soleus and plantarflexor weakness. Conditioning consisted of two 3×10 maximal plantarflexor concentric contractions at 30 °/s daily for a period of 6 weeks. The patients used the trace of the moment, which was recorded on a storage scope, as a visual feedback.

Testing revealed that compared with the uninvolved leg, plantarflexor performance in the involved leg was markedly depressed before the conditioning program. With a test velocity spectrum of 30–180 °/s, the involved/uninvolved strength ratio was between 52 and 68% in one patient, and between 53 and 63% in the other.

After conditioning this ratio was improved to between 82 and 90% for the first patient, and 61 and 88% for the second. The more limited success with the second patient could be attributed to chronic muscular variations after 4 postoperative years. These strength gains persisted, though not fully, 3 months after the conditioning program. The angular delays in reaching the peak moment were definitely improved, attesting to a better recruitment of the plantarflexors. It was also noted that the improved mechanical performance was accompanied by normalization of the cross-sectional profile and area of the myopathic soleus fibers, as shown by biopsies, pre- and post conditioning.

Whether a levelling-off of the strength scores had indeed taken place was not explicitly mentioned in the paper, but the final strength gains should be noted. It appears that the maximal involved/uninvolved values, around 90%, may serve as a landmark for discontinuing conditioning. As mentioned before, deficiencies of up to 20% are commonly observed in patients long after surgical treatment of Achilles tendon rupture without disturbance to normal activities.

REFERENCES

Backman E, Oberg B 1989 Isokinetic muscle torque in the dorsiflexors of the ankle in children 6–15 years of age. Scandinavian Journal of Rehabilitation Medicine 21: 97–103

Bobbert M F, Van Ingen Schenau G 1990 Mechanical output about the ankle joint in isokinetic plantar flexion and jumping. Medicine and Science in Sports and Exercise 22: 660–668

Cawthorn M, Cummings G, Walker J R, Donatelli R 1991 Isokinetic measurement of foot invertor and evertor force in three positions of plantarflexion and dorsiflexion. Journal of Orthopaedic and Sports Physical Therapy 14: 75–81

Diffrient N, Tiley A, R, Bardagjy J C 1974 Humanscale 7/8/9. The MIT Press, Cambridge, Massachusetts

Fischer R D 1982 The measured effect of taping, joint ROM and their interaction upon the production of isometric ankle torques. Athletic Training 17: 218–223

Frankel V, Nordin M 1980 Basic biomechanics of the skeletal system. Lea & Febiger, Philadelphia

Fugl-Meyer A R 1981 Maximum isokinetic ankle plantar and dorsiflexion torque in trained subjects. European Journal of Applied Physiology 47: 393–404

Fugl-Meyer A R, Nordin G, Sjostrom M, Wahlby L 1979 Achilles tendon injury: a model for isokinetic strength training using biofeedback. Scandinavian Journal of Rehabilitation Medicine 11: 37–44

Fugl-Meyer A R, Sjostrom M, Wahlby L 1979 Human plantarflexion strength and structure. Acta Physiologica Scandinavica 107: 47–56

Fugl-Meyer A R, Gustavsson L, Burstedt Y 1980 Isokinetic and static plantarflexion characteristics. European Journal of Applied Physiology 45: 221–234

Fugl-Meyer A R, Mild K H, Hornsten J 1982 Output of skeletal muscle contraction: a study of isokinetic plantarflexion in athletes. Acta Physiologica Scandinavica 115: 193–199

Fugl-Meyer A R, Gerdle B, Eriksson E, Jonsson B 1985 Isokinetic plantarflexion endurance. Scandinavian Journal of Rehabilitation Medicine 17: 47–52

Garrick J G 1977 The frequency of injury, mechanism of injury and epidemiology of ankle sprains. American Journal of Sports Medicine 5: 241–242

Gerdle B, Fugl-Meyer A R 1985 Mechanical output and iEMG of isokinetic plantar flexion in 40–64-year-old subjects. Acta Physiologica Scndinavica 124: 201–211

Gerdle B, Fugl-Meyer A R 1988 Rank order of peak amplitude of EMG between the three muscles of triceps surae during maximum isokinetic contractions. Scandinavian Journal of Rehabilitation Medicine 20: 89–92

Gerdle B, Hedberg B, Angquist K, Fugl-Meyer A R 1986 Isokinetic strength and endurance in peripheral arterial insufficiency with intermittent claudication. Scandinavian Journal of Rehabilitation Medicine 18: 9–15

Gross M T, Brugnolotti J C 1992 Relationship between multiple predictor variables and normal Biodex eversion–inversion peak torque and angular work. Journal of Orthapaedic and Sports Physical Therapy 15: 24–31

Herlant M, Delahaye H, Voisin Ph, Bibre Ph, Adele M F 1992 The effect of anterior cruciate ligament surgery on the ankle plantar flexors. Isokinetics and Exercise Science 2: 140–144

Inman V T 1976 The joints of the ankle. Williams & Wilkins, Baltimore

Karnofel H, Wilkinson K, Lentell G 1989 Reliability of isokinetic muscle testing at the ankle. Journal of Orthopaedic and Sports Physical Therapy 11: 150–154

Lentell G, Cashmnan P A, Shiomoto K J, Spry J T 1988 The effect of knee position on torque output during inversion and eversion movements at the ankle. Journal of Orthopaedic and Sports Physical Therapy 10: 177–183

Leslie M, Zachazewski J, Browne P 1990 Reliability of isokinetic torque values for ankle invertors and evertors. Journal of Orthopaedic and Sports Physical Therapy 12: 612–616

Manter J T 1946 Distribution of compression forces in joints of the human foot. Anatomical Record 96: 313–324

McPoil T G, Knecht H G 1985 Biomechanics of foot in walking: a functional approach. Journal of Orthopaedic and Sports Physical Therapy 7: 69–72

Miller P J 1985 Assessment of joint motion. In: Rothstein J M (ed) Measurement in physical therapy. Churchill Livingstone, New York, pp 104–109

Nickson W 1987 Normative isokinetic data on the ankle invertors and evertors. Australian Journal of Physiotherapy 33: 85–90

Nistor L 1981 Surgical and non-surgical treatment of Achilles tendon rupture. Journal of Bone and Joint Surgery 63A: 394–399

Norkin C C, Levangie P K 1983 Joint structure and function: a comprehensive analysis. F A Davis, Philadelphia, pp 341–346

Oberg B, Bergman T, Tropp H 1987 Testing of isokinetic muscles strength in the ankle. Medicine and Science in Sports and Exercise 19: 328–332

Osternig L, Bates B, James S 1980 Patterns of tibial rotatory torque in knees of healthy subjects. Medicine and Science in Sports and Exercise 12: 195–199

Reinking M F 1992 The effect of concentric and eccentric training on the strengthening of tibialis anterior. Isokinetics and Exercise Science 2: 193–201

Seymour R J, Bacharach D W 1990 The effect of position and speed on ankle plantarflexion in females. Journal of Orthopaedic and Sports Physical Therapy 12: 153–156

Shields C L, Kerlan R K, Jobe F W, Garter V S Lombardo S J 1978 The Cybex II evaluation of surgically repaired Achilles tendon ruptures. American Journal of Sports Medicine 6: 369–372

Simoneau G G 1990 Isokinetic characteristics of ankle evertors and invertors in female control subjects using the Biodex dynamometer. Physiotherapy Canada 42: 182–187

Sjostrom M, Fugl-Meyer A R, Wahlby L 1978 Achilles tendon injury: plantar flexion strength and structure of the soleus muscle after surgical repair. Acta Chirurgica Scandinavica 144: 219–226

Smith R W, Reischl S F 1986 Treatment of ankle sprains in young athletes. American Journal of Sports Medicine 14: 465–471

Soutas-Little R W, Beavis G C, Verstraete M C, Markus T L 1987 Analysis of foot motion during running using a joint coordinate system. Medicine and Science in Sports and Exercise 19: 285–293

Sutherland D H, Cooper L, Daniel D 1980 The role of the ankle plantar flexors in normal walking. Journal of Bone and Joint Surgery 62A: 354–363

Svantesson U, Ernstoff B, Bergh P, Grimby G 1991 Use of a Kin-Com dynamometer to study the stretch–shortening cycle during plantar flexion. European Journal of Applied Physiology 62: 415–419

Wong D L, Glasheen-Wray M, Andrews L F 1984 Isokinetic evaluation of the ankle invertors and evertors. Journal of Orthopaedic and Sports Physical Therapy 5: 246–252

Wennerberg D 1991 Reliability of an isokinetic dorsiflexion and plantar flexion apparatus. American Journal of Sports Medicine 19: 519–522

Isokinetics of the trunk muscles

In contrast to all other major muscle–joint systems, where isokinetic evaluation and conditioning assumed a clinical dimension relatively late, trunk isokinetics was targeted almost from the start at a clinical problem: low-back dysfunction (LBD).

Due to the enormous cost of this disorder in human suffering and economically, it has had a unique impact on isokinetic technology. Currently there are several models of isokinetic dynamometers intended solely for the evaluation and treatment of the dysfunctional lower back. These sometimes replace the use of special trunk attachments with ordinary dynamometers.

Simulated isokinetic lift dynamometry, which measures the combined capacity of trunk, hip and knee extensors, has recently become an attractive option for trunk testing to the extent that special norms have been developed for users of this technology (Timm 1988). Obviously within-patient bilateral comparisons of the crucially important sagittal exertions cannot be made, and thus normative databases are essential. However, these apply only to a given dynamometer and test position, as findings from different systems are notoriously incompatible.

Consequently, it is strongly advised that the choice of a trunk testing system should not rest only on financial considerations or on the range of options offered. Rather, clinicians are urged to explore the availability of published material, such as articles in peer review journals, which describe particular systems, their method of operation and the process of data collection and interpretation. Some of the trunk testing systems, which are well described in the scientific literature, offer considerable potential for research and clinical applications.

PART 1
GENERAL ISSUES

IMPORTANCE OF SAGITTAL MOTION

The trunk is capable of performing three major rotations, commonly defined as the sagittal movements of flexion and extension and the coupled movements of lateral flexion and axial rotation. By far the most important among these is the sagittal movement in the lumbar spine intricately related to sagittal motion at the hip joint.

In contrast with sagittal flexion–extension, lateral flexion and axial rotation have attracted very limited attention. This is partly because of the serious technical difficulty of effectively isolating and accurately aligning the relevant segments during lateral flexion and axial rotation testing. This is illustrated by the complexity of the Cybex trunk rotation unit.

Furthermore, research, not exclusively isokinetic, has found that performance, as shown in the strength curves, of antagonistic lateral flexion and axial rotation muscle groups is basically symmetrical (Thorstensson & Nilsson 1982), and this symmetry is preserved in LBD patients (Thorstensson & Arvidson 1982, Mayer & Gatchel 1988). Although there may be a reduction of up to 25% in rotatory strength in LBD, compared with controls, this is less dramatic than the deficit in sagittal flexion–extension strength (Mayer et al 1985). The clinical benefit of axial rotation testing may thus be questionable.

Finally, isokinetic test-lift instruments have been used so far to test sagittal plane motions, only. However by creative use of these instruments, lifts in a plane which is not strictly sagittal could be devised, and here lateral extension and axial rotation would also be tested. Nevertheless, this Chapter generally describes the testing, interpretation and clinical applications if sagittal isokinetic motions of the trunk.

MECHANISMS OF TRUNK MOVEMENT

The mechanisms responsible for moving the 'aggregate' of the head, arms and back are neither limited to the lumbar region nor are they exclusively muscular in nature. Calculations, based on simulations of the trunk in extension, demonstrate that the intricate system of lumbar extensors cannot by itself generate sufficient tension to 'lift' the trunk when it is heavily loaded (Farfan 1978).

In order to account for the required additional force, two theories have been proposed. One claimed that the extra force was derived from intraabdominal pressure, but the body of evidence against the hypothesis precluded wide acceptance (Macintosh & Bogduk 1987).

The second theory suggested that the prime mover role for forceful trunk extension belonged to the hip extensor mechanism, comprising the gluteus maximus, gluteus medius and the hamstrings. This system, it was argued, was capable of developing the amount of force needed to extend the trunk, provided that a 'force transmission element', stretching from the pelvis to the thorax, was available. This element has been identified as a combination of noncontractile structures i.e. the zygapophyseal joint capsules, the posterior ligaments and the posterior layer of the thoracolumbar fascia, known collectively as the posterior ligamentous system (Macintosh & Bogduk 1987).

According to this theory, hip extensors contribute the initial thrust, when the moment of the external resistance plus that of the weight of the trunk is high. As extension progresses the moments of these forces diminish and hence the required muscular balancing moment may be produced increasingly by the lumbar extensors. Since maximal isokinetic exertions are by definition highly demanding it is clear that if the second theory holds, the initial phase of lifting depends critically on hip muscle activity. Consequently, blocking pelvic motion during trunk testing, which in turn may limit hip extensor output, should help to show more precisely the net contribution of the lumbar extensors.

CONCENTRIC AND ECCENTRIC ACTIVITY

The mode of muscle contraction under evaluation is of paramount importance in the trunk region.

Until the mid 1980s isokinetic studies of trunk performance were almost exclusively limited to concentric contractions. These studies emphasized the 'active' component of extensor performance namely, extension of the trunk from a flexed position. Additionally, based on the controversial 'abdominal balloon' theory, the abdominal muscles were considered a key factor in extending the spine, so measuring their concentric activity was as integral to comprehensive trunk testing as measuring that of the extensors.

Importance of eccentric activity

However, simple kinesiological analysis shows that except when trunk flexion is performed against gravity, e.g. in a forward rise from a supine position, it is generally assisted by it. Therefore, as soon as the trunk moves anteriorly, possibly due to a brief, low-level contraction of the hip flexors, eccentric contraction of the extensors is required to control the otherwise 'free fall' of the trunk.

This activity becomes even more crucial where handling a load is concerned, particularly when it has to be carefully lowered onto a platform. When this eccentric activity is both forceful and slow, it may provoke pain (Dvir et al 1991) with obvious implications for LBD patients.

It is for this reason that, for a comprehensive trunk evaluation, it is at least as important to test the eccentric performance of the extensor mechanism as to test its concentric performance. Moreover, comparing the shapes of concentric and eccentric strength curves for trunk extensor function may yield significant information, particularly in the clinical setting. Although eccentric testing of trunk muscle performance is still at an early stage, it is possible that it will play an increasing role within the foreseeable future. In line with other joint systems, to exclude the eccentric component may limit the scope of the assessment, and any conclusions drawn from it.

HARDWARE IN TRUNK ISOKINETICS

Uniaxial isokinetic trunk testing technology developed along two lines. One used slight modifications to the basic system, fitting special attachments or even incorporating the dynamometer within a to-

tally reconstructed frame. The other approach was to use entirely originally designs, culminating in special purpose dynamometers.

Special attachments

Special attachments/frames, normally used in conjunction with a Cybex dynamometer, were reported in a number of studies. Hause et al (1980), Smidt et al (1980, 1983), Thorstensson & Nilsson (1982) and Thorstensson & Arvidsson (1982) tested subjects, both with and without LBD in the supine, side-lying and supine and side-lying positions. Langrana & Lee (1984) and Marras & Mirka (1989) tested subjects in the seated and upright positions. The systems used in these studies generally required a great deal of mechanical design work and ingenuity.

There are a number of special attachment designs which lock onto the mainframe and allow testing in the seated position. One such design, the Biodex Back Attachment (Fig. 8.1), consists of a reclined seat, in which the subject is partially reclined but otherwise in almost full body extension, and stabilized. This attachment does not seem to offer accurate alignment since the actuator is connected directly to the seat hinge, which is fixed at the lumbar region. It does however afford a full range of trunk flexion and hyperextension. Another

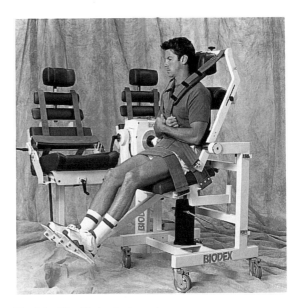

Fig. 8.1 The Biodex back attachment.

advantage is that Biodex is an active system and hence enables eccentric testing or conditioning, in addition to all other modes.

A more recent model, the trunk attachment by KinCom also operates on the stand-alone attachment principle. However, there is a striking difference in alignment procedure between this and the Biodex attachment. In the KinCom design, the positions of both the force pad and the mechanical axis are adjustable, using a fairly elaborate assembly of sliding blocks for the pad. The initial position of the subject is sitting, with hips semiflexed. The KimCom is also an active system, enabling eccentric testing/conditioning.

Special purpose dynamometers

Two manufacturers have produced special purpose dynamometers. The Cybex trunk extension and flexion (TEF) unit was the first special purpose trunk machine. The subject is tested in a standing position, and concentric performance may be measured.

This company also produced another special purpose trunk dynamometer, the Torso Rotation Device, which tested torsional trunk muscle performance in the seated position. This machine has not acquired popularity, probably because of the studies of Mayer et al (1985b), as well as its bulk and price. The indications concerning the limited value of trunk rotation testing have recently been significantly reinforced by Newton et al (1993). The authors claimed that rotational testing did not add any useful clinical information to findings based on sagittal measurements.

The Lido isokinetic sagittal tester is a passive special purpose dynamometer system, which allows testing in the standing as well as the sitting position, an option which is exclusive to this design.

MULTIJOINT TESTING

Alongside the uniaxial devices conventionally used for analysis of trunk isokinetic performance, recent years have seen the development of so-called multijoint systems, in which the force pad does not necessarily move in a rotatory fashion. These systems generally incorporate the closed kinetic chain (CKC) principle. Because of the greater

number of moving body segments their motion profile may be less repeatable and therefore the test scores could be less reproducible.

The spine itself is a multijoint structure, but the term multijoint testing is somewhat inadequate, as for this particular purpose, the spine is considered a single-segment-single-joint system.

The operation of a typical multijoint trunk apparatus is based on a cable which unwinds at a preset linear velocity. The adjustments of the displacement of the handle, by which the cable is pulled, and its linear speed is carried out in a fashion similar to that of conventional testing. Subjects may assume any of the accepted test positions e.g. straight knees and bent back, or alternatively bent knees and a slightly flexed back. Figure 8.2 illustrates a multijoint system (Lift simulator) manufactured by Biodex.

The test consists of pulling up the handle, exerting a submaximal or maximal effort. The test findings show the total force and cannot discriminate trunk muscle output from that of other segments. Hence, although this isokinetic testing method is more nearly functional, its inability to locate deficiencies at the individual joint/s level is a weakness. Moreover, unlike the situation in uniaxial flexion-extension testing, the subject cannot be accurately positioned, and proven testing practices cannot be followed.

In the following sections, isokinetics of the trunk

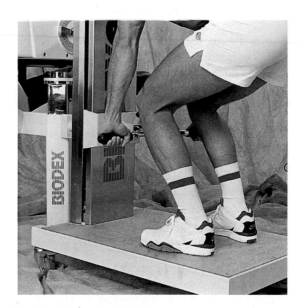

Fig. 8.2 The Biodex lift simulator.

will be discussed in terms of general testing procedures, normative databases, interpretation of findings and clinical applications. Where relevant, these sections will separately consider uniaxial versus multijoint isokinetics.

PART 2
TESTING PROCEDURES FOR THE TRUNK

Trunk evaluation poses particular problems, particularly with respect to LBD patients. Since LBD may be directly or indirectly associated with muscle dysfunction, patients suffering from this syndrome must be tested with extreme care. For those involved in assessing/treating LBD, the thought of provoking an acute episode of back pain in a patient who has been misinstructed to exert maximal effort, verges on nightmare. Moreover, if the patient is a woman who suffers from osteoporosis, such an effort carries a certain risk.

Therefore, clinicians are advised not to urge patients to attempt maximal effort until they are well into the recovery period, or unless they are absolutely confident that there is a residual risk-free potential which the patient does not exercise.

It has been pointed out (Mayer et al 1985a) that patients may not produce their maximal force output for fear of injury or pain. It is therefore advisable to extensively use the feedback force/moment signals, available in most systems, both as a means of motivation and instruction. The present author would also suggest that pain scales be used during the tests, so that the examiner is fully aware of any ominous sign.

The issues dealt with in this section are:

1. Alignment of the biological and mechanical axes
2. Positioning and stabilization
3. Range of motion
4. Test velocities
5. Gravity correction
6. Strength normalization.

ALIGNMENT OF THE BIOLOGICAL AND MECHANICAL AXES

Trunk motion during isokinetic testing involves a large number of joints including the lumbosacral, the intervertebral (up to the thoracic articulations) and potentially the hip. Consequently, the optimal alignment of the biological and mechanical axes is not as straightforward as is the case with, for example, the knee joint. Consistent alignment is of course a normal prerequisite for repeatability; in the trunk, inconsistency is also liable to lead to differing contributions from the various muscle groups.

Hip joint versus midlumbar alignment

In an early attempt to define the extent of the problem, Thorstensson & Nilson (1982) compared the effect of aligning the force actuator of the dynamometer with the greater trochanter (hip joint) level, with alignment with an imaginary axis passing through the L2–L3 intervertebral junction.

It was indicated that the peak moment, in both flexion and extension was significantly higher when the axis was aligned with the L2–L3 level compared to the trochanteric level. Furthermore, the difference was greater for flexion than for extension, and resulted in significantly lower extension/flexion ratios, when alignment was made with respect to L2–L3. The authors suggested that these differences could be attributed to hip flexor function and hence use of the term 'abdominal' strength was inappropriate.

LBD patients and controls

In another study (Thorstensson & Arvidson 1982) it was found that the strength of trunk flexion, when the axes were aligned at the hip joint level, was significantly lower in LBD patients compared with control subjects. No significant differences were noted at the L2–L3 level alignment, suggesting a selective hip flexor deficiency in the former group.

Anterior and posterior superior iliac spine, and hip joint aligments

In a more recent study the effect of axis alignment on measured trunk strength was assessed in the seated position, at three velocities, using the Biodex dynamometer (Grabiner et al 1990). Alignment was made with respect to the anterior superior iliac spine, the posterior superior iliac spine and the greater trochanter.

While the statistical analysis did not demonstrate the superiority of any alignment, the data based on the anterior superior iliac spine were associated with the smallest variability overall. Because of the test position and lack of stable pelvic restraint, these findings may be applicable to the Biodex back attachment only.

Lumbosacral versus midlumbar alignment

It should be emphasized that in most studies alignment has been made with respect to the lumbosacral joint, L5–S1 (Langrana & Lee 1984, Langrana et al 1984, Marras et al 1984, Smith et al 1985, Mayer et al 1985a,b, Marras & Mirka 1989, Jerome et al 1991) possibly due to ease of location.

This practice was challenged by Stokes (1987) using a simulation of the movement of T12 about a fixed pelvis. It was demonstrated that under normal conditions, the motion of the instantaneous center of rotation of T12 was similar to that of L3 along the total simulated ROM in both flexion and extension. It was therefore suggested that the mechanical axis should be aligned with the L3 vertebra, and pelvic as well as thoracic motion should be maximally controlled. It was also argued that: 'failure to observe these precautions would tend to make the motion of the lumbar spine nonisokinetic and, thus, interfere with angular measurement of spinal motion'. Unfortunately no error analysis was performed, and hence the significance of misaligning the axes at the level of L5–S1 rather than L2–L3 was not determined.

Consistency and correctness

A consistent, as well as a correct alignment, is crucial for a reliable isokinetic test score. Even though L5–S1 may not be the optimal axis, as long as it is accurately located and aligned with the dynamometer axis, the error resulting from misaligning the axes is constant and, in principle, there will be no effect on the test–retest correlations.

Conversely, even though L2–L3 is the optimal axis, the error made in locating this vertebral level is liable to adversely affect the repeatability of the findings.

Consequently, clinicians who are comfortable in locating spinal landmarks are advised to align the axes at the midlumbar level. Otherwise, the lumbosacral level and even more so the iliac crest level (Delitto et al 1990), which corresponds approximately to the L4–L5 interspace, lend themselves to more accurate location. In this case sacrificing correctness for consistency may prove a more practical solution. Where possible, it is also advisable to record the position of the mechanical axis, using its height from the floor or support platform, if further evaluations are envisaged.

POSITIONING AND STABILIZATION

Positioning for uniaxial motion

Among procedural parameters, the positioning and stabilization of subjects for trunk evaluation occupy a central role. Different methods of positioning have been studied over the years and the experience gathered has been incorporated in a number of commercial trunk systems. Early studies used side-lying positions, thus cancelling the effect of gravity (Smidt et al 1980, 1983, Thorstensson & Nilsson 1982). However, this position was not only non-functional, but complex methods were needed to interface the dynamometer with the frame which supported the subject. More recent solutions concentrated on standing or sitting test positions but these meant that the gravitational effect had to be accounted for (see below).

Langrana & Lee (1984)

To examine the effect of test position on flexion and extension strength, Langrana & Lee (1984) designed a special isokinetic system which permitted tests both standing and sitting. In a group of 25 men, the average extension strengths were 253 and 313 N m, for sitting and standing, respectively with an extension/flexion ratio of 1.18. (These data were probably not corrected for gravitational effect). On the other hand the corresponding figures for flexor strengths were 125 and 220 N m respectively with an extension/flexion ratio of 1.97.

These results showed that both the extensors and flexors exert greater effort in standing compared to sitting, and the sitting position had however a greater effect on flexor strength, reducing the latter to some 50% of its capacity in standing. This effect was attributed to the involvement of the iliopsoas in the standing position.

The authors also mentioned that testing in the sitting position was tolerated better than in the standing position. This finding echoed those of an earlier study (Smidt et al 1983), in which it was noted that the sitting position, compared to standing, allowed greater ROM, both in flexion and extension, and hence was the preferred testing position.

Conclusion

It therefore seems that the optimal test position is sitting though the final decision rests with the clinician who should consider the health status of the subject/patient, her/his work environment, the need to compare findings derived from the two positions, as well as the availability of an adequate testing system.

Positioning for multijoint motion

Isokinetic testing of multijoint trunk motion is carried out basically in one position, i.e. standing. However, even within this position the initial configuration of the joints may differ as mentioned earlier. Furthermore, the distance between the feet and the external force vector is another factor which ought to be taken into account when setting the test parameters.

Porterfield et al (1987) have studied the effect of these parameters on the total work, in two age groups of LBD-free male subjects. The two initial positions were first, squatting arms straight as possible and head looking forward, and second, knees locked and trunk fully curled forward. The foot positions were toes in a line with the exit point of the cable, or toes 10 cm behind this point. It was indicated that the amount of work generated from the squatting position was greater than that from the straight-leg position, and the same applied for the toe-forward compared with toe-backward position. These findings may serve as general guidelines for multijoint isokinetic trunk testing. Because of the high stresses that are likely to be exerted by the lumbar extensors, lifting activity has to be closely monitored and controlled. For this purpose, and particularly in the case of subjects with or prone to

LBD, the test must be preceded by a warm-up session consisting of stretch manoeuvres and then submaximal lifts.

Stabilization in trunk testing

Stabilization of body segments, particularly the pelvis, is the next essential step after the selection of test position. Failure to adequately stabilize the segments below the force application point may result in substitution with variations in moment output.

Effect of level of stabilization

Smidt et al (1983) compared the effect of three levels of stabilization on the spatial movement of the spinous process of L5, during testing in the sitting position. Rigorous stabilization was ensured by placing rigid pads in firm contact with the anterior shank (pointing against the tibial tuberosity), anterior thigh, anterior superior iliac spine and immediately below the level of L5–S1. For medium stabilization, the thighs and feet were strapped and for minimal stabilization only the feet were strapped leaving the pelvis, in both cases, unstabilized. It was indicated that although all modes of stabilization were effective in preventing side (lateral) movements, anteroposterior and vertical movements increased with relaxation of strapping.

Another systematic study which examined the effect of several levels of stabilization on trunk flexion and extension strength, was conducted by Timm (1991) using a Cybex TEF system. The ankle, knee, and hip/pelvis regions were independently stabilized. Blocking motion in all of these regions resulted in a configuration of 'maximal stabilization'. The footplate which served to stabilize the ankle could be removed, resulting in 'no ankle stabilization', or the anterior knee pads could be removed resulting in 'no knee stabilization'. Finally, the lowest level of stabilization (minimal) consisted of blocking of hip/pelvic motion only.

The results demonstrated highly significant differences between the above configurations. Analysis revealed significant differences between maximal stabilization and all the others; between minimal stabilization and no ankle stabilization; between minimal stabilization and no knee stabilization, but not between no ankle and no knee stabilization.

The importance of these findings is that they indicate not only that the level of stabilization has a direct bearing on trunk muscle strength, but that this effect is not necessarily 'linear'. In other words, a more distal stabilization is not directly correlated with a higher force input and vice versa. Therefore, in order to maximize trunk muscle strength in normal subjects stabilization should be applied to all major joint system distal to the axis of alignment.

RANGE OF MOTION

ROM in uniaxial motion

The literature concerning this topic is not particularly extensive and some studies even fail to specify the ROM. However, in most cases an angular range of some 80–100° is quoted as relevant for trunk testing. For pain-free subjects, the following ROMs were typically used: – 10° of 'hyperextension' to 90° of flexion (Delitto et al 1989), or 0–80° flexion (Smidt et al 1985, Hazard et al 1988, Jerome et al 1991). Langrana & Lee (1984) used a range of 110° in standing and 50° in sitting, even though Smidt et al (1983) noted that a greater ROM in sitting could be better tolerated, particularly by patients.

The isokinetic testing ROM for LBD patients is obviously more limited. Mayer et al (1985a) used 45° for pain-free LBD patients and reduced this range to 30° when clear limitations of motion were noted.

It should be emphasized that if performance is to be assessed by the peak moment only, a flexion of 50° is sufficient. This guideline is based on findings relating to the angle of peak moment (Thorstensson & Nilsson 1982) which have shown that this parameter peaks at about 30° of flexion for extension and less for flexion. The same conclusion, based on their own experience was reached by Smith et al (1985).

ROM in Multijoint motion

The available information regarding multijoint testing is very limited as this is a rather novel technology. Moreover, since the motion of the end segment is linear, the normalizing effect of angular motion is no longer relevant. The 'ROM' in multijoint tests

depends on the linear dimensions of the subject; given the same angular joint displacements, a tall subject would obviously have to pull the handle a proportionally greater distance than a shorter one. Hence, even if the peak moment is the same for both subjects, the work output may not be comparable.

Since the starting position assumed by the subject depends on personal preference to a great extent, care should be taken to record knee angle, handle height and feet position relative to the handle, in order to ensure ROM repeatability if retesting is envisaged.

TEST VELOCITIES

Uniaxial testing

The issue of test angular velocities is more complex and the variations in this case are wider. Goniometry-based measurements of trunk velocities have indicated that these could reach a maximum of 200–300 °/s (Thorstensson & Nilsson 1982) while in walking and running the range was 15–75 °/s. This observation also fits well with another study (Parnianpour et al 1988) which indicated that the velocity of 60 °/s closely approximated the flexion and extension velocities in a number of activities of daily living.

The kinematic behavior or the trunk in LBD and control groups was studied by Marras & Wongsam (1986) using a lumbar motion monitor. It was found that LBD patients differed significantly from controls, presenting with dramatically reduced velocities in flexion and extension. These differences were particularly marked in hyperextension, where patients did not exceed 10 °/s both in normal and maximal velocity, versus averages of 35 and 65 °/s in the control group. In flexion and extension from flexion, the velocities in the LBD group were within the 30 °/s range, whereas the figures for control subjects were roughly between 50–100 °/s for flexion and 30–75 °/s for flexion from reextension.

In a more recent study, ROMs, velocities and accelerations in the sagittal as well as off-sagittal planes were measured in 85 subjects (Marras et al 1990). It was indicated that the average velocity in both flexion and extension was 100 °/s, and that there was a significant reduction in flexion and extension velocities for motion in the off-sagittal planes.

Broader performance indices

Alongside the measurement of the strength of the different muscle groups involved in trunk function, there is as growing school of researchers who are looking into broader aspects of trunk muscle performance (see the section on Interpretation for a more detailed analysis). Parameters such as average power and total work at the medium velocities of 120 and 150 °/s have been used, in order to arrive at a single performance parameter: the muscle performance index (MPI) devised by Jerome et al (1991), or the average performance deficit (APD) suggested by Timm (1992). Using an alternative approach, Grabiner & Jeziorowski (1992) tested LBD and control subjects at 60, 120 and 180 °/s and demonstrated the crucial value of adding the latter velocity to the test protocol. It should be emphasized, however, that the testing of patients in this study took place 8 years, on average, after the initial injury, permitting the incorporation of this relatively high velocity.

Recommended angular velocities

The selection of the appropriate velocities for trunk testing depends primarily, therefore, on the ability of the subject/patient to generate and maintain a maximal moment, while isokinetic conditions prevail through a substantial sector of the tested ROM. Secondly, the purpose and the timing of the test are essential factors.

Clearly in view of the studies mentioned earlier, flexion and extension testing of patients at velocities above 60 °/s, and during a relatively early period postinjury/attack, may be hampered by their inability to perform isokinetically. Consequently, if testing is for follow-up of patient progress, a single test velocity at the lower end of the spectrum, that is 60 °/s, may suffice.

On the other hand, normal subjects and well-healed LBD patients can be tested at higher velocities, i.e. 90–180 °/s. If in addition a comprehensive performance index is sought, a spectrum of velocities should be used.

Velocities in multijoint testing

The velocities employed in multijoint testing have normally been quoted in inches per second (ips). Since the metric system is adopted throughout this book, metric units will be used for this parameter also. For some reason, the 'quantal speed unit' reported in most studies has been 15 cm/sec (6 ips). Thus for instance Mayer et al (1985a) tested subjects at 45, 75 and 90 cm/s, speeds which have also been used by Hazard et al (1988). A wide spectrum of testing velocities was reported by Timm (1988): 15, 30, 45, 60, 75 and 90 cm/s.

Prescribing a multijoint testing velocity in this case is a more difficult undertaking, not only because of the paucity of data, but also on account of individual differences. For instance, given the same angular excursion, a velocity of 15 cm/s may be reasonable for a short subject but unsafe for a very tall one. Subject comfort as well as pain levels should therefore be carefully checked and recorded before initiating a maximal effort multijoint test.

GRAVITY CORRECTION

Due to the mass of the trunk, 63 and 67% of bodyweight in women and men respectively (Diffrient et al 1978), its gravitational moment can be considerable. The magnitude of this moment depends on the location of the trunk's center of mass which is a function of individual anthropometry. In any case the fact that isokinetic trunk testing is regularly performed either in the standing or sitting position necessitates consideration of the gravitational effect.

For a rough estimate of the significance of the gravity factor consider the following example which uses data from different sources. Calculations based on the antropometric tables of Diffrient et al (1978) indicate that for an adult male, with an 'average' build whose height and weight are 180 cm and 80 kg respectively, the gravitational moment at 30° of trunk flexion is approximately 90 N m. At this flexion angle, the peak moment-based extension/flexion ratio, for subjects in a side-lying position with L2–L3 alignment and at a velocity of 30 °/s, was 2.93 (Thorstensson & Nilsson 1982). Consider now the corresponding extension/flexion ratio of Delitto et al (1991), calculated without incorporating a gravity correction. Measured at a velocity of 60 °/s, the average male trunk strength, was 223 and 305 N m for flexion and extension respectively, giving an extension/flexion ratio of 1.36. The average weight of the participants in the study of Delitto et al was 80 kg and therefore as a post hoc 'gravity correction', one should add and subtract 90 N m, to the peak extension and flexion moments respectively. The ratio then becomes $(305 + 90)/(223 - 90)$, i.e. 2.96 which is almost identical to the 'zero gravity' ratio of 2.93 obtained by Thorstensson & Nilsson (1982). This is drastically different, by a factor of more than 100%, from the ratio of 1.36.

The above arithmetic exercise serves to underline the importance of introducing gravity corrections to trunk muscle performance analysis. Clearly, those studies where the contribution of gravity was ignored, have seriously underrated extensor strength and conversely overrated that of the flexors. This has obvious clinical implications besides making comparison difficult between data which do or do not include a correction. In spite of some problems in applying the gravity correction procedure for trunk performance (Cale-Benzoor et al 1992), clinicians are strongly advised to incorporate this procedure routinely, wherever possible, in trunk testing.

STRENGTH NORMALIZATION FOR BODYWEIGHT

In a growing number of studies strength, hitherto expressed in newton-meters (N m) or foot-pounds (ft-lb), is quoted relative to the subject's bodyweight. The unit of measurement is therefore newton-meters per kilogram (N m/kg) of bodyweight or ft-lb/lb. This practice is based on the assumption that individual weight differences partly account for variance in isokinetic measurements.

This assumption was not supported in three consecutive papers. In a study by Delitto et al (1989), it was indicated that though weight and strength were positively related, the correlation was not significant in women, and in men it accounted for less than 20% of the peak moment variance. Delitto therefore concluded that normalizing strength by bodyweight cannot be justified in women, and that in men, the range of expected values is quite wide. For instance, based on the findings collected in this study, trunk extensor

strength could be regarded deficient if the subject developed 64% or less of her/his own body weight. It was suggested that if factors other than weight namely age and activity level were added, the variance could be reduced.

These observations were supported by a later study (Jerome et al 1991) which indicated that bodyweight indeed exerted a major effect, greater than that of age or height, on the variance, but increased weight was not necessarily correlated with an increase in strength. The findings of Newton et al (1993) are much the same as those of Delitto et al (1989). In this study of patients with low back dysfunction and normal subjects, gender-based analysis indicated that consistent correlations between bodyweight and isokinetic measurements associated with trunk flexion, extension and rotation were apparent only in normal men. However, even in this individual group, there was no significant correlation between bodyweight and the moment developed during multijoint motion (linear lift). No correlations between bodyweight and any of the isokinetic measurements were found in the male and female patient groups. The authors have therefore concluded that there are no grounds for presenting trunk isokinetic measurements in terms of bodyweight. This recommendation is well supported by the above-mentioned papers and should hence guide users of trunk isokinetic systems when quoting relevant figures.

PART 3
REPRODUCIBILITY OF TRUNK TESTING

UNIAXIAL MOVEMENT AND REPRODUCIBILITY

This issue was studied for the first time by Smidt et al (1980) with respect to the side-lying position. In a later study by this group (Smidt et al 1983) consistency and reproducibility of strength scores were investigated for the sitting position. Scores from 24 subjects were used in the consistency analysis. It was indicated that the intraclass correlation coefficients. (ICCS) for concentric flexion and extension were good to excellent ranging from 0.88 to 0.99. Four subjects were retested a week later and the average reproducibility variations in concentric flexion and extension were 13 and 21%

respectively. These relatively low figures could be partly attributed to the very small sample size.

Smith et al (1985) have tested and retested, within a period of 7–14 days, a group of 15 subjects, using Cybex TEF and axial rotation prototype dynamometers. Consistency as judged by Pearson's r was 0.80–0.99 for flexion, 0.88–0.99 for extension and greater than 0.90 for rotation. Reproducibility which was determined using Pearson product–moment correlations ranged 0.74–0.96 for extension, 0.76–0.77 for flexion and 0.77–0.90 for rotation. These are generally modest to good or excellent figures.

Study of Smidt et al 1989

Using the KinCom back attachment, Smidt et al (1989) calculated the reproducibility of a very large number of variables which they divided into kinetic, electromyographic and trunk angle categories. Using a small group ($n = 7$) and a retesting period of 3 days, it was discovered that:

1. None of the measured variables demonstrated significant variations on retesting.
2. The kinetic parameters, peak moment, range of moment rise and decay (between 25 and 75% of maximum), impulse and work were highly reproducible.
3. Reproducibility of extension/flexion ratios for the concentric and eccentric peak moment and work were excellent ($r > 0.90$)
4. There was good reproducibility of the eccentric/concentric ratio in extension but it was poor in flexion.

It should be mentioned that in this outstanding study, tight control of stabilization and axis alignment, as well as the position of testing (sitting), probably played a decisive role in reducing intertest variations to a minimum.

Delitto et al (1991)

Delitto et al (1991) used another dynamometer, the Lidoback, to test the reproducibility of the normalized peak moment, extension/flexion ratio and average work/repetition, using velocities of 60, 120 and 180 °/s. A total of 62 asymptomatic subjects were tested three times with intervals of a week and 2 weeks between the initial and retesting sessions respectively. The tests were performed

standing and did not include gravity corrections. Intraclass correlations coefficients (ICCs) varied from 0.74 to 0.88, and 0.88 to 0.93, for the peak moment measures and work respectively. However, the standard error of the mean increased with the increase in test velocity. The authors concluded that: 'isokinetic measurements of muscle function offer … sensitive and reliable measurements of trunk muscle performance'. In one of the most comprehensive studies so far, Newton et al (1993) tested trunk muscle performance in a group of 70 normal subjects and 120 low back pain (LBP) patients using sagittal and rotational movements. For the reproducibility and learning effect study, a subgroup of 21 normal and 20 patients was selected and tested on four consecutive occasions, 2–3 days apart. Reproducibility was assessed using intraclass correlation coefficients (ICCs) which, in view of an apparent learning effect, referred to the tests carried out on days 2–4. (The learning effect refers to the variation in the strength scores which cannot be attributed to changes in the actual performance of the muscle/s but to the acquisition of skill or familiarity with the testing procedures. Thus the first testing day was dropped from the analysis.) The spectrum of velocities for testing extension and flexion consisted of 60, 90 and 120 °/s, and for rotations the velocities were 60, 120 and 150 °/s.

The peak moments in all test conditions proved to be highly reliable, with ICCs ranging from 0.93 to 0.98 for the 'interobserver' situation and 0.84 to 0.96 and 0.85 to 0.98 for the two intraobserver situations respectively. On the other hand, isokinetic ratios such as flexion/extension, left/right rotations, endurance or recovery, were shown to be unreproducible. It was hence claimed that these ratios could not be used for clinical purposes. Additionally, the average points variance (APV), which was used in the context of identifying consistency of effort, was not a reproducible parameter. There was a considerable learning effect expressed in increments in the measured variables, ranging from 2 to 16% between day 1 and 2. The authors recommended therefore that isokinetic performance should be assessed on the second test session, on a different day. Though this is an important reflection, it is doubtful whether such advice can be effectively carried out.

The findings derived from the above studies indicate that peak moment, work and probably impulse are reproducible within the context of uniaxial sagittal tests. This statement may be extended to the peak moment in rotational tests. In both cases it refers, however, to the low/medium end of the velocity spectrum.

MULTIJOINT MOTION AND REPRODUCIBILITY

The reproducibility of this type of motion has recently been examined using the Cybex Liftask apparatus (Hazard et al 1993). A group of symptom-free women and men were tested twice over a period of 3–30 days. The protocol consisted of practice pulls followed by three maximal pulls to waist height. The linear velocity of the handle was not specified. The ICC of the peak force was 0.96 with a standard error of the mean of 58 N. The latter figure is very agreeable, considering the mean and SD of peak force in the first and second test sessions were 948 and 379, and 926 and 374, respectively. On the evidence of this study, multijoint test findings are reproducible. However, it is not possible to specify the range of relevant velocities since the test velocity was not quoted.

PART 4
REPRESENTATIVE VALUES

Considering data from isokinetic uniaxial and multijoint testing of normal subjects and LBD patients, in terms of population size, only a few studies stand out as adequate sources for a so-called normative data base. Indeed, except for the studies by Timm (1988) and Freedson et al (1993), which were based on close to 2700 and 4500 subjects respectively, none of the studies qualify in the strict statistical sense, for this purpose. This is quite surprising, considering the economic significance of LBD and the specific role strength testing plays in assessment of back function. Thus although 'strength is the most tangible aspect of lumbar spine function' (Saal et al 1990) judgements concerning the functional capacity or degree of impairment, are still made on a 'local' basis.

On the other hand, the studies mentioned below excelled in controlling the relevant variables (ex-

cept for gravity correction), and used a sufficiently large number of subjects to form a reasonable frame of reference.

As pointed out by Delitto et al (1989) the addition of activity level and age could substantially contribute to a better definition of trunk performance profiles. Smith et al (1985) did mention activity level, but since almost all their subjects were characterized by the same level, this parameter was not introduced into the calculations. Currently, normative data refer to women and men, although some insight into the impact of age has been obtained through the studies of Langrana & Lee (1984), Smith et al (1985) and Mayer et al (1985a, b).

UNIAXIAL TESTING: CONCENTRIC PERFORMANCE

Sagittal trunk motion only, is considered, since this has received almost exclusive attention in work on trunk performance. After the studies by Smith et al (1985) and Mayer et al (1985b) which also dealt with trunk muscle rotational performance, interest in this motion seems to have dwindled quite considerably. The same applies to lateral flexion (side-bending).

Normal trunk muscle performance

Tables 8.1–8.4 outline data on trunk muscle performance for normal women and men. In certain instances, data were presented graphically, notably in the series of papers by Mayer and his colleagues. In these cases, the numerical values of the normalized peak moments as given in the text have been used (Smith et al 1985).

Performance in LBD

Table 8.5 outlines findings of trunk performance for male and female LBD patients from Suzuki & Endo (1983), Mayer et al (1985a) and Reid et al (1991). It should be emphasized that the test positions described by Suzuki & Endo (1983), prone for extension and supine for flexion, are no longer used for testing. The findings from this study are cited to enable the comparison of LBD and control subjects

Table 8.1 Mean normal trunk flexion and extension strength in women

	Nordin et al (1987)	Langrana et al (1984)	Smith et al (1985)	Delitto (1991)
n	101	26	63	32
Position	Sitting	Sitting	Standing	Standing
Units	N m	N m	%ft-lb/lb	%ft-lb/lb
Velocity				
30 °/s				
Flexion	111	60	68	
Extension	122	98	94	
60 °/s				
Flexion	107		68	58
Extension	108		92	82
120 °/s				
Flexion			61	49
Extension			79	73
180 °/s				
Flexion				32
Extension				50

Table 8.2 Mean normal trunk flexion and extension strength in men

	Suzuki & Endo (1983)	Langrana et al (1984)	Smith et al (1985)	Delitto et al (1991)
n	50	50	63	32
Position	Prone/supine	Sitting	Standing	Standing
Units	N m	N m	%ft-lb/lb	%ft-lb/lb
Velocity				
30 °/s				
Flexion	87	137	94	
Extension	157	212	124	
60 °/s				
Flexion			94	81
Extension			121	111
120 °/s				
Flexion			90	79
Extension			110	99
180 °/s				
Flexion				65
Extension				82

Table 8.3 Normative values (N m) for extension in women at 60 °/s, based on Freedson et al (1993)

Percentile	Age (years)				
	< 21	21–30	31–40	41–50	> 50
90	176.3	183.3	199.5	173.6	164.1
70	147.4	155.9	163.1	150.1	116.3
50	130.2	138.3	143.7	137.6	107.1
30	117.0	122.6	124.8	116.5	102.2
10	99.1	104.4	100.3	99.0	84.6

Table 8.4 Normative values (N m) for extension in men at 60 °/s, based on Freedson et al (1993)

Percentile	Age (years)				
	< 21	21–30	31–40	41–50	> 50
90	320.0	333.6	325.4	330.5	259.9
70	272.3	284.8	280.4	276.6	254.4
50	244.1	254.9	248.1	243.4	222.4
30	212.9	223.7	219.7	211.5	197.2
10	173.6	184.4	183.6	180.3	167.9

performance (Table 8.1). Particularly notable is the similarity between the findings of Mayer et al (1985a) and those based on the submaximal effort group of Reid et al (1991).

NORMS IN MULTIJOINT TESTING

In terms of sample size, the most authoritative source on multijoint testing in normal subjects is the work of Timm (1988), in which the descriptive

Table 8.5 Mean trunk strength with low back dysfunction (LBD) in women and men

	Mayer et al (1985a)	Reid et al (1991)		Suzuki & Endo (1983)
		Maximal effort	Submaximal effort	
Women				
n	108	29	16	
Position	Standing	Standing	Standing	
Units	%ft-lb/lb	%ft-lb/lb	%ft-lb/lb	
30 °/s				
Flexion	39			
Extension	36			
60 °/s				
Flexion	32*	65*	38*	
Extension	28*	62*	25*	
120 °/s				
Flexion	13			
Extension	12			
Men				
n	178	86	24	90
Position	Standing	Standing	Standing	Prone/supine
Units	%ft-lb/lb	%ft-lb/lb	%ft-lb/lb	N m
30 °/s				
Flexion	55			70
Extension	49			134
60 °/s				
Flexion	53	90*	53*	
Extension	44	105*	43*	
120 °/s				
Flexion	28			
Extension	22			

* determined from graphical data.

statistics of 1236 women and 1452 men were outlined. Another important study which referred to normal subjects as well as LBD patients is that of Kishino et al (1985). Both studies utilized the Cybex Liftask device, initially positioning subjects in the flexed knees/flexed trunk configuration. The test velocities, given in inch/s (ips), were 6, 12, 18, 24, 30 and 36 ips in Timm (1988) and 18, 30 and 36 ips in Kishino et al (1985).

Table 8.6 is based on Timm's paper and outlines the overall performance parameters versus speed. There was a general decrease in the overall performance with increases in test velocity and age. Timm's study produced some 20 tables relating performance to gender and velocity. Women performed at a level which was generally about 50% that of men.

Table 8.7 combines data from the Kishino et al and Timm studies. The findings for normal subjects in the Kishino study were generally compatible with those of Timm. Differences were somewhat higher scores and a more moderate slope of

Table 8.6 Isokinetic lifting: across age performance parameters*, based on Timm (1988)

Speed, cm/s	Peak force, newtons	Peak force × 100 / Bodyweight	Average force, newtons	Average force × 100 / Bodyweight	Average power, watts	Total work, joules
15	261 (81)	106 (39)	162 (54)	65 (26)	102 (29)	693 (212)
30	245 (77)	99 (37)	149 (51)	60 (24)	143 (59)	638 (231)
45	227 (74)	92 (35)	129 (46)	52 (22)	185 (79)	558 (205)
60	205 (77)	83 (36)	113 (49)	46 (23)	219 (109)	485 (220)
75	197 (82)	79 (39)	108 (49)	44 (24)	266 (147)	475 (236)
90	181 (79)	73 (37)	95 (47)	38 (25)	307 (118)	421 (217)

* Rounded to integers, mean (SD).

Table 8.7 Mean lifting force in lbs in normal and LBD subjects. Data in parentheses are normalized units, % lb/lbs body-weight

			Velocity, cm/s	
	n	45	75	90
Women				
Kishino et al (1985)				
LBD	25	70* (53)	62* (45)	55* (40)
Normal	42	105* (78)	95* (72)	90* (68)
Timm (1988)†				
Normal	1001	105 (61)	77 (55)	69 (48)
Men				
Kishino et al (1985)				
LBD	43	140* (68)	130* (63)	120* (57)
Normal	23	210* (115)	200* (110)	195* (107)
Timm (1988)†				
Normal	1110	200 (107)	173 (86)	161 (79)

* Figures determined from the graphical data.
† Figures based on the average of the four decade groups 20–59.

the force–velocity curve. The same gender performance ratios were indicated. The findings also demonstrated a difference of some 25–30% between control and LBD subjects.

UNIAXIAL TESTING: CONCENTRIC AND ECCENTRIC PERFORMANCE NORMS

None of the available studies which compare concentric and eccentric exertions, provide normative data. Smidt et al (1980) reported findings based on 11 subjects, tested at 13 °/s. In a more recent study by Smidt et al (1989) the findings, from a group of seven subjects tested at 20 °/s, indicated that the concentric and eccentric flexion torque were 156 and 174 N m respectively whereas for extension the figures were 270 and 330 N m. The authors did not distinguish between women and men. In the same paper, the approximate preconditioning peak moment scores of 45 subjects, 24 women and 21 men, were as follows: 130 and 140 N m in concentric and eccentric flexion, and 220 and 280 N m for concentric and eccentric extension. In this case also, all findings were pooled.

In another study by Marras et al (1989) the peak concentric and eccentric moments at 30 °/s were calculated to equal approximately 150 and 160 N m, whereas the figures at 10 °/s were 160 and 150 N m respectively.

No eccentric performance scores were available for LBD patients at the time this book went into press.

PART 5
INTERPRETATION OF TRUNK ISOKINETIC TEST FINDINGS

GENERAL GUIDELINES

The interpretation of findings from isokinetic trunk sagittal performance of patients suffering from LBD, is more difficult than that for other major joint systems. Difficulty arises not only from the complexity of the trunk, but also from the absence of a symmetric contralateral segment. Therefore, unless performance records from the preinjury/LBD period are available, one has to rely on normative databases. The latter, however, are not always adequate and intra- or extrapolation is normally needed to put individual findings in the correct clinical perspective.

Starting therefore with data from symptom-free subjects, the following general guidelines are used:

1. Men are significantly stronger than women, hence findings should be treated according to gender, even if bodyweight is accounted for.

2. Trunk extensors are stronger than flexors throughout the normally used velocity spectrum.

3. There are significant differences in the strength output between the most commonly used test velocities and hence findings from tests at different velocities may not be compared. Furthermore, the typical relationship of moment versus angular velocity and force versus distance are maintained during concentric contractions.

4. The range of the ratio: peak extension/peak flexion moment is 1.2–1.4. However, considering discrete points along the strength curve, the ratio of extension/flexion moments is highly variable, and reflects the individual mechanical behavior of the flexors and extensors.

5. While the eccentric to concentric strength ratio is in most cases greater than unity, there is a difference between the flexor and extensor muscle groups. The ratio for the flexors seems to be smaller than that for the extensors 1.1 and 1.25 respectively.

6. There are discrepancies between sources concerning the effect of age. One study indicated that age had a negative effect on uniaxial trunk muscle performance, and that variations were more

conspicuous between the third and fifth decade (Langrana & Lee 1984). Multijoint tests confirmed this effect but show that the overall performance increases from the second to the third decade and henceforth decreases through the eighth decade (Timm 1988). On the other hand Smith et al (1985) and Mayer et al (1985a) suggested that trunk performance remained basically the same throughout the decades relevant for LBD.

STRENGTH-BASED (SINGLE PARAMETER) INTERPRETATION

Reduction in strength in LBD

Consideration of the common features in LBD patients, shows that the most conspicuous among them is a general reduction in strength, which may be evident from the peak moment level in uniaxial as well as multijoint exertions. (Although this observation was not supported by either Thorstensson & Arvidson (1982) or Suzuki & Endo (1983), the testing positions employed in these studies, which could decisively influence the test outcome, are no longer in use, and these will not be further discussed). It should be borne in mind that LBD results from a variety of causes and this is a general rather than specific observation. Moreover, since pain itself has a directly inhibitory effect on muscle tension production, the test may reflect patient tolerance as well as muscle capacity (see also below).

Comparison of Tables 8.1 and 8.2 with Table 8.5 and examination of Table 8.7 highlight this reduction. Clearly, the extensors demonstrate a significantly greater strength deficit, compared to the flexors, which has been universally reported. This conclusion is also illustrated by Table 8.8, which gives the ratios obtained by dividing the average strength of LBD patients by that of normal subjects. The figures shown in this Table were calculated from the original papers by Smith et al (1985) and Mayer et al (1985a). Since the raw data were not available to this author, these ratios may be interpreted as estimates only, but they indicate that the relative decline in the extensor strength was without exception greater than that experienced by the flexors.

The proportionately much higher reduction in extensor strength has been attributed to muscle atrophy and neuromuscular inhibition (Mayer et al 1985a). The neuromuscular inhibition was claimed to play a 'substantial role' in the observed strength deficit, and it is possible that it was instrumental in bringing about the muscle atrophy.

On the other hand, pain was not implicated alone for inconsistent curve shapes (Mayer et al 1985a). The possible variations in the strength curves of some muscle groups brings forward the issue of maximal versus non-maximal effort.

Effort characteristics

As pointed out in Chapter 3, effort is a multifaceted construct, comprising physiological, behavioral and performance elements. The individual effort during isokinetic trunk testing may be judged according to the presence or absence of, for example, exaggerated autonomic signs (physiological), compliance and/or pain complaints (behavioral), and variations in the fundamental performance criteria such as peak moment, curve shape or the ability to duplicate the curve in three trials (Mayer et al 1985a).

Effort was rated by Mayer and his colleagues using the qualitative categories: excellent, good, fair and poor. It was indicated that 'effort was not ideal in many of these patients and this was a factor in the lower strength test results for the chronic LBD patients'.

Reid et al (1991) used curve shape reproducibility as a criterion for classifying chronic LBD patients into maximal and submaximal effort subgroups; the

Table 8.8 Ratios of trunk strength: LBD/normal subjects, as percentage, calculated from studies by Mayer et al (1985a) and Smith et al (1985)

	30 °/s		60 °/s		120 °/s	
	Flexion	Extension	Flexion	Extension	Flexion	Extension
Women	57	38	47	30	21	15
Men	59	40	56	37	31	20

maximal effort group developed significantly greater extension and flexion moments, as well as a greater extension flexion ratio compared with the submaximal group. Moreover, it is patently clear from Table 8.5 that for women and men alike, the average extension and flexion strength in the submaximal groups closely resembled the findings by the Mayer group. Again, comparing the data of Reid et al from the maximal effort group with the data of the control group in the same study, as well as with the normal subjects of Smith et al (1985), there is a great similarity in flexion strength but a reduction in extension.

These comparisons support the suggestion of Mayer et al (1985a) that fear of injury, rather than an intention to mislead, was behind the lower 'nonideal' effort. This conclusion was related to the fact that 'vast majority' of the patients demonstrated reasonable reproducibility, and hence low variability, of the strength curves. On the other hand, Reid et al regarded over 25% of the patients as manifesting submaximal effort using reproducibility as a criterion. The issue of curve reproducibility in LBD patients versus normal subjects has recently been investigated using the average points variance (APV) parameter (Newton et al 1993). It was strongly indicated that there was no evidence to support the contention that consistency of curves in isokinetic testing could serve as a criterion for maximal or submaximal effort. This conclusion, which indirectly supports those reached by Mayer et al (1985a), seems to put to rest, at least for the time being, the issue of curve reproducibility as a basis for determination of optimality of effort as it relates to the *trunk muscles' isokinetic performance*. It should, however, be pointed out that this statement does not detract from the significance of curve reproducibility in analyzing sincerity of effort relative to limb muscle performance.

Implications for interpretation

It follows from the above discussion that a significant reduction in trunk performance is not a sufficient basis for a clinical decision and consistency of reproduction of the strength curves should be studied. If they do not show a reasonable degree of overlapping then the performance parameters evidently reflect a nonoptimal effort. It the curves demonstrate reasonable consistency, the observed reduction should be judged against the general effort made by the patient, using behavioral parameters, particularly pain scales/questionnaires.

Only when one has become convinced that there is a firm basis for the low strength scores, may a decision for further treatment or other recommendation be made. As pointed out by Beimborn & Morrissey (1988), the use of pain measurement tools as an integral component of isokinetic testing could serve to define criteria for continuing/discontinuing the latter.

Interpretation of reduction in strength

What should then be considered a significant reduction in trunk strength? The answer depends on:

1. the reference normative data base
2. the test parameters
3. the degree of effort.

As the most comprehensive database available is still that of Mayer's group, it is suggested that a combination of findings based on the latter, together with those by Reid et al (1991), would furnish the optimal frame of reference.

For example a 41-year-old, LBD woman patient, has the following performance scores, from a standing position test at 60 °/s: peak flexion and extension strength are 55 and 48 ft-lb/ft. At this velocity, a normal woman is expected to produce, according to Mayer et al (1985a) approximately 70 and 95 flf (SDs were were about 5 flf) for flexion and extension respectively. Thus, according to the accepted standards, this patient is presenting with reduced strength of both muscle groups, approximately 20 and 50% for flexion and extension respectively. In addition the inversion of the extension/flexion ratio is typical of LBD.

If she is exerting a submaximal effort, one would expect this patient to be capable of improving her scores, probably eliminating the need for attention to the flexors, and concentrating on the extensor performance. Conversely, if the subject demonstrates cooperation and motivation, and the effort results in good curve reproducibility, these scores indicate a general reduction in performance.

EFFECT OF TEST VELOCITY

The impact of test velocity on muscle performance is most conspicuous in uniaxial testing of LBD patients. This effect, 'high velocity drop-off', takes the form of a steeper decline of the moment–velocity curve, in both genders and for all age groups, relative to controls (Mayer et al 1985a). In that study, it was indicated that whereas in flexion, the mean moment/bodyweight (in ft-lb/lb) for male patients was about 60% of the control mean at the lowest test velocity (30 °/s), it dropped to 30 °/s of the control mean at the highest velocity (120%). In extension, the drop-off in absolute, though not in relative, terms was even greater, going down from 40 to 20%.

These figures should be compared with the normal drop-off in men (Table 8.2): increasing the test velocity from 30 to 120 °/s resulted in a decrease of approximately 4 and 11% in flexion and extension strength respectively (Smith et al 1985), whereas the change from 60 to 180 °/s (Delitto et al 1991) meant a reduction of 20 and 26% respectively. Similar figures were noted for women. Although Mayer et al (1985a) have suggested that the dramatic drop-off, particularly in the extensors could be partially explained by their lower content of fast twitch fibers compared to the flexors, these findings may primarily be interpreted in terms of neuromuscular inhibition. As the prescribed test velocity increases, so does the acceleration and a higher initial force is necessary. This higher force may in turn be imposed on vulnerable structures which in certain circumstances is liable to provoke pain. This is probably part of the explanation for the fear of injury.

On the other hand, it has been shown (Dvir et al 1991) that in the knee, a slower effort was correlated with a greater degree of pain, because of a longer exposure to the mechanical stresses as well as a stronger contraction intensity. Therefore, if this pain duration model is equally valid for trunk exertions, the so-called higher drop-off may reflect an adaptation to the initial high stresses rather than to those that take place along the full ROM.

In this respect, velocity ramping (isoacceleration) could offer a creative solution to the patient's discomfort/anxiety. This again emphasizes the importance of adopting slow rather than fast velocities in clinical trunk isokinetics.

MULTIPLE-PARAMETER INTERPRETATION

Recent studies have attempted to incorporate other mechanical parameters such as work and power, in addition to strength, in order to arrive at a composite muscle performance index (Jerome et al 1991, Timm 1992). These indexes are said to be:

a. More reflective of trunk muscle capacity, as they give equal weight to the peak moment and average power which are maximal at low and high velocities respectively.

b. More stable than the peak moment in the sense that they are unaffected by the testing velocity and need not be adjusted for age, height and weight.

The muscle performance index

In order to produce a performance index, test protocols consist of a combination of several velocities. Table 8.9 outlines the original protocol used in the study by Jerome et al (1991).

A muscle performance index (MPI) was defined by Jerome et al (1991) using the following formula:

$$\text{Muscle performance} = 0.125\,(PM_{L1} + PM_{L2} + AP_{H1} + AP_{H2} + BW_{L1} + BW_{L2} + BW_{H1} + BW_{H2})$$

where: PM, peak moment (torque in the original paper); AP, average power; BW, best work repetition; H_1, H_2, highest and second highest velocity respectively, and L_1, L_2, lowest and second lowest velocity respectively.

Table 8.10 outlines the MPI scores obtained in the study from a group of 160 healthy subjects (83 women, 77 men).

Interpretation of performance index

In interpreting the scores some considerations should be borne in mind.

Table 8.9 Test protocol for trunk performance index, based on Jerome et al (1991)

Protocol I: low velocity					
Velocity (°/s)	30	60	90	120	60
Repetitions	5	5	5	5	5
Rest time (s)	30	30	30	30	30
Protocol II: intermediate velocity					
Velocity (°/s)	60	90	120	150	90
Repetitions	5	5	5	5	5
Rest time (s)	30	30	30	30	30
Protocol III: high velocity					
Velocity (°/s)	90	120	150	180	120
Repetitions	5	5	5	5	5
Rest time (s)	30	30	30	30	30

Table 8.10 Mean muscle performance (MP) indices, based on Jerome et al (1991)

Protocol		MP-Flexion	MP-Extension	MP-Flexion*	MP-Extension*
I	Men	197	240	183	227
	Women	110	127	127	147
	Pooled	148	177	152	182
II	Men	202	233	186	218
	Women	119	133	137	150
	Pooled	163	186	164	186
III	Men	218	269	190	239
	Women	164	197	137	155
	Pooled	158	186	162	194

* Adjusted for age, height and weight.

1. The MPI is based on a combination of parameters which do not share a unified unit. Thus although both peak moment and best work repetition are newton-meters (or in foot-pounds) the former is a moment unit whereas the latter is a unit of work also known as the joule. Moreover, power is given in terms of watts (joules per second). Hence the number obtained from the MPI is meaningless insofar as it is assumed to stand for a single mechanical entity.

2. As no significant differences, within gender, were noted among the MPIs of the three protocols, the selection of the protocol is left to the discretion of the examiner

3. Currently, this index may only apply to flexion–extension analysis, as its applicability to, for example, axial rotations, has not so far been demonstrated.

4. Similarly, the MPI was derived from a sample of normal subjects, and its value for LBD patients has yet to be proven

While the full implications of the MPI are not known, its single most important advantage is the simultaneous incorporation of muscle performance indices at different velocities. On the other hand, since trunk performance is often expressed relative to norms, the latter must first be established.

The use of the MPI: an example

A male subject, of 42 years, was tested for trunk extension using protocol II (intermediate velocity, see Table 8.10) and produced the test scores shown in Table 8.11. The MPI was thence calculated:

$$MPI = 0.125 (130 + 120 + 250 + 180 + 120 + 95$$
$$+ 65 + 50)$$
$$= 126.25$$

Table 8.11 Scores produced by a 42-year-old man tested for trunk extension, using protocol II (see Table 8.10)

	Velocity; °/s			
	60	90	120	150
Peak moment (ft-lb)	130	120	110	90
Average power (ft-lb/s)	80	140	180	250
Best work repetition (ft-lb)	120	95	65	50

If the findings quoted in Jerome et al (1991) represent norms, this score would have translated to about a 42% reduction in performance.

The average performance deficit

Another performance index, the average performance deficit (APD), incorporates, in addition to peak moment, average power and total work the endurance ratio which is defined as the work comparison between the first and last half of the set of test repetitions (Timm 1992). Conversion formulae enable the calculation of APD from MPI and vice versa.

Discrimination of normal and LBD subjects

The use of multiple indicators for discriminating normal subjects from LBD patients was demonstrated in an excellent study by Grabiner and Jeziorowski (1992). All subjects were asked to exert maximal extensor effort at three velocities, 60, 120 and 180 °/s. A set of nonstandard isokinetic parameters were extracted, based on the graphic representation as illustrated in Figure 8.3. A mathematical expression, using these parameters correctly discriminated between all control and LBD subjects. All the parameters were derived from the two

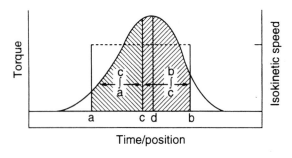

Fig. 8.3 Stylized extraction of isokinetic variables; a, onset of isokinetic motion; b, end of isokinetic motion; a–b, isokinetic range; c, midrange moment; d, peak moment; shaded area a–c ($\int_a^c$), work from onset of isokinetic motion to midrange moment; shaded area c–b ($\int_c^b$) work from midrange moment to offset of isokinetic motion. Trunk angles are taken from the X-axis, —— moment, ---- isokinetic velocity. X axis refers to the angular position of the lever arm which is also the displacement of the trunk relative to the initial position. The true isokinetic range is reached past the transient (nonisokinetic) motion. (From Grabiner & Jeziorowski 1992 Clinical Biomechanics 7: 195–200, with permission of Butterworth-Heinemann.)

higher velocities, emphasizing the significance of muscle power as a major component in trunk muscle performance.

As pointed out, at the time of writing this book, the use of multiple-parameter analysis is still in its infancy. However, it seems to be a promising development in the application of isokinetics to trunk assessment. The present author believes that once test protocols and norms are established, the interpretation of tests will become more thorough and cogent. This will no doubt help practitioners to provide rational rehabilitation programs.

EXTENSION/FLEXION RATIOS

Extension to flexion (E/F) ratios occupy a special niche in trunk performance, isometric as well as isokinetic. Because of the lack of bilateral comparisons, additional parameters were required for a better understanding of trunk performance characteristics. Thus the rationale behind the interest in the extension/flexion ratio was that a deviation from the so-called normal proportion indicated a specific disorder in trunk function.

Though reduction of the extension/flexion ratio, from approximately 1.3 to less than unity among LBD patients was noted (Mayer et al 1985a), its

relevance was later questioned by Delitto et al (1991), who indicated a low test–retest reliability.

In another study, Reid et al (1991) failed to demonstrate such an inversion in maximal effort male LBD patients although it did appear in the maximal effort female group. On the other hand, this 'inversion' phenomenon was typical of both men and women belonging to the submaximal effort group. The significance of the effort factor is clearly evident. Since powerful extension is probably threatening to LBD patients, those that are more anxious avoid, consciously, or even subconsciously, exerting high stresses on the lumbar spine.

Hence the change in the ratio reflects first and foremost a reduction in the extensor capacity as mentioned earlier. Therefore when interpreting the significance of this ratio, one should pay particular attention to the degree of effort exerted by the patient.

CONCENTRIC AND ECCENTRIC RELATIONSHIPS

The question of eccentric versus the concentric strength of the trunk muscles has received relatively little attention. One reason for the importance of this topic is the empirical observation that the onset of low back pain, in a substantial number of cases, takes place during an eccentric activity, that is, lowering the trunk to pick up or manipulate an object. Furthermore, LBD patients perform extension at a significantly slower rate compared with control subjects (Marras & Wongsam 1986), probably attempting to minimize the dynamic loads imposed on the lumbar spine. These loads obviously tend to increase as flexion progresses and may reach thousands of newtons.

The commonly held impression that the moment output during eccentric contractions is higher than in concentric contractions has been challenged in a study of trunk extensors by Marras & Mirka (1989). In this study, subjects were tested in the sagittal as well as off-sagittal planes and maximal moments were recorded as a function of the contraction mode, and angular position and velocity. It was indicated that the eccentric moments were greater than the concentric moments only in the forward flexion position of 40°. It was also demonstrated that at 22.5° the tension output of the extensors is greater than at both ends of the tested ROM, suggesting the angle of choice for determination of the extensor eccentric/concentric ratio.

Although a study comparing the eccentric with the concentric performance of trunk muscles in LBD patients could not be located at the time of writing this book, the implications of such a study are obvious. In analogy to other studies which emphasized the possible connection between pain and eccentric activity (Bennett & Stauber 1986, Dvir et al 1991), it may not be unreasonable to expect similar patterns in trunk extensor function. Furthermore, with the alleviation of pain these patterns may vary, allowing for less restrained motion in terms of velocity and rhythm, and providing a more comprehensive basis for interpretation.

MULTIJOINT TESTING AND INTERPRETATION

Though published studies concerning interpretation of clinically-related data were not available at the time of writing, it is quite certain that isokinetic lift simulation will become an important tool. The subject of materials handling has received considerable attention because of the possible association with LBD (Andersson 1991), and the possibility of simulating this activity and extracting information from the force–distance curve is particularly appealing.

Significance of isokinetic lift testing

As an example for the value of isokinetic lift versus isokinetic trunk flexion–extension testing, consider the following case presented by Rowinski & McGorry (1992) using a Biodex lift apparatus.

The performance of a normal subject (Fig. 8.4) is contrasted with that of a patient with a hemivertebra. The patient's flexion and extension performance during early rehabilitation, after an acute episode of instability and inflammation (Fig. 8.5), is compared with that of 1 month later (Fig. 8.6). A significant peak moment increase, from about 200 ft-lb to 260 ft-lb, was apparent, indicating the recovery of near normal values.

Comparison of this patient's lift performance (Fig. 8.7), at the same time as the test shown in

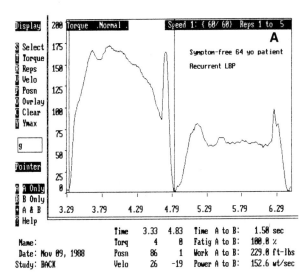

Fig. 8.4 Normal trunk flexion/extension MAP curves. (From Rowinski & McGorry 1992, with the permission of Biodex Corp.)

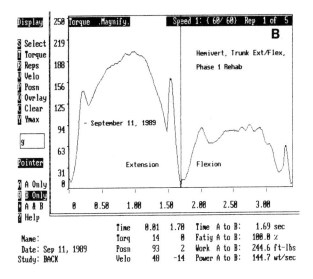

Fig. 8.5 Trunk flexion/extension MAP curve of a patient with a hemivertebra during the subacute phase. (From Rowinski & McGorry 1992, with the permission of Biodex Corp.)

Figure 8.6, with that of a normal subject (Fig. 8.8) demonstrated a severe reduction in his ability to sustain lifting in mid-range, in spite of the fact that extensor strength was almost entirely recovered. Therefore, the functional integration of strength had not yet been achieved. This important observation of Rowinski & McGorry emphasizes the especial significance of functional integration in trunk rehabilitation.

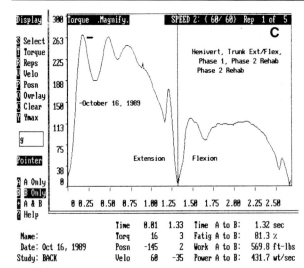

Fig. 8.6 Same patient during the chronic phase. Improvement in strength, total work, power and development of moment (rising phase) was evident with symptom resolution and stabilizing exercise program. Moment values consistent with normative values for the patient's age group. (From Rowinski & McGorry 1992, with the permission of Biodex Corp.)

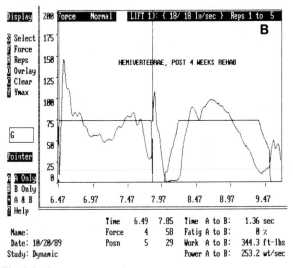

Fig. 8.7 Same patient performing a dynamic lift simulation during the same stage of rehabilitation as in Figure 8.9. Note severe depression in ability to sustain lifting force in mid-range, even though trunk extension musculature had been appropriately strengthened. (From Rowinski & McGorry 1992, with the permission of Biodex Corp.)

PART 6
ISOKINETIC CONDITIONING PROTOCOLS

The question of isokinetic trunk conditioning can be described as terra incognita. Although the prin-

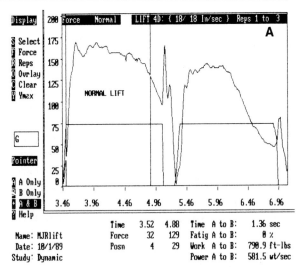

Fig. 8.8 Matched normal subject performing a dynamic lift simulation. (From Rowinski & McGorry 1992, with the permission of Biodex Corp.)

ciples governing conditioning of muscles in other joint systems may be equally relevant in LBD, almost all clinical literature concerns testing and evaluation rather than treatment.

The indications for trunk muscle conditioning were clearly presented by Mayer and his colleagues in their classical series of papers. Later, in a book on restoration for spinal disorders (Mayer & Gatchel 1988), the authors coined the term the 'deconditioned spine' which referred to measurable deficits in performance, that is, ROM, strength and endurance, and functional abilities.

As far as muscle capacity is concerned, a significant and selective reduction in extensor performance in maximal effort patients was shown in these studies. Flexion was also compromised in patients performing at a submaximal level, but the main deficit still rested with the extensors. Consequently, the main target in reconditioning of the spine should arguably be the extensors.

A concentric conditioning program

Timm (1987) described the use of concentric isokinetic conditioning of trunk flexors and extensors in the rehabilitation of two back patients. One patient was referred following spinal surgery while the other patient had suffered a right cardiovascular accident. These events had taken place 6 months and 2 years, respectively, before the initiation of the treatment program. Both patients complained of lumbar pain and problems with sitting.

A pyramidal velocity spectrum protocol was used, consisting of 10 repetitions of flexion and extension progressing from 30 to 60, 90, and 120 °/s and regressing back down to 30 °/s through a ROM of 45°. One minute of rest was allowed between speeds and patients were instructed to perform to personal tolerance while emphasizing the extension component. The ROM was progressively increased to up to 90° of flexion and 10° hyperextension.

The author quoted consistent improvement in extension and flexion strength during the treatment periods, which lasted typically 2 months, until a complete resolution of the symptoms.

It is, however, difficult to judge the findings of this paper as the strength values quoted by the author were grossly outside the expected capacity of patients, even those who demonstrate outstanding restoration of strength. For instance, one patient whose weight was 179 lb, was reported to reach peak moments of 250 and 291 ft-lb, in flexion and extension respectively, at 30 °/s. These numbers translate into 140 and 163 %ft-lb (!), figures attributable to very strong normal males. Though the moments quoted for the other patient were smaller, they too were far from what could reasonably be expected. Thus besides wondering whether the system was properly calibrated one cannot draw any significant conclusion from this study.

However, some elements of the above treatment protocol may be incorporated within a general protocol.

GUIDELINES FOR ISOKINETIC TRUNK CONDITIONING

As far as the isokinetic component of conditioning of low back musculature is concerned, the following considerations should be taken into account:

1. Assessment of passive compliance following nonisokinetic warm-up. Most systems are currently equipped with the passive mobility option which requires no effort from the patient to be exerted against the machine. By gradually varying the passive trunk ROM and following the resulting changes in the moment curves one may be able to determine 'failure points'. These may either signify painful sectors of the arc of motion or a disproportionate increase/decrease in soft tissue compliance. These points may consequently serve both as clinical indicators and motion limits.

2. Proportionately larger emphasis on extension. The input ratio, in terms of contractile activity, should not be less than 2:1 in favor of extension relative to flexion. Though this is an arbitrary 'rule', the present author believes this to be a more clinically sound proportion. This should be compared with a protocol dictating flexion–extension concentric activity cycles which conform to no particular activities of daily living (ADL) need.

3. Incorporation of upper force (moment) limits. Though patients may be their own best judges, it is advisable to set these limits, whenever possible. This option is readily available in all modern systems, and it helps in ensuring that the patient does not inadvertently exceed safety values. Such a limit may be based on the peak moment recorded during prior testing (single exertion).

4. A spectrum of concentric velocities limited to 90 °/s. This holds unless a special employment skill, or other activity in which a patient is often engaged, dictates otherwise. The pyramidal increase and decrease of velocities can be used efficiently with a 'quantal' step of 30 °/s as used by Timm (1987). The velocities used should be compatible with the allowed ROM; it is useless to prescribe a 90 °/s exercise when the total ROM is only 20°.

5. Gradual incorporation of eccentric activity. The stage of incorporation depends on factors which have been discussed in detail before as well as on the patients tolerance. The velocities used should not exceed 60 °/s since in certain circumstances these may result in unacceptable loads. Force or moment limits should be applied throughout.

REFERENCES

Andersson G B 1981 Epidemiologic aspects of low back pain in industry. Spine 6: 53–60

Beimborn D S, Morrissey M C 1988 A review of the literature related to trunk muscle performance. Spine 13: 655–660

Bennett G, Stauber W 1986 evaluation and treatment of anterior knee pain using eccentric exercise. Medicine and Science in Sports and Exercise 18: 526–530

Biering-Sorensen F 1984 Physical measurements as risk indicators of low back troubles over a one year period. Spine 9: 106–119

Cale-Benzoor M, Albert M, Grodin A, Woodruff L D 1992 Isokinetic trunk muscle performance characteristics of classical ballet dancers. Journal of Orthopaedic and Sports Physical Therapy 15: 99–105

Delitto A, Crandell C E, Rose J 1989 Peak torque-to-body weight ratios in the trunk: a critical analysis. Physical Therapy 69: 138–143

Delitto A, Rose S J, Crandell C C Strube M J 1991 Reliability of isokinetic measurements of trunk muscle performance. Spine 16: 800–803

Diffrient N, Tilley A R, Bardagjy J C 1978 Humanscale 1/2/3. MIT Press, Cambridge, Massachusetts

Dvir Z, Halperin N, Shklar A, Robinson D 1991 Quadriceps function and patellofemoral pain syndrome. Part 2: pain provocation during concentric and eccentric activity. Isokinetics and Exercise Science 1: 26–30

Farfan H F 1975 Muscular mechanism of the lumbar spine and the position of power and efficiency. Orthopaedic Clinics of North America 6: 135

Farfan H F 1978 The biomechanical advantage of lordosis and hip extension for upright activity. Man as compared with other anthropoids. Spine 3: 336

Freedson P S, Gilliam T B, Mahoney T, Maliszewski A F, Kastango K 1993 Industrial torque levels by age group and gender. Isokinetics and Exercise Science 3: 34–42

Grabiner M D, Jeziorowski J J 1992 Isokinetic trunk extension discriminates uninjured subjects from subjects with previous low back pain. Clinical Biomechanics 7: 195–200

Grabiner M D, Jeziorowski J J, Divekar A D 1990 Isokinetic measurements of trunk extension and flexion performance collected with the Biodex clinical data station. Journal of Orthopaedic and Sports Physical Therapy 11: 590–598

Gracovetsky S, Farfan H F, Lamy C 1977 A mathematical model of the lumbar spine using an optimized system to control muscles and ligaments. Orthopaedic Clinics of North America 8: 135

Hause M, Fujiwara M, Kikuchi S 1980 A new method of quantitative measurement of abdominal and back muscle strength. Spine 9: 171–175

Hazard R G, Reid S, Fenwick J, Reeves V 1988 Isokinetic trunk and lifting strength measurements: variability as an indicator of effort. Spine 13: 54–57

Hazard R G, Reeves V, Fenwick J W, Fleming B C, Pope M H 1993 Test-retest variation in lifting capacity and indices of subject effort. Clinical Biomechanics 8: 20–24

Jerome J A, Hunter K, Gordon P, McKay N 1991 A new robust index for measuring isokinetic trunk flexion and extension: outcome from a regional study. Spine 16: 804–808

Kishino N D, Mayer T G, Gatchel R J, McCrate Parrish M, Anderson C, Gustin L, Mooney V 1985 Quantification of lumbar function. Part 4: isometric and isokinetic lifting simulation in normal subjects and low-back dysfunction patients. Spine 10: 921–927

Langrana N A, Lee C K 1984 Isokinetic testing. Spine 9: 171–175

Langrana N A, Lee C K, Alexander H 1984 Quantitative assessment of back strength under isokinetic testing. Spine 9: 287–290

Macintosh J E, Bogduk N 1987 The anatomy and function of the lumbar back muscles and their fascia. In Twomey L T,

Taylor J R (eds) Physical therapy of the low back. Churchill Livingstone, New York, pp 103–134

Marras W S, Mirka G A 1989 Trunk strength during asymmetric trunk motion. Human Factors 31: 238–249

Marras W S, Wongsam P E 1986 Flexibility and velocity of the normal and impaired lumbar spine. Archives of Physical Medicine and Rehabilitation 67: 213–217

Marras W S, King A I, Joynt R L 1984 Measurement of loads on the lumbar spine under isometric and isokinetic conditions. Spine 9: 176–187

Marras W S, Rongarajulu S L, Wongsam P E 1987 Trunk force development during static and dynamic lifts. Human Factors 29: 19–29

Marras W S, Ferguson S A, Simon S R 1990 Three dimensional dynamic motor performance of the normal trunk. International Journal of Industrial Ergonomics 6: 211–224.

Mayer T G, Gatchel R J 1988 Functional restoration for spinal disorders: the sports medicine approach. Lea & Febiger, Philadelphia

Mayer T G, Smith S S, Keeley J, Mooney V 1985a Quantification of lumbar function. Part 2: sagittal plane trunk strength in chronic low-back pain patients. Spine 10: 765–772

Mayer T G, Smith S S, Kondraske G, Gatchel R J, Carmichael T W, Mooney V 1985b Quantification of lumbar function. Part 3: preliminary data on isokinetic torso rotation testing with myoelectric spectral analysis in normal and low-back pain subjects. Spine 10: 912–920

Mostardi R A, Noe D A, Kovacik M W, Porterfield J A 1992 Isokinetic lifting and occupational injury a prospective study. Spine 17: 189

Newton M, Thow M, Somerville D, Henderson I, Waddell G 1993 Trunk strength testing with iso-machines part II: experimental evaluation of the Cybex II back testing system in normal subjects and patients with chronic low back pain. Spine 18: 812–824

Nordin M, Kahanovitz N, Verderame R, Parianpour M, Yabut S, Viola Greenidge N, Mulvihill M 1987 Normal trunk muscle strength and endurance in women and the effect of exercise and electrical stimulation. Part 1: normal endurance and trunk muscle strength in women. Spine 12: 105–111

Parnianpour M, Nordin M, Kahanovitz N, Frankel V 1988 The triaxial coupling of torque generation of trunk muscles during isometric exertions and the effect of fatiguing isoinertial movements on the motor output and movement patterns. Spine 9: 982–992

Porterfield J A, Mostardi R A, King S, Ariki P, Moats E, Noe D 1987 Simulated lift testing using computerized isokinetics. Spine 12: 683–687

Rowinski M J, McGorry R 1992 Lift simulation. Biodex Evaluation and Management, Shirley, New York

Reid S, Hazard R G, Fenwick J W 1991 Isokinetic trunk strength deficits in people with and without low-back pain: a comparative study with consideration of effort. Journal of Spinal Disorders 4: 68–72

Saal J S, Lerman R M, Keane J P 1990 Objective assessment of lumbar spine function. Critical Reviews in Physical Medicine and Rehabilitation 2: 25–38

Smidt G L, Amundsen L R, Dostal W F 1980 Muscle strength at the trunk. Journal of Orthopaedic and Sports Physical Therapy 1: 165–170

Smidt G L, Hering T, Amundsen L, Rogers M, Russel A, Lehmann T 1983 Assessment of abdominal and back extensor function: a quantitative approach and results for chronic low-back patients. Spine 8: 211–219

Smidt G L, Blanpied P R, White R W 1989 Exploration of mechanical and electromyographic responses of trunk muscles to high-intensity resistive exercises. Spine 815–830

Smith S S, Mayer T G, Gatchel R J, Becker T J 1985 Quantification of lumbar function Part 1: isometric and multispeed isokinetic trunk strength measurements in sagittal and axial planes in normal subjects. Spine 10: 757–764

Stokes I A F 1987 Axis for dynamic measurement of flexion and extension torques about the lumbar spine: a computer simulation. Physical Therapy 67: 1230–1233

Stokes I A F, Gookin D M, Reid S, Hazard R G 1990 Effects of axis placement on measurement of isokinetic flexion and extension torque in the lumbar spine. Journal of Spinal Disorders 2: 114–118

Suzuki N, Endo S 1983 A quantitative study of trunk muscle strength and fatigability in the low-back pain syndrome. Spine 8: 69–75

Thompson N N, Gould J A, Davies G J 1985 Descriptive measures of isokinetic trunk testing. Journal of Orthopaedic and Sport Physical Therapy 7: 43–49

Thorstensson A, Arvidson A 1982 Trunk muscle strength and low back pain. Scandinavian Journal of Rehabilitation Medicine 14: 69–75

Thorstensson A, Nilsson J 1982 Trunk muscle strength during constant velocity movements. Scandinavian Journal of Rehabilitation Medicine 14: 61–68

Timm K E 1987 Case studies: use of the Cybex extension flexion unit in the rehabilitation of back patients. Journal of Orthopaedic and Sports Physical Therapy 8: 578–581

Timm K E 1988 Isokinetic lifting simulation: a normative data study. Journal of Orthopaedic and Sports Physical Therapy 9: 156–166

Timm K E 1991 Effect of different kinetic chain states on the isokinetic performance of the lumbar muscles. Isokinetics and Exercise Science 1: 153–160

Timm K E 1992 Lumbar spine testing and rehabilitation. In: Davies G E (ed) A compendium of isokinetics in clinical usage. S & S Publishers, Onalaska, Wisconsin, p 497–532

Isokinetics of the shoulder muscles

Apart from few studies in the late 1970s, evaluation of shoulder muscle performance using isokinetic dynamometry did not begin in earnest before the 1980s. This was because of the overriding interest in knee evaluation and rehabilitation, and the particular suitability of common isokinetic systems to knee testing. The latter may still be the methodological reason for the relative dearth of information about the highly intricate relationships of the shoulder complex muscles. Thus for instance there are no standard examination positions. Consequently, it is difficult to establish norms according to which patient status and/or progress may be judged except by using bilateral comparisons.

Moreover, the particular vulnerability of several glenohumeral structures to the high loads which may sometimes obtain during isokinetic efforts, might have given rise to some reluctance among clinicians to test or treat the shoulder using isokinetic systems (Walker et al 1987).

The following subjects are discussed in this chapter: general principles of shoulder isokinetics; isokinetic testing procedures; representative values, and interpretation and clinical applications.

PART 1
GENERAL PRINCIPLES OF SHOULDER ISOKINETICS AND TESTING PROCEDURES

GENERAL PRINCIPLES

The most striking feature of the shoulder complex is the extensive range of movement it affords the arm and hand. Arm motion may be described in terms of three independent movements: swing, elevation and axial rotation. Swing is defined in terms of the angle spanned by the arm as it moves within a plane defined at a given angle of arm elevation and relative to an initial position. For instance if the angle of arm elevation is 90° and its initial position is that of maximal horizontal adduction, a maximal swing of the arm would result in a position of maximal horizontal abduction.

Elevation and scapation

Elevation is probably the most complex among the three movements. It is the movement of the arm away from the body along a plane described by the swing angle/s, and therefore its classification according to the usual anatomical planes seems to have no kinematical merit.

On the other hand, elevation in the scapular plane, also known as scapation (Townsend et al 1991) is of particular significance. Performed at a swing angle of about 20–30° relative to the coronal plane, scapation is characterized by a relatively smooth rotation of the scapula over the rib cage. If no axial rotation of the arm is present, the juxtaposition of the articular surfaces of the humeral head and the glenoid is better than in any other plane. Moreover, the joint capsule is exposed to a minimal amount of stretch. Therefore, evaluation of shoulder muscle performance is best carried out in this plane, especially in patients who suffer from disorders of the rotatory mechanism and/or the capsule (Greenfield et al 1990, Warner et al 1990).

Change in position of the glenohumeral joint

During elevation, the position of the glenohumeral joint proper is not fixed (Walmsley 1993a, 1993b). This situation results from the extensive movement which takes place in the shoulder girdle. Therefore, alignment of the dynamometer actuator axis with that of the arm cannot in fact be achieved.

Moreover, when shoulder evaluation is carried out in unstabilized standing positions, compensatory trunk movements make it even more difficult to align the mechanical and biological axes. Hence effective stabilization of the patient is essential.

Relationship of arm elevators and shoulder girdle elevators

The importance of the relationship between the muscles responsible for elevating the arm, and those which elevate the shoulder girdle is generally overlooked in isokinetic studies (Dvir & Berme 1978). The latter, principally the trapezius (particularly in elevations up to 90–100°) and serratus anterior, rotate the girdle and ensure the stabilization of the acromion. The rotation of the girdle, particularly the scapula, greatly increases humeral ROM, while acromial stabilization prevents the loss of effective deltoid length. The force couple created by the simultaneous activity of these muscles is essential to elevation, since the mass of the upper limb exceeds by a large margin that of the girdle. In the absence of this couple the scapula could override the humerus and no elevation would be possible. Therefore, isokinetic examination of the glenohumeral elevators is to a large extent an examination of the entire mechanism of elevation.

The present author could find no study investigating the separate contributions to elevation of the two muscle groups. Such information could cast light on the mechanism of elevation.

Given the theoretical importance of muscle balance, that of, for instance the internal versus the external rotators of the glenohumeral joint, imbalance of girdle rotators and humeral elevators, might explain phenomena such as deltoid insufficiency, limited ROM and even impingement due to overriding. Measurement of the concentric activity of the girdle elevators against a superiorly positioned isokinetic resistance might provide information about this.

ISOKINETIC TESTING OF SHOULDER MUSCLES

PREPARATION

Because of the risk of injury to the complex shoulder mechanisms, the safety and comfort of the patient must be the prime consideration. Following trauma, surgical intervention or rotator cuff dysfunction, maximal effort testing should not be attempted before submaximal efforts are well tolerated; normally not less than 1 month after the injury or procedure (Albert & Wooden 1991). Moreover, after the first dislocation of a shoulder, there should be a much longer period before any isokinetic testing because of the need for strict immobilization (Reid et al 1991).

Where joint motion must be limited, for instance, because of instability or pain, the mechanical stops should be placed with great care, either manually or using the software.

Warm-up

Warm-up is an essential part of maximal effort isokinetic testing. It should consist preferably of upper limb repetitive low-load isotonics (Albert & Wooden 1991) or submaximal aerobics lasting up to 5 minutes, so that the test scores are not adversely affected by fatigue. Preparatory submaximal repetitions on the dynamometer could then be performed, at a comfortable speed of 120 °/s (see below). The following procedural issues should be considered: the test ROM; patient positioning and stabilization; alignment of the biological and mechanical axes; plane-specific versus diagonal movements; test angular velocities, and the types of muscle contraction involved.

TEST ROM

This depends on the clinical status of the subjects and the parameter to be measured. For instance, the ROM for a patient with impingement should not extend above shoulder level, or if the measured parameter is strength, a ROM may be used outside of which strength does not vary unpredictably, as far as is known.

In an isokinetic study of shoulder musculature, Shklar & Dvir (1994) examined the MAP curves for concentric and eccentric contractions. Testing was

carried out with the subjects seated and the findings are outlined in Table 9.1. There were two basic curve shapes, 'inverted-U' and 'flat'. For muscle groups presenting with the former curve shape, identification of the peak moment angle and hence isokinetic ROM is straightforward. Obviously for the 'flat' curves the strength was practically the same throughout the range. In this case the test angular velocity would be taken into account as a greater ROM is required in higher velocities.

POSITIONING AND STABILIZATION

Shoulder test positions, primarily for evaluation of the rotator musculature, have been described in terms of whole body and upper limb postures. The elbow joint was maintained at 90° of flexion in all studies. The positions used have been:

1. Standing with the arm at a slight elevation. This position is also known as the standing/neutral.
2. Seated with the arm in either slight elevation (seated/neutral) or in any other combination of swing and elevation.
3. Supine with either extended or partly flexed hip and knee joints, with the shoulder in 90° abduction.
4. Prone with the arm hanging freely below the supporting surface.

Movements other than humeral rotation, that is elevation or the more complex diagonal motions, are preferably tested using the supine or seated positions.

Effect of posture on rotator performance

The effect of posture on the performance of the

Table 9.1   Angle of peak moment for shoulder muscles, measured in degrees from the neutral position. Based on Shklar & Dvir (1994)

	Mode	Flexors	Extensors	Abductors	Adductors	Internal rotators	External rotators
Women	Concentric	0–120*	0–105	0–105	0–105	45	0–105
	Eccentric	45	90	60	30	60	0–105
Men	Concentric	0–105	75	75	0–105	60	0–105
	Eccentric	60	60	75	45	75	0–105

* Flat curve; values refer to the tested range.

rotator mechanism has been the subject of a number of studies.

Soderberg & Blaschak (1987)

These authors used three angular velocities, 60, 180 and 300 °/s to test subjects in six different seated examination positions. In the neutral position, the arm hung freely with 0° abduction or flexion. The arm positions at 45°, and then 90°, of abduction were defined as the 'midabduction' and 'full abduction' positions. The corresponding positions, at 45 and 90° of flexion were termed 'midflexion' and 'full flexion' positions. The arm position at 45° of flexion and abduction was termed midposition. Stabilization was provided only for the forearm, using a V-shaped padded trough to support the elbow. Gravity correction was not performed.

The differences in the mean peak moment between the six positions were found to be significant. The order of positions for decreasing strength for the internal rotators was: neutral, full flexion, full abduction, midabduction, midposition and midflexion. For the external rotators it was: full abduction, neutral, midposition, midabduction, full flexion and midflexion.

The authors suggested that the differences were caused by: gravitational factors, which were not accounted for; variations in the length–tension relationships of the rotator cuff and other muscles, and variations in the ligament and capsule structures which provide the fulcrum. They did not explain why the highest internal rotation moment was produced in the neutral position; the muscles involved are not necessarily at their optimal length in this position.

On the other hand the fact that full abduction led to the maximal external rotation moment agreed with the length pattern of teres minor and infraspinatus. It was concluded that the neutral position for both internal and external rotators was optimal.

Hageman et al (1989)

Hagemen et al (1989) compared the 45° abduction and 45° flexion positions in both concentric and eccentric test conditions. No stabilization other than elbow support was used. They found that the 45° abduction position resulted in significantly higher concentric and eccentric strength values for external rotation for both women and men, and generally comparable results in internal rotation.

Walmsley & Szybbo (1987), Hinton (1988) and Reid et al (1989)

Walmsley & Szybbo (1987) compared the concentric internal and external rotatory strength in three positions: standing with the arm at 15° abduction (neutral) seated with arm flexed at 90° and supine with the arm at 90° abduction. While the elbow was supported in all positions there seems to have been no stabilization in the standing position, but straps were used in the supine position. Their findings indicated that the preferred positions for internal and external rotation were standing/neutral and seated/flexed respectively.

A study by Hinton (1988) supported the findings with respect to testing internal rotators but indicated that the supine/90° abduction position was significantly better for external rotation.

Using basically the same test positions, Reid et al (1989) failed to support these observations, finding that peak concentric moments did not differ significantly between standing and supine positions.

Greenfeld et al (1990), Hellwig & Perrin (1991)

The effect on rotator strength of two variants of the standing position, that is, the arm elevated at 45° in the frontal or the scapular plane, and without proper stabilization, was investigated by Greenfield et al (1990). It was concluded that the scapular plane was the more suitable, as in this plane, the joint was in a loose-packed position, allowing unrestricted motion during rotation. It was therefore better suited for patients with various dysfunctions of the shoulder joint, such as rotator cuff impingement or chronic dislocations.

Recently another study compared rotator performance in the scapular and frontal planes (Hellwig & Perrin 1991). Using the seated, stabilized, 90° abducted arm position, and also evaluating eccentric performance, the authors failed to demonstrate significant differences between the two planes although they recommended testing in the scapular plane.

Test position and activity pattern

Particular positions may be more suitable for specific subjects, as has been indicated in a study which examined rotator testing in prone and supine positions in a group of swimmers (Falkel et al 1987). It was shown that rotator strength in the prone position was significantly higher than in the supine, by 20–40%. These findings reflect the importance of the correspondence between the test position and the general activity pattern of the joint under consideration.

Diagonal movements

Since evaluation of rotator function is carried out in positions which are not optimal for elevation and vice versa, diagonal patterns of arm motion have been recommended as a general testing position (Albert & Wooden 1991) (Fig. 9.1). These movements are performed in the supine or seated position, either on the supporting surface of the system or on a special apparatus like the Cybex UBXT. The actuator is placed at an angle relative to the coronal and sagittal planes of the subject, so that the full

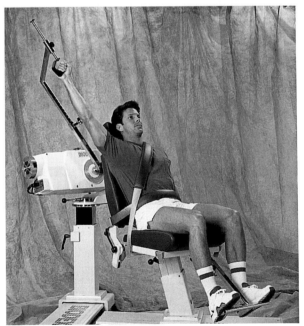

Fig. 9.1 Diagonal movements testing attachment. The plane of motion is determined using rotation/tilt of the dynamometer head and plinth. A supine position is very commonly used also.

potential of the arm ROM may be realized.

These patterns have two variants. The first diagonal, also known as D1, consists of the simultaneous combination of flexion, adduction and external rotation and its opposite sequence extension, abduction and internal rotation. The second diagonal, D2, corresponds to flexion, abduction, external rotation and its opposite, extension, adduction and internal rotation.

STABILIZATION

As with alignment, no systematic study on the effect of stabilization on shoulder muscle performance could be found. Stabilization is particularly important because of the large number of muscles involved in the execution of even simple movements. Clearly, there is a direct association between the magnitude of the moment developed by the muscle/s and the degree of stabilization required; submaximal, compared with maximal contractions may not require very rigorous stabilizing.

As mentioned earlier stabilization has two purposes: to portray, as faithfully as possible, the length–tension relationships of the muscles under consideration; and to maintain at a minimal level, or even to exclude, contributions from other muscles. Thus, prone positioning for rotator cuff testing calls for minimal stabilization as friction and gravity limit postural demands. However, the upright position, often used for rotator cuff testing, requires stabilization at nearly all the major joint systems, particularly at the spine and pelvis.

Methods of stabilization

Various methods of stabilization have been described. The least rigorous consists of supporting the elbow only. At the other extreme, Wilk et al (1991) describe stabilization of the trunk, while the subject is in the seated position, using a combination of a pelvic strap and a pair of straps which cross each other diagonally at midsternum level. Other studies, using the supine position describe the application of two straps, at midthoracic and pelvic levels.

Conclusions

In view of the foregoing discussion, there does not seem to be an acceptable formula concerning the selection of position and method of stabilization. The use of diagonal patterns may not be ideal for evaluating the rotator cuff, however appealing this method in terms of expediency or functionality. Also there is for instance no indication whether the same extent of stabilization is needed in treatment sessions as in testing. Since most shoulder activities are performed with the trunk vertical, functionality is not served by horizontal positioning, although the latter improves stabilization. On the other hand, testing/treating the shoulder while the patient stands means that, because of the design of most isokinetic dynamometers, shoulder movement other than rotations cannot be assessed. Also, this position almost precludes effective stabilization and may not be comfortable for longer periods of conditioning.

Consequently, considering all of the commonly tested/treated shoulder motions, it seems that the optimal position is seated. The trunk should remain upright or very slightly inclined, and stabilized, mainly during testing, according to the method described by Wilk et al (1991). This procedure is particularly valid for rotators (Figs 9.2 and 9.3).

The arm position depends on the movement to be tested. Rotators should be tested with the arm in the scapular plane and elevated to approximately 45°, with elbow flexed at 90° and supported. This position also does not interfere with the vascular supply for the supraspinatus. If the external rotators are being investigated, the arm should be elevated to 90° and another test performed.

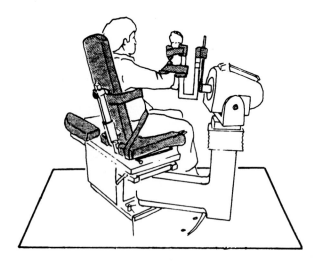

Fig. 9.3 Testing glenohumeral rotators using a special attachment.

For the purpose of treating rotator cuff function, the stabilization may be slightly relaxed; supporting the elbow may be sufficient, as long as the contralateral arm is stabilized, either actively or passively.

Elevation and/or depression may be tested in the sitting (Fig. 9.4) or in the side-lying position (Fig. 9.5) with the arm outstretched and preferably in the scapular plane. A different swing plane may be indicated depending on the particular needs.

Diagonal patterns. The testing of diagonal patterns might prove to be less reproducible in the

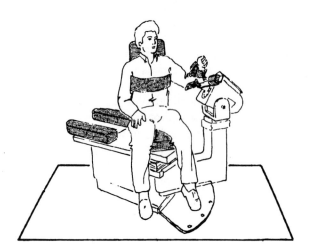

Fig. 9.2 Testing glenohumeral rotators.

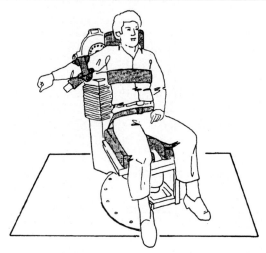

Fig. 9.4 Testing arm elevation and depression muscles in the seated position.

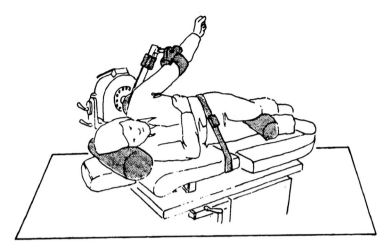

Fig. 9.5 Testing arm elevation and depression muscles in the side-lying position.

seated position since a large degree of misalignment is associated with motion of the shoulder girdle. Therefore, for testing, the supine position is probably more suitable than the seated. For treatment both positions may be equally appropriate.

ALIGNMENT OF THE BIOLOGICAL AND MECHANICAL AXES

The alignment of the biological and mechanical axes concerns three distinct movements:

1. Elevation or depression in a fixed swing plane namely abduction and adduction of flexion and extension
2. Elevation and depression in a variable swing plane, typical of diagonal patterns
3. Internal and external rotations

An excellent recent study is the only source for assessing the effect on test findings of the alignment of the shoulder joint 'axis' with that of the lever-arm (Walmsley 1993a, 1993b). Using a special optoelectronic system for tracking anatomical landmarks, attached to the subject's shoulder region, it was found that in both flexion and abduction the glenohumeral joint moved superiorly, by 8 cm on average. Thus the resulting moment in the motion of flexion/extension had to be corrected because of the variations in the effective distance between the force pad and the axis of rotation of the joint.

Elevation/depression in a fixed swing plane

For testing abduction, adduction, flexion or extension, the common practice is to position the axis of the actuator against a point which is roughly 2–3 cm below the inferior lip of the acromial arch.

Whatever the magnitude of error in this alignment, certain motions may increase it. These would typically consist of large ROM elevations and/or swings where the scapula underwent considerable deviations from its initial position, for instance in diagonal movements.

Diagonal movements alignment

The optimal alignment in diagonal movements depends on the purpose of testing. This may demand, for instance, the minimization of the cumulative error throughout the ROM, or the error made in the vicinity of the peak moment.

As no systematic study of this issue is available at the time of writing, clinicians are advised to align the axis of the actuator against the point already mentioned, when the arm is in the midposition of the total ROM.

Alignment for rotator testing

Alignment for testing the rotators of the shoulder joint is less difficult since both scapular and glenohumeral motions are relatively limited. The axis of the actuator is made co-linear with that of the humerus, through the olecranon (Wilk et al 1991).

PLANE-SPECIFIC AND DIAGONAL MOVEMENTS

A comprehensive isokinetic evaluation of the shoulder ought to include independent testing of the three principal motions of the shoulder joint, axial rotation, elevation/depression and swinging of the arm. The latter should be performed at elevations comfortably below shoulder level. As already mentioned, in specific cases additional tests will be required. Undoubtedly where attention had been focused on a particular movement component, such as rotation, individual examination of the rotators would be mandatory.

However, in the clinical situation such comprehensive evaluations may become very expensive, mainly due to the time factor, and at times 'unmanageable' (Albert & Wooden 1991). The idea of using diagonal movements as a single combined replacement for all of the above motions has been forcefully advocated by these authors. The reasons given were enhanced functionality, incorporation of shoulder complex joints other than the glenohumeral, loading of a larger number of muscles and shorter testing time.

These are important considerations and one would not hesitate to recommend the use of diagonal movements particularly for treating patients with strength deficits. However, diagonal motion testing may not be clinically relevant as the findings are not specific, and hence cannot assist in revealing the source of a problem.

Moreover, the present author could find no study of the reproducibility of findings based on diagonal movement, and therefore margins of error cannot yet be determined with any assurance. Consequently it is suggested that baseline and predischarge evaluations, at least, be performed in as rigorous a manner as possible.

TEST ANGULAR VELOCITIES

Arbitrary choice of velocities

This topic is of central importance to the assessment of the shoulder but has received surprisingly little attention. Although modern isokinetic systems allow fine control of the actuator's angular velocity, research into shoulder muscle performance has popularized the use of 60 °/s and/or its multiples.

Though this practice certainly helps to standardize the tests, no study has ever demonstrated its biomechanical or clinical rationale. Also, kinematic analysis of the arm during isokinetic motion would reveal that the component angular velocities, those of swing, elevation and rotation are rarely equal. Hence, to use the same velocities for assessing muscle performance in, say, rotation and elevation, may be erroneous.

Clearly, the current choice of velocities is arbitrary rather than scientific.

Very high functional velocities

The shoulder joint angular velocities attained during certain sporting activities, such as pitching in baseball, have been reported to reach thousands of degrees per second (Pappas et al 1985). This figure is an order of magnitude above the maximal velocity of all dynamometers in clinical usage, and raises questions concerning the applicability of isokinetic shoulder muscles testing/conditioning in certain groups of sportsmen.

It should however be pointed out that these extremely high velocities occur through a very limited arc of motion. Therefore even if a suitable dynamometer were to become available, the chance of recording a reproducible force of any significant magnitude would be low.

Obviously the problem facing the athlete is that of accelerating the segments of the upper limb, requiring a system of strong, rapidly recruitable and highly coordinated muscles. Measurement of some of these factors may be achieved satisfactorily with existing systems.

Velocities used in research

Though in a few instances only one test velocity has been used for measuring performance (Reid et al 1989, Otis et al 1990, Greenfield et al 1990, Magnusson et al 1990) most studies have employed a protocol using either two (Ivey et al 1985, Cook et al 1987, Walker et al 1987, Connelly Maddux et al 1989, Hageman et al 1989, Warner et al 1990, McMaster et al 1991) or three (Soderberg & Blaschak 1987, Walmsley & Szybbo 1987, Brown et al 1988, Ellenbecker 1991, Schexneider et al 1991, Walmsley & Hartsell 1992) distinct velocities. The velocities most often used were 60, 180 and 300 °/s.

High speed test

The question of whether a high speed test, 300 °/s or above, should be incorporated, has been addressed incidentally by Cook et al (1987) who studied the moment ratios of extensors/flexors and internal/external rotators in baseball pitchers and nonpitchers. The test velocities were 180 and 300 °/s. It was assumed that strength imbalances would be more conspicuous in the faster test since pitchers were accustomed to moving their arm at higher speeds.

However, it was found that 300 °/s was too fast for both groups, supporting another study (Wallace et al 1984) which suggested that the optimal speed for testing of flexion and extension was 120 °/s.

Recommended test velocities

What, then, should be the recommended test velocity? For the purpose of obtaining a baseline as well as a comprehensive picture of the moment–velocity relationship, a three-velocity protocol, which includes a high speed test is indicated. Such a protocol would also help to expose potential deficits, (compared with normative values).

Alternatively, if the main interest is in muscle imbalance, and a frequent appraisal of the patient's status is required, a two-velocity, or even a single velocity test, performed preferably at a medium velocity of 120 °/s, should suffice. Shoulder treatment protocols are obviously different and will be discussed in the last section of this chapter.

CONCENTRIC AND ECCENTRIC PERFORMANCE

Importance of eccentric contractions

Following its introduction some 10 years ago, eccentric 'capacity' features in most leading isokinetic systems. As far as the shoulder is concerned, this feature is particularly appealing. Because of the instability of the shoulder joint, its dynamic stabilizers, particularly the rotator cuff, are called into action during almost every movement of the upper limb. Their mode of contraction may often be eccentric, increasingly so where deceleration of the arm is needed. For instance during the phase of follow-through in the tennis serve or other similar

overhead activities, the cuff's external rotators are contracting eccentrically in order to prevent the mediosuperior gliding of the humeral head. This motion, if unchecked, could result in impingement of suprahumeral structures on the coracoacromial arch (Ellenbecker et al 1988).

The range of velocities

The question arises whether the spectrum of velocities used in concentric testing is equally applicable for eccentric testing. In one of the first studies which addressed this question Hageman et al (1989) indicated that the variations in the eccentric peak moments between 60 and 180 °/s were generally nonsignificant. These findings were supported in a recent analysis of concentric and eccentric muscle function in the shoulder (Shklar & Dvir 1994), not only with respect to joint rotation but also for elevation and depression in the coronal and sagittal planes.

It therefore seems that for eccentric testing one velocity would furnish the required information. Given the problems associated with high velocity eccentric contractions, a medium velocity of 120 °/s seems to be suitable. It is suggested that this velocity should serve as a standard for short protocol isokinetic shoulder joint testing.

Muscle strength ratios

A second question concerns the commonly used strength ratios, particularly with regard to the combined function of internal rotation and swing versus external rotation and swing. As mentioned above, in fast arm activities that involve relatively large inertial forces, antagonists often work in opposite modes; when one group contracts concentrically the other, stabilizing group, contracts eccentrically. These reciprocal contractions can also be found in other joints, such as the knee, which require significant dynamic stabilization.

In patients suffering from an ACL-deficient knee the use of the ratio, eccentric strength of the stabilizer (hamstrings)/concentric strength of the agonist (quadriceps), also known as H_{ecc}/Q_{con} (see Chapter 6), has been shown to have a significantly higher differentiating power compared with the common H_{con}/Q_{con} ratio (Dvir et al 1989). By analogy it is suggested that future studies and clinical analyses of shoulder antagonistic muscle function also consider strength ratios of reciprocal mode contractions.

PART 2
REPRESENTATIVE VALUES IN SHOULDER ISOKINETICS

GENERAL CONSIDERATIONS

The range of options involved in testing the shoulder is an obstacle to establishing normative values. Though the database has increased in recent years, a standard procedure is notably lacking leading to incompatible data. Moreover, the number of subjects in the studies quoted in this Chapter, except for that of Freedson et al (1993), was small, rarely exceeding 30 in one homogeneous group. Findings derived from such groups can hardly serve as a basis for generalization. An attempt will be made here to put these findings into an acceptable perspective.

As with other joint systems, normative values for shoulder isokinetic performance should normally be based on three factors: gender, age and general activity level.

Gender differences

Concerning gender, the usual difference in muscle strength is maintained and is highly significant. However, normalization to bodyweight tends to diminish the factor by which men are stronger than women. Thus for instance, calculations based on the peak moment, derived from concentric testing at 60 °/s (Ivey et al 1985) show that on average women have about 55% the strength of men. When normalized to bodyweight this figure is about 72%. In a recent study (Shklar & Dvir 1994) the figures for concentric testing at 60 °/s were 53 and 66% for the absolute and normalized ratios respectively. This study also investigated eccentric muscle performance and the ratios at 60 °/s were 55 and 72% respectively.

Age range

The age range in all the studies was typically adolescence to the middle of the fourth decade and therefore any large variations in measured strength would not be a result of this factor.

Activity level and the effect on dominance

Participation in athletic activities, specifically those that incorporate forceful arm motions, does account for significant bilateral performance differences. Among these activities, asymmetrical sports have a particular significance, highlighting the issue of side dominance and its effect on bilateral ratios of muscle strength. Shoulder muscles of the dominant side in baseball pitchers (Cook et al 1987, Brown et al 1986, Hinton 1988) and water polo players (McMaster et al 1991) were found to be significantly stronger than their nondominant counterparts. Moreover, although dominance was examined with particular emphasis on the rotator cuff, at least two studies (McMaster et al 1991, Ellenbecker et al 1988) indicated that in athletes the dominance effect also encompassed other major muscle groups. Consequently, care should be taken when interpreting bilateral strength ratios of athletes who use their upper limbs in an asymmetrical manner.

Findings based on normal subjects (Ivey et al 1985, Connelly-Maddux et al 1989, Reid et al 1989, Otis et al 1990, Shklar & Dvir 1994) did not indicate any effect of dominance. On the other hand, two studies (Warner et al 1990, Cahalan et al 1991) did indicate a significant dominance effect regarding a number of selected movement planes and test velocities. It should, however, be noted that poor stabilization and positioning in the former study and splinting of the elbow at 90° of flexion (overstabilization) in the latter could account for the findings. Therefore, whether the same degree of caution in interpreting bilateral differences is warranted with respect to the healthy nonathletic population is debatable.

ORDER AND MAGNITUDE IN SHOULDER MUSCLE STRENGTH

The strength order of shoulder muscles has been investigated using concentric testing at 60 and 180°/s (Ivey et al 1985) and at 60, 180 and 300°/s (Cahalan et al 1991). In the former study it was indicated that the strongest muscle group was the adductors followed by the extensors, flexors, abductors, internal rotators and external rotators (ERs). In the latter study this order was changed in only one respect, namely the extensors were found to be stronger than the adductors. The same strength order was later indicated by Shklar & Dvir (1994, see below). These findings were supported by other studies of concentric performance which, however, did not include all six groups of muscles. Adductors were stronger than abductors (McMaster et al 1991, Reid et al 1989); extensors were stronger than flexors and flexors were stronger than abductors (Otis et al 1990). These muscle groups were in turn stronger than the rotators, for which all studies to date have shown the internal rotators to be stronger than the external rotators.

CONCENTRIC AND ECCENTRIC PERFORMANCE VALUES

In a comprehensive analysis (Shklar & Dvir 1994) of the shoulder the concentric and eccentric performance parameters of the major muscle groups were measured. The order mentioned above was true for all velocities, for the two contraction modes and for women and men alike. Differences in positioning and stabilization and, particularly, the application of a gravity correction procedure in the latter study could account for the change in order.

Indeed, in a recent study (Perrin et al 1992), gravity correction exerted a highly significant effect on the strength findings of the rotator group. It was argued that the internal rotators were assisted by gravity whereas the opposite was true for the external rotators. Adopting the same line of reasoning, in the above studies, the adductors were reinforced by gravity more than the extensors, leading to the reversal in the strength order when a gravity correction was applied.

Tables 9.2–9.7 show findings from the Ivey et al (1985), Cahalan et al (1991) and Dvir & Shklar (1994) studies which were based on mixed samples of 31, 50 and 30 normal nonathletic subjects, respectively. The systems used were Cybex UBXT (Ivey et al 1985), Cybex II (Cahalan et al 1991) and KinCom II (Shklar & Dvir 1994). Attention is drawn to the fact that Cahalan et al (1991) have used an orthoplast splint for stabilizing the elbow, whose weight could be one of the reasons for the limited compatibility of their findings with those derived from the other two studies. Comparison of the norms derived from these studies show a close agreement in flexor, extensor and abductor strength, a fair agreement for internal and external rotators and up to a 47% difference in adductor strength.

In a recent study (Freedson et al 1993) 4541 women and men, shoulder flexor and extensor

Table 9.2 Representative values for abductor group concentric and eccentric strength (in N m). The data are based on Ivey et al (1985), Cahalan et al (1991)* and Shklar & Dvir (1994) using 31, 50 and 30 nonathletic subjects respectively. In Tables 9.2–9.7 data from Cahalan et al 1991 are reproduced by permission of J.B Lippincott Co.

	60 °/s			120 °/s	180 °/s			300 °/s
	Ivey	Caln	S&D	S&D	Ivey	Caln	S&D	Caln
Concentric								
Men								
Mean	56.6	52.9	50.5	50.5	42.4	44.7	43.6	36.6
SD	15.5	12.2	13.0	13.0	14.0	12.2	11.9	10.8
Women								
Mean	29.4	27.1	28.4	26.6	21.1	17.6	24.8	10.9
SD	9.0	5.4	4.6	11.9	6.9	5.4	3.5	4.1
Eccentric								
Men								
Mean			64.8	67.9			73.1	
SD			18.2	17.3			18.3	
Women								
Mean			37.3	38.9			41.8	
SD			6.1	7.5			7.2	

* = dominant side; Ivey = Ivey et al; Caln = Cahalan et al; S&D = Shklar & Dvir

Table 9.3 Representative values for adductor group concentric and eccentric strength (in N m). The data are based on Ivey et al (1985), Cahalan et al (1991)* and Shklar & Dvir (1994) using 31, 50 and 30 nonathletic subjects respectively

	60 °/s			120 °/s	180 °/s			300°/s
	Ivey	Caln	S&D	S&D	Ivey	Caln	S&D	Caln
Concentric								
Men								
Mean	89.6	108.5	72.9	69.8	74.8	99.0	66.1	88.1
SD	22.3	21.7	19.6	15.2	23.1	19.0	17.4	19.0
Women								
Mean	50.4	52.9	34.4	31.0	41.6	46.1	29.4	38.0
SD	9.1	8.1	6.9	5.3	7.5	9.5	4.4	10.8
Eccentric								
Men								
Mean			95.2	92.7			97.5	
SD			28.0	27.8			22.3	
Women								
Mean			46.7	47.5			50.2	
SD			8.9	9.0			8.2	

* = dominant side; Ivey = Ivey et al; Caln = Cahalan et al; S&D = Shklar & Dvir.

Table 9.4 Representative values for external rotator group concentric and eccentric strength (in N m). The data are based on Ivey et al (1985), Cahalan et al (1991)* and Shklar & Dvir (1994) using 31, 50 and 30 nonathletic subjects respectively

	60 °/s			120 °/s	180 °/s			300 °/s
	Ivey	Caln	S&D	S&D	Ivey	Caln	S&D	Caln
Concentric								
Men								
Mean	32.4	35.3	25.6	22.9	28.7	25.8	21.2	19.0
SD	7.9	6.8	7.9	6.4	9.2	5.4	5.7	5.4
Woman								
Mean	18.9	19.0	16.3	14.1	15.2	9.5	13.5	5.4
SD	4.1	8.1	2.5	2.6	3.1	4.1	3.2	2.7
Eccentric								
Men								
Mean			32.0	30.9			31.3	
SD			8.1	8.5			7.8	
Women								
Mean			19.9	19.8			19.6	
SD			4.6	4.6			4.4	

* = dominant side; Ivey = Ivey et al; Caln = Cahalan et al; S&D = Shklar & Dvir.

Table 9.5   Representative values for internal rotator group concentric and eccentric strength (in N m). The data are based on Ivey et al (1985), Cahalan et al (1991)* and Shklar & Dvir (1994) using 31, 50 and 30 nonathletic subjects respectively

	60 °/s			120 °/s	180 °/s			300 °/s
	Ivey	Caln	S&D	S&D	Ivey	Caln	S&D	Caln
Concentric								
Men								
Mean	49.5	62.4	42.7	38.2	44.5	54.2	37.1	46.1
SD	16.6	19.0	13.4	11.9	15.0	17.6	11.4	17.6
Women								
Mean	26.7	29.8	27.4	26.1	23.3	23.1	26.3	19.0
SD	3.9	5.4	6.2	6.4	4.1	5.4	6.6	5.4
Eccentric								
Men								
Mean			47.4	46.5			45.2	
SD			14.8	15.1			15.8	
Women								
Mean			27.4	26.1			26.2	
SD			6.2	6.4			6.6	

★ = dominant side; Ivey = Ivey et al; Caln = Cahalan et al; S&D = Shklar & Dvir.

Table 9.6   Representative values for extensor group concentric and eccentric strength (in N m). The data are based on Ivey et al (1985), Cahalan et al (1991)* and Shklar & Dvir (1994) using 31, 50 and 30 nonathletic subjects respectively

	60 °/s			120 °/s	180 °/s			300 °/s
	Ivey	Caln	S&D	S&D	Ivey	Caln	S&D	Caln
Concentric								
Men								
Mean	80.4	118.0	84.9	82.4	64.8	103.1	73.3	86.8
SD	20.1	24.4	20.5	21.1	17.7	23.1	19.0	20.3
Women								
Mean	43.0	54.2	38.7	38.0	33.7	43.4	35.5	25.8
SD	9.5	5.4	9.1	6.9	7.5	9.5	7.5	8.1
Eccentric								
Men								
Mean			112.2	113.5			113.8	
SD			30.0	33.1			30.2	
Women								
Mean			56.3	58.1			59.8	
SD			8.2	9.6			8.2	

★ = dominant side; Ivey = Ivey et al; Caln = Cahalan et al; S&D = Shklar & Dvir.

Table 9.7 Representative values for flexor group concentric and eccentric strength (in N m). The data are based on Ivey et al (1985), Cahalan et al (1991) and Shklar & Dvir (1994) using 31, 50 and 30 nonathletic subjects respectively

	60 °/s			120 °/s	180 °/s			300 °/s
	Ivey	Caln	S&D	S&D	Ivey	Caln	S&D	Caln
Concentric								
Men								
Mean	62.3	67.8	61.2	57.1	51.0	59.7	53.8	48.8
SD	12.5	16.3	13.3	9.8	11.4	16.3	10.3	14.9
Women								
Mean	35.6	29.8	36.5	35.5	39.1	23.1	32.3	16.3
SD	8.7	6.8	6.1	6.4	7.5	8.1	5.8	6.8
Eccentric								
Men								
Mean			72.4	75.2			77.1	
SD			18.0	18.4			18.1	
Women								
Mean			43.1	45.7			47.7	
SD			7.7	8.8			8.7	

* = dominant side; Ivey = Ivey et al; Caln = Cahalan; S&D = Shklar & Dvir.

strength was measured in two velocities, using the seated position. No gravity correction was appar ently performed. These findings provided probably the only normative data base and are presented in terms of percentiles, age and gender, as outlined in Tables 9.8 and 9.9

The findings of Alderink & Kuck (1986), though comprehensive, were based on a group of young men and adolescent boys all of whom were baseball pitchers.

PERFORMANCE RATIOS

Performance ratios are obtained by dividing one performance parameter by another, for instance peak concentric by peak eccentric moment. Con

cerning the shoulder muscles the ratio which has received most attention is that of the concentric strengths of antagonist groups, notably the gleno-humeral rotators. Attempts have been made to correlate disorders of the joint, such as instability and impingement, with extreme values of this ratio.

Because of its significance, the ratio 'external rotator/internal rotator strength' has been examined in terms of different populations, genders, testing positions and health status. Table 9.10 outlines the major findings. Except for two studies, research indicated that the range of this ratio was consis-tently 0.6–0.7 with apparently no significant veloc-ity effect. The proportions for eccentric contrac-tions stayed within this range. Ratios relating abductor and adductor, as well as flexor and exten-

Table 9.8 Normative values (N m) for flexion (F) and extension (E) in men. From Freedson et al (1993) Isokinetics and Exercise Science 3: 34–42, with permission of Butterworth-Heinemann

	Percentile	< 21 years		21–30 years		31–40 years		41–50 years		> 50 years	
		F	E	F	E	F	E	F	E	F	E
60 °/s	90	75.4	117.3	81.4	123.4	77.3	119.7	78.0	115.7	67.7	108.1
	70	63.7	102.4	69.2	107.1	66.4	104.4	65.8	104.4	57.0	94.6
	50	57.6	92.9	61.7	98.3	59.7	95.6	59.0	96.3	51.5	84.8
	30	50.2	84.8	54.2	88.8	52.3	86.8	52.9	85.3	46.8	78.5
	10	41.4	73.2	46.1	75.9	45.4	75.9	44.6	72.5	39.7	62.1
180 °/s	90	61.0	95.6	65.1	101.0	61.0	97.6	60.3	94.6	52.5	90.9
	70	48.8	82.7	52.9	86.8	50.2	84.1	49.5	84.6	42.0	74.6
	50	42.7	73.9	46.1	78.0	44.1	75.9	44.1	76.6	38.0	68.5
	30	37.3	65.8	40.7	69.2	38.6	68.6	38.6	67.8	32.1	63.1
	10	29.8	55.6	32.5	57.6	31.2	57.8	29.8	54.1	29.2	48.4

Table 9.9 Normative values (N m) for flexion (F) and extension (E) in women. From Freedson et al (1993) Isokinetics and Exercise Science 3: 34–42, with permission of Butterworth-Heinemann

	Percentile	< 21 years F	< 21 years E	21–30 years F	21–30 years E	31–40 years F	31–40 years E	41–50 years F	41–50 years E	> 50 years F	> 50 years E
60 °/s	90	38.0	63.1	40.7	65.1	43.4	67.0	40.0	63.6	34.2	54.4
	70	32.5	54.9	33.9	56.0	36.6	58.3	34.6	55.5	30.1	51.0
	50	28.5	49.5	30.5	51.6	32.3	52.2	29.8	50.2	26.4	46.6
	30	25.4	45.0	27.8	46.6	28.5	46.8	26.4	45.7	22.0	40.8
	10	21.7	38.8	23.1	41.4	22.4	40.0	21.2	40.8	18.2	34.6
180 °/s	90	28.5	48.8	30.5	52.9	32.5	53.6	28.5	48.1	23.5	42.6
	70	23.6	42.0	25.8	47.7	26.4	45.4	24.4	41.3	20.3	35.0
	50	20.3	38.0	22.4	40.0	23.1	40.7	20.3	38.0	15.5	32.5
	30	17.2	33.2	19.0	35.9	19.0	32.3	17.1	32.1	12.2	27.0
	10	13.6	27.3	14.9	29.8	13.6	28.5	13.6	30.5	4.5	19.4

sor strength, have also been computed and representative scores are given in Table 9.10.

PART 3
INTERPRETATION AND CLINICAL APPLICATIONS

In this section, the interpretation of findings based on isokinetic evaluation of patients who suffer from shoulder dysfunction is considered. This is followed by a discussion of protocols of treatment.

INTERPRETATION

Whatever the disorder or intervention, isokinetic testing of the shoulder should not be attempted before the whole complex is capable of withstanding and tolerating the loads imposed on it, through the tested range of motion. This means that: 'fractures, dislocations, muscle tears and other soft tissue injuries should be well healed, stable and past the acute stage' (Albert & Wooden 1991).

Bearing in mind the options afforded by the available isokinetic system, the decision concerning the exact method of testing should take into account:

1. Postoperative considerations, if relevant.
2. All the factors mentioned in the section on 'isokinetic testing procedures'.
3. The optimal ROM within the pain-free arc.

The various methods of interpreting isokinetic test data will be described in the light of clinical studies of shoulder dysfunction. A few leading papers will be reviewed.

BILATERAL COMPARISONS

The study of Walker et al (1987)

This method was used by Walker et al (1987) who studied the strength patterns of shoulder muscles after surgical repair of a torn rotator cuff.

A total of 33 and 24 patients were tested 6 months and 1 year postoperatively, respectively, using concentric testing at 60 and 180 °/s. The peak moments of muscle groups on the operated side were compared with their counterparts on the unoperated side. It should be emphasized that this approach implicitly assumed that dominance had no effect.

Agonist-antagonist comparisons

The strengths in the operated side, of the adductors, extensors and internal rotators was not significantly different from those of the abductors, flexors and external rotators, respectively. As mentioned earlier, each of these muscle groups is normally stronger than its antagonist.

Whether this finding was associated with a higher exercise dosage for the glenohumeral elevators, and external rotators, or with a faster recovery rate for these muscles was not considered by the authors. However this finding may be a pointer to selective strength conditioning in this disorder.

Bilateral differences

The second major finding related to the bilateral difference between the abductors, flexors and

Table 9.10 Shoulder muscles peak moment ratios

Source	Gender	Mode	Ordinary/athletic	n	Abductors/adductors	Flexors/extensors	External rotators/internal rotators
Alderink & Kuck (1986) 90, 120, 210, 300 °/s	M	Concentric	Athletic	24	0.50–0.70	0.48–0.55	0.68–0.76
Brown et al (1988) 180, 240, 300 °/s	M	Concentric	Athletic	41	—	—	0.61–0.72
Connelly Maddux et al (1989) 60, 180 °/s	F, M	Concentric	Ordinary	17, 20	—	—	0.67, F, 0.62, M
Cook et al (1987) 180, 300 °/s	M	Concentric	Ordinary, athletic	19	—	0.70–0.99	0.70–0.87
Ellenbecker (1988) 90, 210, 300 °/s	M	Concentric	Athletic	22	—	0.76–0.82	0.65–0.72
Hinton (1988) 90, 240 °/s	M	Concentric	Athletic	26	—	—	0.55–0.63
McMaster et al (1991) 30, 180 °/s	M	Concentric	Ordinary, athletic	25	0.48–0.69	—	0.55–0.78
Reid et al (1989) 60 °/s	M	Concentric	Ordinary, athletic	80	0.50 (ordinary only)	—	0.53–0.66
Shklar & Dvir (1993) 60, 120, 180 °/s	F, M	Concentric / Concentric / Eccentric / Eccentric	Ordinary	30	0.85–0.90, F / 0.68–0.71, M / 0.81–0.85, F / 0.71–0.77, M	0.92–0.97, F / 0.71–0.75, M / 0.77–0.80, F / 0.67–0.69, M	0.67–0.74, F / 0.59–0.62, M / 0.75–0.79, F / 0.69–0.74, M
Soderberg & Blaschak (1987) 60, 180, 300 °/s	M	Concentric	Ordinary	20	—	—	0.57–0.69

external rotators. Six months postoperatively the strength in the muscles of the operated shoulder was approximately 35% less than that of the parallel groups in the sound side. This would generally be considered a significant difference. Six months later the deficit was reduced, on average, to 20%, an improvement that was statistically significant ($p < 0.05$). It was therefore concluded that 'continuing rehabilitation beyond 6 months was advisable in many patients'. Whether or not a deficit of 20% is a reasonable criterion for discontinuing strength conditioning is a legitimate question. However the use of this figure is one example of how isokinetic findings may be interpreted.

The flexor mechanism

Another important finding concerned the impact of this operation on the flexor mechanism. The isokinetic strength of the flexors was compromised, although no such effect would be expected. The conclusion drawn from this finding, that extreme care should be exercised in dissection and retraction of the deltoid, could only have been derived from bilateral comparisons.

Size and type of tear

Finally, the authors grouped patients into those with small tears and those with large (avulsed) tears. It was demonstrated that the size and type of the tear generally did not affect strength.

This is probably the first example of analysis and comparison of shoulder isokinetic findings based on a division into clinical subgroups. It is highly significant as it shows that the prognosis after repair of large tears is no worse than that after repair of small tears, providing adequate physical therapy is administered.

Walmsley & Hartsell (1990)

In a recent study which also used bilateral comparison, Walmsley & Hartsell (1992) examined a group of 24 subjects a minimum of 1 year following surgical repair of the rotator cuff because of degenerative processes. All six movement patterns were tested for concentric strength, at 60, 120 and 180 °/s. Significant bilateral deficits were noted only for flexors and external rotators.

Warner et al 1990

In a clinical study of rotator performance, interpretation was based on bilateral comparisons of strength and total work ratios, and comparison with control values. Three groups, healthy individuals and patients with either instability or impingement syndrome, were concentrically tested at 90 and 180 °/s (Warner et al 1990). In asymptomatic subjects, internal rotator strength of the dominant side was approximately 30% higher than on the other side, leading to a parallel difference in the internal/external rotator ratios. The latter were expressed in terms of both the peak moment and total work (calculated from five consecutive repetitions).

Patients were divided into those who had involvement of the dominant side (the 'dominant' group) and those whose involved side was nondominant (the 'nondominant' group). Findings from the dominant and nondominant groups were than compared with those derived from the dominant and nondominant sides of the control subjects.

In the dominant group, significant differences in the internal rotator/external rotator strength ratios were demonstrated between patients with instability and patients with impingement. Patients with instability had a ratio close to 100%, whereas for those with impingement it was nearly 200%. In the nondominant group there was a parallel but statistically nonsignificant trend. Analysis of the absolute internal and external rotator strength, failed to reveal weaknesses in either of these groups.

The authors suggested that the relatively low internal rotator/external rotator ratio in the instability group indicated an 'association between relative imbalance of internal rotator strength and anterior instability'. On the other hand, the relatively high value of this ratio in the impingement group could not be interpreted in terms of the available data. The authors nevertheless suggested that a relative weakness of the external rotators was an important factor in impingement.

COMPARISON OVER TIME

Another form of interpretation uses unilateral comparison over a period of time. Comparison over time was used by Walker et al (1987) (see above) but rather than comparing a given muscle group with itself, a bilateral ratio was the parameter.

This form of interpretation should be applied very carefully because of the dearth of studies confirming the reproducibility of shoulder isokinetic findings. In the study (Magnusson et al 1990) addressing this issue, the margin of error with respect to the abductors was found to be 19%. However it seems that in this study positioning and stabilization were not carefully monitored and a gravity correction was not carried out.

The same test conditions, including the time of day, must be maintained if test–retest is the protocol of choice.

THE MOMENT GENERATION CAPACITY

A performance parameter which has not gained much attention concerns the moment generation capacity (MGC) of the muscle. This may take into account the time required to reach the maximal moment, or to reach 50% of the maximal moment, or may include other moment/work/power-based values.

One of the MGC derivatives, the work done by the contracting muscles during the first 1/8 second has been termed the Torque Acceleration Energy (TAE). As an exclusive basis for interpretation, the TAE may be doubtful.

However, the present author believes that, combined with other performance parameters, MGC-related parameters could serve as a basis for judging the neuromotor integrity of shoulder musculature, especially of the rotator mechanism.

THE SHAPE OF THE ISOKINETIC CURVE

Finally, rather than considering the numerical findings, it is possible, and indeed advisable to examine the shape of the isokinetic curve. As mentioned earlier, it is notoriously difficult to transform these curves into a mathematically meaningful entity. On the other hand, an experienced clinician can quite clearly distinguish a curve which looks 'normal' from one that may be associated with some dysfunction. For instance, given the same conditions a steeper curve during the initial phase indicates a more rapid fiber recruitment, whereas a break in the curve (Dvir et al 1991) may indicate pain.

Two recent case studies (Engle 1991, Engle & Faust 1991) attempted to interpret findings using curve shape. In the Engle & Faust study, which related to evaluation of posterior glenohumeral subluxation, a significant break in the curve during the performance of a D1 motion was recorded. The break started at 70° of flexion and lasted for the next 40°. On moving the arm in the opposite direction a reproducible deficit occurred at about 85°. Motions, in both directions, within the 70–110° arc, which were symptomatic preoperatively, produced neither pain nor clicking postoperatively.

Engle (1991) described the isokinetic curves of a patient who suffered tears of the acromioclavicular and coracoclavicular ligaments as well as a disruption of the upper trapezius attachment to the clavicle. Curves at 6 and 2 weeks postoperatively demonstrated improvements in moment and work.

Unfortunately, the curves shown in both these papers were not calibrated, either for angle or moment, and thus the full significance of the graphical findings could not be judged.

ISOKINETIC CONDITIONING PROTOCOLS

In principle, the rationale of treatment protocols for the shoulder should not differ from that for other major joint systems. It is based on velocity-dependent muscle overloading. Under isokinetic conditions, concentric and eccentric alike, the available, sometimes the maximal, muscle tension is accommodated by the resistance of the system. The physiological load imposed on the joint is equally important. This load is expressed in newton-meter seconds (N m s), corresponding to the time for which the moment is acting, or the contraction impulse (Sale 1991). A large number of shoulder problems require attention to the possible impact of glenohumeral (or other) joint loading and thus the impulse is a cardinal factor in protocol design.

It should also be mentioned that all factors concerned with the safety of the patient in isokinetic testing also hold for isokinetic conditioning.

Principles of rehabilitation

The published literature on the general use of isokinetic treatment procedures for the shoulder is particularly scanty. Most of the papers are based on case studies and their findings may not be generalized. However, from its initiation and through its progression, shoulder rehabilitation follows two principles (Davies 1992) in initiation and progression:

1. Arm motion is initially very limited, that is, contractions are performed at fixed angles; this followed by short arc motion, and then movements spanning the full ROM.
2. The shoulder muscle contraction mode is initially isometric, followed by concentric and then eccentric. The magnitude of these contractions varies from submaximal to maximal.

Velocities in rehabilitation

The choice of speeds used in treatment sessions depends primarily on the patient's tolerance. If tolerance is assured, the speed/s in which significant deficits are indicated require particular attention.

It should be emphasized that lower speeds mean higher impulse, and therefore an increase of joint loading and, frequently, pain. Consequently higher speeds are better as a conditioning input. On the other hand these speeds involve higher accelerations which may lead to significant inertial forces. The solution in this case is to employ the damping procedure, an option the present author has used quite liberally in isokinetic conditioning. Limiting the arc of motion is another method of containing pain but this applies generally.

Albert & Wooden (1991) suggest another guideline for speed selection, the '25% rule': if strength deficit at the low testing speed of 60 °/s is greater than 25%, rehabilitation at this speed is indicated; otherwise it should be at the medium/high speed of 180 °/s.

Velocity spectrum rehabilitation protocols

The use of velocity spectrum rehabilitation protocols (VSRPs) has been advocated for other joints, and the shoulder is no exception. Because of the high angular velocities attainable by the arm, the 'velocities pyramid' may shift to the right, i.e., the lowest velocity is 60 °/s or even higher, whereas the apex of the pyramid, the highest speed, may reach hundreds of degrees per second.

In a case study of a functional subluxation of the shoulder joint, the VSRP for the internal and external rotators started at 180 °/s and proceeded up to 450 °/s at 30 °/s intervals (Engle 1991). Ten repetitions at each of these speeds with 20 s of interset rest were performed. No upper limit to the number of repetitions at the highest speed was set, and the patient was directed to reach fatigue.

However, in view of the guideline set by Wallace et al (1984) it seems that the value of very high speeds is questionable. Moreover, the present author doubts if such high speeds induce a genuine isokinetic effort. Thus in a more relevant VSRP, the peak would be set at velocities around 200 °/s.

Concentric and eccentric conditioning

The use of concentric and eccentric conditioning protocols, in the case of chronic anterior shoulder instability, has been advocated in an excellent paper by Glousman et al (1988). This study centered on dynamic electromyography of shoulder muscles, comparing baseball pitchers with chronic instability to a control group. It was demonstrated how muscle imbalance, because of weak internal rotators (subscapularis, pectoralis major and latissimus dorsi) and scapular protractors (serratus anterior) on one hand, and their sound antagonists on the other, may cause or aggravate the instability.

The authors pointed out that: 'during a muscle strengthening program, improper synchrony and decreased muscle activity must be corrected. Often, asymmetrical or subtle differences cannot be appreciated'. The last sentence almost prescribes the use of isokinetic testing since this is the only method through which such differences may be discovered.

The incorporation of eccentric conditioning raises the questions 'when' and 'how?' A possible protocol which is fairly functional could consist of submaximal D2 patterns, attempted relatively late in the rehabilitation process. These would involve eccentrically contracting the internal rotators against the actuator's induced flexion, abduction and external rotation. A concentric, maximal effort return movement to the initial position should then follow, thus exerting a medium to high demand on the muscles. The present author would recommend using, at this stage, low/medium eccentric speeds, 90–120 °/s, and medium/high, 180–240 °/s concentric speeds. At the very last stage, high speed concentric and eccentric motions may be

attempted, providing the safety of the patient is ensured.

REFERENCES

Albert M S, Wooden M J 1991 Isokinetic evaluation and treatment of the shoulder. In: Donatelli R (ed) Physical therapy of the shoulder, 2nd edn. Churchill Livingstone, Edinburgh

Alderink G J, Kuck D J 1986 Isokinetic shoulder strength of high school and college-aged pitchers. Journal of Orthopaedic and Sports Physical Therapy 7: 163–172

Bassett R W, Browne A O, Morrey B F 1990 Glenohumeral muscle force and movement mechanics in a position of shoulder instability. Journal of Biomechanics 23: 405–415

Brown L P, Niehues S L, Harrah A, Yavorsky P, Hirschman H P 1988 Upper extremity range of motion and isokinetic strength of the internal and external rotators in major league baseball players. American Journal of Sports Medicine 16: 577–585

Cahalan T D, Johnson M E, Chao E Y S 1991 Shoulder strength analysis using the Cybex II isokinetic dynamometer. Clinical Orthopaedics and Related Research 271: 249–257

Connelly Maddux R E, Kibler W B, Uhl T 1989 Isokinetic peak torque and work values for the shoulder. Journal of Orthopaedic and Sports Physical Therapy 10: 264–269

Cook E E, Gray V L, Savinar-Nogue E, Medeiros J 1987 Shoulder antagonistic strength ratios: a comparison between college level baseball pitchers and nonpitchers. Journal of Orthopaedic and Sports Physical Therapy 8: 451–461

Davies G J 1992 Compendium of isokinetics in clinical usage. S & S Publications, La Crosse, Wisconsin

Dvir Z, Berme N 1978 Elevation of the arm in the scapular plane: a mechanism approach. Journal of Biomechanics 11: 98–103

Dvir Z, Eger G, Halperin N, Shklar A, 1989 Thigh muscle activity and anterior cruciate ligament insufficiency. Clinical Biomechanics 4: 87–91

Dvir Z, Halperin N, Shklar A, Robinson D 1991 Quadriceps function and patellofemoral pain syndrome. Part II: the break phenomenon during eccentric activity. Isokinetics and Exercise Science 1: 31–35

Ellenbecker T S 1991 A total arm strength isokinetic profile of highly skilled tennis players. Isokinetics and Exercise Science 1: 9–22

Ellenbecker T S, Davies G E, Rowinski M J, 1988 Concentric versus eccentric isokinetic strengthening of the rotator cuff: objective data versus functional test. American Journal of Sports Medicine 16: 64–69

Engle R P 1991 Isokinetic analysis in acromioclavicular joint rehabilitation: a case study. Isokinetics and Exercise Science 1: 49–55

Engle R P, Faust J S 1991 Isokinetic evaluation in posterior shoulder subluxation. Isokinetics and Exercise Science 1: 72–74

Falkel J E, Murphy T C, Murray T F 1987 Prone positioning for testing shoulder internal and external rotation on the Cybex isokinetic dynamometer. Journal of Orthopaedic and Sports Physical Therapy 8: 368–370

Freedson P S, Gilliam T B, Mahoney T, Maliszeski A F, Kastango K 1993 Industrial torque levels by age group and gender. Isokinetics and Exercise Science 3: 34–42

Glousman R E, Jobe F W, Tibone J E, Moynes D, Antonelli D, Perry J 1988 Dynamic electromyographic analysis of the

throwing shoulder with glenohumeral instability. Journal of Bone and Joint Surgery 70A: 220–226

Greenfield B H, Donatelli R, Wooden M J, Wilkes J 1990 Isokinetic evaluation of shoulder rotational strength between the plane of the scapula and the frontal plane. American Journal of Sports Medicine 18: 124–128

Hageman P A, Mason D J, Rydlund K W, Humpal S A 1989 Effect of position and speed on eccentric and concentric isokinetic testing of the shoulder rotators. Journal of Orthopaedic and Sports Physical Therapy 11: 64–69

Hellwig E V, Perrin D H 1991 A comparison of two positions for assessing shoulder rotator peak torque: the traditional frontal plane versus the plane of the scapula. Isokinetics and Exercise Science 1: 202–206

Hinton R Y 1988 Isokinetic evaluation of shoulder rotational strength in high school baseball pitchers. American Journal of Sports Medicine 16: 274–279

Inman V T, Saunders J BdeC M, Abbott L C 1944 Observations on the function of the shoulder joint. Journal of Bone and Joint Surgery, 26: 1–30

Ivey F M, Calhoun J H, Rusche K, Bierschenk J 1985 Isokinetic testing of shoulder strength: normal values. Archives of Physical Medicine and Rehabilitation 66: 384–386

Jobe F W 1990 Comments on Warner et al's paper. American Journal of Sports Medicine 18: 375

Jobe F W, Jobe C M 1983 Painful athletic injuries of the shoulder. Clinical Orthopaedics and Related Research 173: 117–124

Magnusson S P, Gleim G G, Nicholas J A 1990 Subject variability of shoulder abduction strength testing. American Journal of Sports Medicine 18: 349–353

McMaster W C, Long S C, Caiozzo V J 1991 Isokinetic torque imbalances in the rotator cuff of elite water polo players. American Journal of Sports Medicine 19: 72–75

Neer C S 1983 Impingement lesions. Clinical Orthopaedics and Related Research 173: 70–77

Otis J C, Warren R F, Backus S I, Santner T J, Mabrey J D 1990 Torque production in the shoulder of the normal young adult male: the interaction of function, dominance, joint angle and angular velocity. American Journal of Sports Medicine 18: 119–123

Pappas A M, Zawacki R M, Sullivan T J 1985 Biomechanics of baseball pitching: a preliminary report. American Journal of Sports Medicine 13: 223–235

Perrin D H, Helwig E V, Tis L L, Shenk B S 1992 Effect of gravity correction on shoulder rotation isokinetic average force and reciprocal group ratios. Isokinetics and Exercise Science 2: 30–33

Poppen N K, Walker P S 1976 Normal and abnormal motion of the shoulder. Journal of Bone and Joint Surgery 58A: 195–201

Reid D C, Oedekoven G, Kramer J F, Saboe L A 1989 Isokinetic muscle strength parameters for shoulder movements. Clinical Biomechanics 4: 97–104

Reid D C, Saboe L A, Burnham R 1991 Common shoulder problems in the athlete. In: Donatelli R (ed) Physical therapy of the shoulder, 2nd edn. Churchill Livingstone, Edinburgh

Sale D G 1991 Testing strength and power. In: MacDougall J D, Wenger H A, Green H J (eds) Physiological testing of the high performance athlete, 2nd edn. Human Kinetics Books, Champaign, Illinois

Schexneider M A, Catlin P A, Davies G J, Mattson P A 1991 An isokinetic estimation of total arm strength. Isokinetics ane Exercise Science 1: 117–121

Shklar A, Dvir Z 1994 Normative values of shoulder muscles performance. Submitted

Soderberg G L, Blaschak M J 1987 Shoulder internal and external rotation peak torque production through a velocity spectrum in differing positions. Journal of Orthopaedic and Sports Physical Therapy 8: 518–524

Townsend H, Jobe F W, Pink M, Perry J 1991 Electromyographic analysis of the glenohumeral muscles during a baseball rehabilitation program. American Journal of Sports Medicine 19: 264–272

Walker S W, Couch W H, Boester G A, Sprowl D W 1987 Isokinetic strength of the shoulder after repair of a torn rotator cuff. Journal of Bone and Joint Surgery 69A: 1041–1044

Wallace W A, Barton M J, Murray W A 1984 The power available during movement of the shoulder. In: Bateman J, Welsh C (eds) Surgery of the shoulder, B C Decker, Philadelphia

Walmsley R 1993a Movement of the axis of rotation of the glenohumeral joint while working on the Cybex II dynamometer. Part I. flexion/extension. Isokinetics and Exercise Science 3: 16–20

Walmsley R 1993b Movement of the axis of rotation of the glenohumeral joint while working on the Cybex II dynamometer. Part II. abduction/adduction. Isokinetics and Exercise Science 3: 21–26

Walmsley R P. Hartsell H 1992 Shoulder strength following surgical rotator cuff repair: a comprehensive analysis using isokinetic testing. Journal of Orthopaedic and Sports Physical Therapy 15: 215–222

Walmsley R P, Szybbo C 1987 A comparative study of the torque generated by the shoulder internal and external rotator muscles in different positions and at varying speeds. Journal of Orthopaedic and Sports Physical Therapy 9: 217–222

Warner J P, Micheli L J, Arslanian L E, Kennedy J, Kennedy R 1990 Patterns of flexibility, laxity and shoulder strength in normal shoulders and shoulders with instability and impingement. American Journal of Sports Therapy 18: 366–375

Wilk K E, Arrigo C A, Andrews J R 1991 Standardized isokinetic testing protocol for the throwing shoulder: the throwers' series. Isokinetics and Exercise Science 1: 63–71

Index